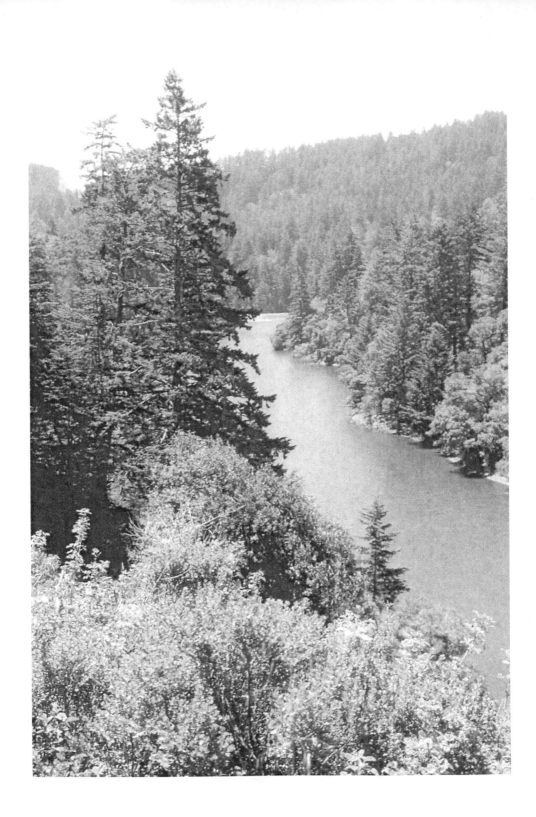

Bay Area Ridge Trail

The Official Guide for Hikers, Mountain Bikers, and Equestrians

JEAN RUSMORE

 WILDERNESS PRESS · BERKELEY, CA

Bay Area Ridge Trail: The Official Guide for Hikers, Mountain Bikers, and Equestrians

1st EDITION 1995
2nd EDITION August 2002
3rd EDITION May 2008

Copyright © 1995, 2002, 2008 by Jean Rusmore

Front cover photos copyright © 2008 by Elizabeth Byers
Interior photos, except where noted, by Jean Rusmore
Maps: Ben Pease, Pease Press
Cover design: Larry B. Van Dyke
Book design and layout: Lisa Pletka
Book editor: Laura Shauger

ISBN 978-0-89997-469-9
UPC 7-19609-97469-7

Manufactured in Canada

Published by: **Wilderness Press**
1345 8th Street
Berkeley, CA 94710
(800) 443-7227; FAX (510) 558-1696
info@wildernesspress.com
www.wildernesspress.com

Visit our website for a complete listing of our books and for ordering information.

Cover photos: *(front top)* Hikers walk up the Ridge Trail toward Mount Wanda in John Muir National Historic Site. *(front bottom)* Hikers take a spur off the Ridge Trail to walk to Mount Wanda's summit in John Muir National Historic Site.

Frontispiece: A glimpse of Pilarcitos Reservoir from Five Points in the San Francisco Watershed

*To Doris Lindfors,
longtime Ridge Trail advocate and dear friend*

❁ ❁ ❁

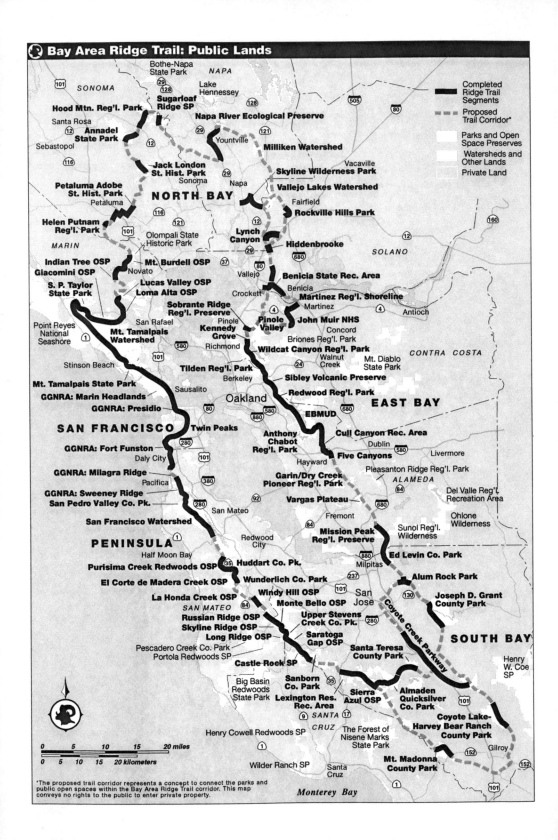

Bay Area Ridge Trail: Public Lands

Legend:
- Completed Ridge Trail Segments
- Proposed Trail Corridor*
- Parks and Open Space Preserves
- Watersheds and Other Lands
- Private Land

SONOMA

Bothe-Napa State Park
NAPA
Lake Hennessey
Hood Mtn. Reg'l. Park
Sugarloaf Ridge SP
Napa River Ecological Preserve
Santa Rosa
Annadel State Park
Sebastopol
Milliken Watershed
Vacaville
Skyline Wilderness Park
Yountville
Jack London St. Hist. Park
Sonoma
Napa
Vallejo Lakes Watershed
Petaluma Adobe St. Hist. Park
Petaluma
NORTH BAY
Fairfield
Rockville Hills Park
Helen Putnam Reg'l. Park
Olompali State Historic Park
Lynch Canyon
Hiddenbrooke
SOLANO
MARIN
Indian Tree OSP
Giacomini OSP
Mt. Burdell OSP
Novato
Vallejo
Benicia State Rec. Area
S. P. Taylor State Park
Lucas Valley OSP
Loma Alta OSP
Crockett
Benicia
Martinez Reg'l. Shoreline
Martinez
Antioch
Sobrante Ridge Reg'l. Preserve
San Rafael
Pinole
Kennedy Grove
Pinole Valley
John Muir NHS
Point Reyes National Seashore
Mt. Tamalpais Watershed
Concord
Briones Reg'l. Park
CONTRA COSTA
Richmond
Wildcat Canyon Reg'l. Park
Walnut Creek
Mt. Diablo State Park
Stinson Beach
Tilden Reg'l. Park
Berkeley
Mt. Tamalpais State Park
GGNRA: Marin Headlands
Sausalito
Sibley Volcanic Preserve
GGNRA: Presidio
Oakland
Redwood Reg'l. Park
EAST BAY
SAN FRANCISCO
Twin Peaks
EBMUD
GGNRA: Fort Funston
Daly City
Anthony Chabot Reg'l. Park
Cull Canyon Rec. Area
Dublin
GGNRA: Milagra Ridge
Pacifica
Five Canyons
Livermore
GGNRA: Sweeney Ridge
San Pedro Valley Co. Pk.
Hayward
Garin/Dry Creek Pioneer Reg'l. Park
Pleasanton Ridge Reg'l. Park
ALAMEDA
San Mateo
Vargas Plateau
Del Valle Reg'l. Recreation Area
San Francisco Watershed
Fremont
Ohlone Wilderness
PENINSULA
Redwood City
Mission Peak Reg'l. Preserve
Sunol Reg'l. Wilderness
Half Moon Bay
Purisima Creek Redwoods OSP
Huddart Co. Pk.
Milpitas
Ed Levin Co. Park
El Corte de Madera Creek OSP
Wunderlich Co. Park
Alum Rock Park
La Honda Creek OSP
Windy Hill OSP
SAN MATEO
Russian Ridge OSP
Monte Bello OSP
San Jose
Joseph D. Grant County Park
Skyline Ridge OSP
Upper Stevens Creek Co. Pk.
Long Ridge OSP
Saratoga Gap OSP
SOUTH BAY
Pescadero Creek Co. Park
Santa Teresa County Park
Portola Redwoods SP
Castle Rock SP
Henry W. Coe SP
Big Basin Redwoods State Park
Sanborn Co. Park
Lexington Res. Rec. Area
Sierra Azul OSP
Almaden Quicksilver Co. Park
SANTA
Coyote Lake-Harvey Bear Ranch County Park
Henry Cowell Redwoods SP
CRUZ
The Forest of Nisene Marks State Park
Gilroy
Mt. Madonna County Park
Wilder Ranch SP
Santa Cruz
Coyote Creek Parkway

0   5   10   15   20 miles
0   5   10   15   20 kilometers

*The proposed trail corridor represents a concept to connect the parks and public open spaces within the Bay Area Ridge Trail corridor. This map conveys no rights to the public to enter private property.

Monterey Bay

Contents

Foreword x

Twenty Years of Success due to Volunteerism and Civic
Commitment xi

Acknowledgments xii

Introducing the San Francisco Bay Area 1

Introducing the Bay Area Ridge Trail 7

How to Use This Book 11

THE NORTH BAY **19**

The Golden Gate Bridge 21

Marin Headlands from the Golden Gate Bridge
to Tennessee Valley 25

Marin Headlands from Tennessee Valley to Shoreline Highway 31

Mount Tamalpais State Park 35

Mount Tamalpais State Park and Golden Gate
National Recreation Area 39

Golden Gate National Recreation Area
and Samuel P. Taylor State Park 43

Samuel P. Taylor State Park to Loma Alta Open Space Preserve. . . . 49

Loma Alta Open Space Preserve to Lucas Valley
Open Space Preserve 53

Lucas Valley Open Space Preserve 56

Indian Tree Open Space Preserve to O'Hair Park 59

Mount Burdell Open Space Preserve 63

Helen Putnam Regional Park and McNear Park
to Petaluma Adobe State Historic Park 69

Jack London State Historic Park. 73

Annadel State Park 79

Hood Mountain Regional Park and Open Space Preserve. 83

Sugarloaf Ridge State Park 86

Yountville Cross Road 91

River-to-Ridge Trail. 93

Skyline Wilderness Park and Napa Solano Ridge Trail 95

Rockville Hills Regional Park 99

Lynch Canyon Open Space................................ 103
Hiddenbrooke Trail...................................... 106
Vallejo-Benicia Buffer.................................... 109
Vallejo-Benicia Waterfront................................ 113

THE EAST BAY.................................... **119**
Al Zampa Memorial Bridge............................... 121
Martinez City Streets to Carquinez Strait Regional Shoreline..... 123
Carquinez Strait Regional Shoreline to John Muir
National Historic Site on the Hulet Hornbeck Trail 127
Mount Wanda Trail...................................... 130
Crockett Hills Regional Park 133
Sobrante Ridge Regional Preserve 135
Kennedy Grove to Tilden Regional Park 139
Tilden Regional Park to Redwood Regional Park.............. 145
Redwood and Anthony Chabot Regional Parks............... 151
Anthony Chabot Regional Park 155
East Bay Municipal Utility District Lands
to Independent School 161
Independent School to Five Canyons....................... 165
Mission Peak Regional Preserve and Ed R. Levin County Park.... 169

THE SOUTH BAY.................................. **175**
Alum Rock Park and Boccardo Trail Corridor 177
Joseph D. Grant County Park............................. 181
Coyote Lake-Harvey Bear Ranch Trail...................... 185
Mount Madonna County Park 188
Sierra Azul Open Space Preserve 193
Coyote Creek Parkway North............................. 195
Coyote Creek Parkway South 199
Santa Teresa County Park and Los Alamitos/Calero Creek Trail .. 201
Almaden Quicksilver County Park......................... 207
Sanborn County Park and Castle Rock State Park............. 211

THE PENINSULA **217**
Saratoga Gap Open Space Preserve to Skyline Ridge
Open Space Preserve.................................... 219
Skyline Ridge and Russian Ridge Open Space Preserves 223

Windy Hill Open Space Preserve 227
Wunderlich County Park to Huddart County Park 231
Purisima Creek Redwoods Open Space Preserve 235
San Francisco Watershed Trail 239
Golden Gate National Recreation Area:
Sweeney Ridge to Milagra Ridge. 243
Mussel Rock to Fort Funston. 249

SAN FRANCISCO **255**
Fort Funston to Stern Grove. 257
Stern Grove to the Presidio. 261
San Francisco Presidio. 267

Appendix 1: Summary of Trail Features 276
Appendix 2: Trail Sampler: Trips for Many Reasons. 286
Appendix 3: Information Sources and Contacts for Parks 298
Appendix 4: Transportation Agencies that Serve the
                       Bay Area Ridge Trail Route 300
Index 302
About the Author 314

Foreword

The preservation of our natural heritage is perhaps the most important legacy we can leave for our children and our children's children, and it is one of the most urgent tasks facing the Bay Area's rapidly growing population. As part of this preservation effort, I am honored once again to write the foreword for *Bay Area Ridge Trail: The Official Guide for Hikers, Mountain Bikers, and Equestrians*. This spectacular 500-plus-mile recreational trail connects parks, people, and communities in the nine Bay Area counties. The Bay Area Ridge Trail Council deserves our admiration and gratitude for its extraordinary vision, leadership, and commitment to this project over the 20 years of its existence. The council partners with more than 200 community groups and land management agencies, a growing number of corporate supporters, and thousands of trail enthusiasts of all ages and interests—no other urban trail in the U.S. has reached this level of complexity.

The Bay Area Ridge Trail is volunteerism at its best. This special mix of people—private citizens, park and trail professionals, and nonprofit and corporate leaders—involved in planning, promoting, and developing the Ridge Trail provides an outstanding example of collaboration toward a common vision. It is only with efforts of this magnitude that completion of this 550-mile trail will be realized. Without the leadership and talent of these hundreds of individual throughout the Bay Area, the trail would not be where it is today, with over 300 miles dedicated so far. We are indeed fortunate to have such loyal volunteers. To each of them I extend my personal and sincere thanks for their tremendous efforts to forever preserve the unique and world-renowned natural beauty of the Bay Area.

A special thanks is also owed to state and federal legislators, especially the Bay Area delegation, who took a leadership role in supporting funding for the Ridge Trail in Sacramento and Washington, D.C. Their commitment to this project has been essential. Thanks also to the voters of California who passed state park bonds (Propositions 12, 40, and 84) that included funds for the Ridge Trail. The State Coastal Conservancy, in allocating those funds, has been a staunch ally of this effort and can be credited with much of the progress in recent years.

I look forward to continuing our work together to meet the goal of completing the Ridge Trail in the next 10 years and honoring our responsibility to leave for the next generations something for which we and they will be proud.

—Congressman George Miller
7th District, California
January 2008

Twenty Years of Success due to Volunteerism and Civic Commitment

Just 20 short years ago, a visionary leader, William Penn Mott, Jr., inspired a small band of citizens and park managers to begin a journey to protect and connect the region's environment and natural beauty by way of a continuous ridgeline trail. As the organization that formed to promote the idea celebrates its 20th anniversary, there is a long string of successes to look back on with pride. Supporters have grown from about 50 to a several thousand-member-strong organization with a staff, dozens of agency partners, landowners, and hundreds of community volunteers all working together to complete the Bay Area Ridge Trail.

These are the folks who scout potential routes; put up with blisters, poison oak, and sore muscles to build sections of the trail; talk with their political representatives to spread the idea; lead group outings; attend local planning committee meetings; host events; raise funds; and take friends and family out to enjoy the ever-growing trail. Because of their collective passion, dedication, and commitment, we have been able to complete 310 miles of trail so far.

What motivates them? The chance to leave a legacy, protect something special, or have a place to go with their children and their children's children to enjoy the outdoors. Some are captivated with the notion of hiking or riding all around the San Francisco Bay on a trail. Still others are motivated by the sheer challenge of creating a trail of this magnitude.

And that challenge continues. Although the 310 completed miles of trail represent significant progress, much more remains to be done. Each day, the Ridge Trail Council—its staff, board, partners, and volunteers—works toward making this guidebook out of date, having set a goal for ourselves to secure another 100 miles of trail for all to enjoy by 2015.

Until then, we are proud to present, in partnership with Wilderness Press, this third edition of *Bay Area Ridge Trail: The Official Guide for Hikers, Mountain Bikers, and Equestrians*. We are especially indebted to Jean Rusmore, whose contributions as a council volunteer have made this book possible. Since 1989, Jean has hiked, researched, and written about each and every leg of the completed Bay Area Ridge Trail.

As you hike, ride, and read about the wonders of the Bay Area Ridge Trail, consider taking up the challenge to help complete the trail—if you haven't already. Join us as we try to reach this inspiring goal! To learn more, to volunteer, or to contribute to the Ridge Trail, contact the Bay Area Ridge Trail Council at www.ridgetrail.org or by phoning (415) 561-2595.

—*Brian O'Neill*
Chairman Emeritus, Board of Directors, Bay Area Ridge Trail Council
Superintendent, Golden Gate National Recreation Area
January 2008

Acknowledgments

Since the Bay Area Ridge Trail concept was first proposed, many people have contributed their efforts and enthusiasm into completing over 300 miles of the trail. Leading this achievement have been the Bay Area Ridge Trail Council's Board of Directors—Brian O'Neill, its first chairman and now emeritus, Marcia McNally, Doug Kerseg, and presently, Bill Long. To these dedicated people and the many board members who have given their energies and talents to guide the Ridge Trail along its successful way, I offer my hearty thanks. I also extend to them my appreciation for approving the idea for the first edition of this book and for endorsing the second and now the third edition.

For the splendid support and considerable skills of the Bay Area Ridge Trail Council staff I am most grateful: Marti Leicester, first executive director; Barbara Rice, who served during its rapidly growing years; interim executive director Mary Burns; Bob Power, who as interim executive director generously piloted the organization through a transitional period and its move to the Presidio; to Holly Van Houten, a recent executive director; and to Janet McBride, the present executive director and former San Francisco Bay Trail Executive Director. It has been a pleasure to know and work with all of them.

The directors, superintendents, and planners of the parks, open space agencies, and water districts through whose lands the Bay Area Ridge Trail trips travel were most cooperative. I extend my appreciation for their specialized knowledge, for their maps and background materials, and for their helpful comments on the trip descriptions. To the rangers, many of whom hiked the trails with me, and to all the field staff who shared their special knowledge of the trails and the natural, historic, and cultural features of their parks, watersheds, and preserves, I offer my thanks. Their love of the lands in their care was truly inspiring.

I salute and thank Larry Orman, Mark Evanoff, and Judy Kanofsky, whose pioneering work at Greenbelt Alliance stimulated Bay Area leaders to reactivate William Penn Mott's dream of a ridgetop trail around San Francisco Bay. Each of them is continuing to work for greenbelt and open space planning and preservation.

It's impossible to mention Greenbelt Alliance without paying tribute to Dorothy Erskine, its founding member and outstanding proponent of preserving the Bay Area's many natural treasures—requiescat in pace.

It's been a pleasure to work with the able members of the County Committees of the Bay Area Ridge Trail Council. I thank all the nine Bay Area County Committees for their volunteer leadership in exploring, planning, and promoting the Bay Area Ridge Trail and for their long-term efforts to complete the Ridge Trail around the Bay Area.

Many friends hiked the trails with me: Doris Lindfors, a special friend and hiking companion, who generously contributed her firsthand knowledge of Bay Area trails and cheerfully joined me on almost every mile of the Bay Area Ridge Trail route described in the book's first and second editions. My monthly hiking friends, the Walkie-Talkies, heartened me with their pleasure in exploring most of the South Bay and the Peninsula segments of the Bay Area Ridge Trail. Bill Long, Elna Cunningham, and J'Anny and Ed Nelson also joined me on several North Bay trips. To these and all who shared the Bay

Area Ridge Trail trips, I extend my appreciation for their company and their delight in the beautiful country we traveled through.

To Ron Brown for his comprehensive mileage data, to Ben Pease for his carefully created maps, to Paula Tuerk for photography assistance, and to volunteer Rollye Wiskerson for his trail-building expertise, my sincere thanks. To Dee Swanhuyser and Bern Smith, the regional Ridge Trail representatives, to the capable office staff, and to Barbara Weitz, Daniel R. Sykes, and Dave Chalk, who reviewed the manuscript for the Marin and North Bay segments, my thanks as well.

To the family of Frances Spangle, I extend my appreciation for her contribution of the original text for four Marin County trips and the Wunderlich to Huddart county parks trip for the first edition.

During the process of producing this guidebook, the staff of Wilderness Press efficiently managed a significant part—my thanks to Caroline Winnett, publisher; Roslyn Bullas, managing editor; and Laura Shauger, editor. To Wilderness Press founding publisher Tom Winnett, now retired, I owe my thanks and appreciation for his unfailing interest in producing excellent outdoor guidebooks.

—*Jean Rusmore*
Palo Alto, California
January 2008

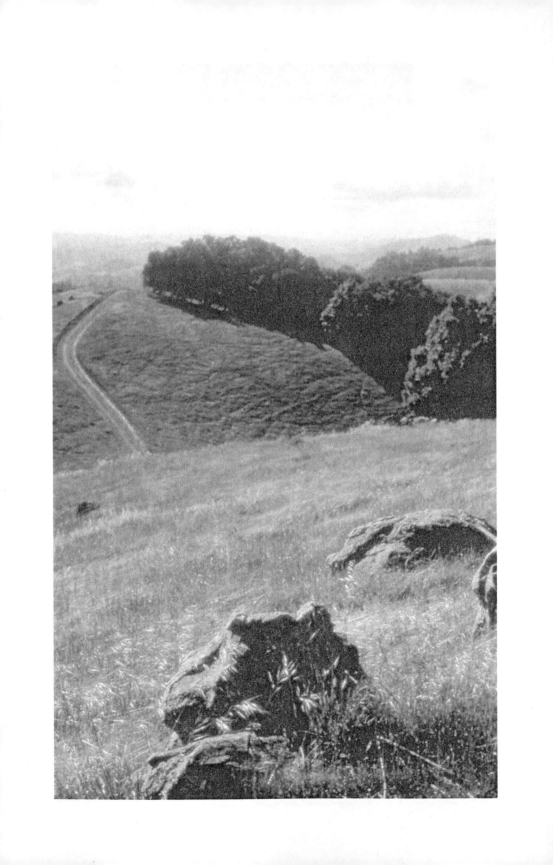

Introducing the
San Francisco Bay Area

The San Francisco Bay Area, with its remarkable juxtaposition of bay, mountains, and sea, is one of the world's premier natural settings. The jewel of this region is San Francisco Bay, one of the largest bays in the U.S. and a unifying feature for the nine counties that ring its shores. Two arms of the Coast Range cradle the bay as they run northwest-southeast along the length of the region. The hills and valleys of the North and South Bay counties loosely connect the inner and outer Coast Ranges.

A wealth of natural beauty resides in the Bay Area's coastal mountains and their rolling foothills—redwood forests, wooded streamsides, oak-studded grasslands, rocky peaks, steep mountainsides, lush meadows, and sunny chaparral slopes. During the last 75 years, public agencies as well as private land trusts have set aside tracts of land in the mountains and foothills that are now parks, open space preserves, and watersheds. Extensive public open space now occupies the land between the Coast Ranges—on shady creek banks, in hillside forests, and in greenspaces within residential areas. In several Bay Area counties this land now forms a continuous open space corridor—a Bay Area greenbelt.

These public open spaces are peaceful backdrops to a bustling urban area—places for adventure, discovery, recreation, and relaxation. Here is "room to breathe," habitat for diverse plant and animal species, and areas for forests to thrive and cleanse our air. Here, too, is the route of the multiuse Bay Area Ridge Trail. When complete, 550 miles of trail will link more than 75 public parks and open spaces and two parcels on private land on the ridgeline surrounding San Francisco Bay.

The route of the Bay Area Ridge Trail lies close to the homes of more than 7 million residents, most of whom live in the valleys of the Coast Range and on the sloping plains that border the bay. From almost any place in the Bay Area, the ridgelands, accented by taller peaks, are visible to Bay Area residents. For them, the sun rises and sets over these mountains, literally and figuratively. Bay Area natives, especially, are fiercely proud and protective of their mountains.

The Bay Area's Heritage of Outdoor Enjoyment

The physical grandeur of this setting and its moderate climate, influenced by the bay and the Pacific Ocean, make the Bay Area ideal for outdoor recreation. You can hike, run, bike, or ride horseback somewhere in the area on almost any day of the year. The area's earliest inhabitants—the Ohlone, Yurock, Pomo, and other Native American tribes—considered this a gentle land. The first explorers marveled at its beauty, great redwood forests, and Mediterranean climate. After the Gold Rush, a wave of settlers arrived to farm and work in its salubrious weather. The first California Geological Survey team report, written by William H. Brewer under the direction of Josiah D. Whitney in the early 1860s, found delight in the variety of terrain and glowingly praised its marvelous scenery. Brewer's book *Up and Down California* describes some Bay Area scenery that is today preserved as parklands in the great Bay Area greenbelt.

As the Spanish built missions and settlements in California, the Spanish government gave large land grants to some colonists as rewards for their service. On vast domains known as *ranchos*, these *rancheros* kept thousands of cattle, which they managed with well-trained horses. The rancheros displayed their fine horses and their equestrian skills at rodeos and games that became important social events. The Spaniards established a tradition of skilled horsemanship and a love for riding that the Mexican rancheros later carried on.

Anglo cattle ranchers blazed trails as they herded their stock and allowed friends—and a relatively small public interested in walking and riding—to cross their lands on these trails, some of which are still in public use. These ranchers also carried on a tradition of fine horsemanship and riding for pleasure.

European immigrants who grew up in the mountains of Germany, Austria, and Switzerland recognized the natural beauty of the Bay Area and took pleasure in walking with friends on weekends. They could wander freely through orchards, along farm roads, through friendly neighbors' meadows, and along hillside animal paths. Mt. Tamalpais was a favorite destination after passenger ferry service from San Francisco reached Marin County in the 1920s.

Eventually many hiking and horseback riding groups sprang up to offer trips in the Bay Area countryside on trails made by the rancheros, cattlemen, early settlers, and weekend explorers. Today, trail enthusiasts can find outings geared for a great variety of skills and interest levels. Trained volunteers for the Bay Area Ridge Trail Council lead trips to many scenic, historic, and cultural sites along the ridges surrounding the bay. Local Sierra Club chapters, as well as sports groups and commercial outfitters, offer outings to many Bay Area destinations.

A Land Conservation Ethic

In 1892, John Muir and others devoted to the outdoors and its natural wonders founded the San Francisco–based Sierra Club. The club grew out its members' dedica-

From high grasslands in Long Ridge Open Space Preserve look for ocean views.

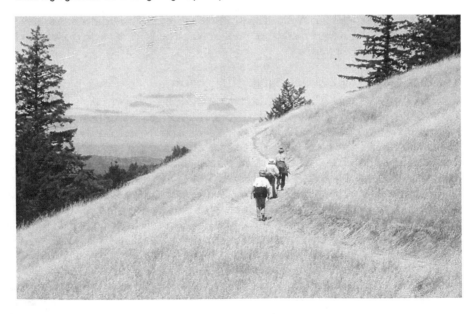

tion to preserving areas of natural beauty and unique wilderness for posterity. It promoted the establishment of many western national parks, including Yosemite National Park in the Sierra Nevada. The Sierra Club continues its conservation mission today at local, national, and international levels. As the Sierra Club grew, local chapters sprang up to lobby for the acquisition of public open space and to support its use. The Bay Area chapters' large membership includes hikers, backpackers, mountain climbers, kayakers, mountain and road bikers, advocates for all types of trail use, and people involved in saving land for parks.

The nine Bay Area counties that border San Francisco Bay have an impetus for cooperation and collaboration. Many government and private reports promote regional unity and planning and preservation of the area's natural resources. The Association of Bay Area Governments, the Metropolitan Transportation Commission, the Regional Air Quality Control Board, the Bay Conservation and Development Commission (BCDC), and the California State Coastal Conservancy seek unity by organizing and managing regional affairs. The Coastal Conservancy has funded the construction of many miles of Ridge Trail, most recently a bridge over a creek on the Tuteur property in Napa County—the Napa Solano Ridge Trail Loop.

Nonprofit grassroots organizations address current needs or glaring deficiencies in government long-range regional planning and land-use problems. The Bay Conservation and Development Commission, for example, brought about by a vigorous grassroots Save the Bay campaign, now regulates use and care of the bay and monitors its shores. The nonprofit Planning and Conservation League, based in Sacramento, works to promote sound legislation for parks, natural resource protection, and land use.

Recognizing that the Bay Area needed a defining greenbelt of open space for its cities, far-sighted citizens and committed activists joined Dorothy Erskine to form a group dedicated to achieving this ideal in the 1960s. First known as People for Open Space, then Greenbelt Congress, and now Greenbelt Alliance, this organization mobilized a regional fight to establish a ring of parks, preserves, open space, farms, and ranches around the Bay Area and continues its mission to this day. As the crusaders grew in numbers, so did the greenbelt around the bay.

Development of Parks and Open Spaces

As the Bay Area population grew, especially in the years following World War II, outdoor lovers began to appreciate the importance of preserving recreation lands for all to enjoy. More and more people gravitated to the outlying hills and valleys to walk or ride horseback freely.

Even before World War II, East Bay citizens began to realize the need for parks adjacent to their growing cities. Inspired and dedicated Alameda and Contra Costa county citizens, aided by civic leaders, launched the East Bay Regional Park District (EBRPD) in 1934 by an overwhelming vote. The EBRPD's first acquisition, Tilden Regional Park, marked the beginning of its present-day 94,500-acre greenbelt of parks, historic units, and recreation complexes.

Other cities and counties eventually followed suit, setting aside small and large areas for parks and open space. Many of these parklands lie on the ridges, mountainsides, and foothills of the Coast Ranges. However, with the recognition that San Francisco Bay was diminishing in size and purity due to landfills and wastewater and garbage dumping, agencies around the bay began establishing shoreline parks to increase stewardship and appreciation of the bay. A notable example is the 30,000-acre Don Edwards San

Francisco Bay National Wildlife Refuge, a unit under the U.S. Fish and Wildlife Service of the Department of the Interior. The refuge seeks to preserve the plant and animal life of the wetlands, to help cleanse bay waters (once an unknown or unheeded need), and to educate the public about these goals. The California Coastal Commission, set up by a statewide ballot initiative that was later resoundingly renewed by public vote, has a mandate to protect the entire state's coastal viewshed and to preserve public access to the shoreline.

As the appreciation of the Bay Area's need for breathing space and stretching room grew, other new agencies also took up the cause. Successful examples include the Marin County Open Space District and the Midpeninsula Regional Open Space District in Santa Clara and San Mateo counties. At the beginning of this decade Sonoma County organized an Agricultural Preservation and Open Space District, and Santa Clara County passed a ballot measure to set up an open space authority. Several cities and counties passed bond measures and initiatives to promote good land use, limit urban sprawl, provide recreational opportunities, and preserve agriculture at city edges. Napa County, for example, adopted land-use regulations designed to protect its world-famous vineyards.

Today, as a result of these many efforts, hundreds of thousands of protected acres in the foothills and mountainsides surround the urbanized bayside, and more acreage edges the bay's shores. In coastal counties—particularly Marin, San Francisco, and San Mateo—thousands of acres are permanently protected by the National Park Service. Local Coastal Plans in Sonoma, Marin, San Francisco, and San Mateo counties afford a measure of protection as well. There is at least one unit of the California State Park System in each Bay Area county, and most Bay Area counties have a county park system; Marin, Sonoma, Alameda, Contra Costa, Santa Clara, and San Mateo counties are blessed with an additional regional park agency.

Many Bay Area parks were established on closed military bases. The military declared Forts Baker, Barry, Cronkhite, and Funston, and Milagra and Sweeney ridges surplus bases during post–World War II downsizing. In 1994, the San Francisco Presidio became a national park under the jurisdiction of the Golden Gate National Recreation Area. A provision of federal law that required these bases to be offered to public entities before the commercial market led to many of the parks that grace our ridgetops and baylands. Alcatraz Island, which formerly housed a high-security federal penitentiary, is now under the supervision of the National Park Service and is a major San Francisco tourist attraction.

Watersheds, too, preserve open space in Marin, Alameda, Contra Costa, Santa Clara, and San Mateo counties. In order to assure a steady water supply for San Francisco's growing population, a group of individuals formed the Spring Valley Water Company in the mid-1880s; the San Francisco Water Department (SFWD) later grew out of this company. Eventually the SFWD began to pipe water from the Sierra Nevada to service the needs of its customers—now more than 1 million—in San Francisco, the East Bay, and on the peninsula.

Other jurisdictions began to develop stable water supplies and to store water in reservoirs. Most of these storage areas are in the foothills surrounding the bay plain. For many years these reservoirs were off-limits to the public. However, with the development of modern purification techniques, some agencies began to open their gates to quiet, passive recreation, such as nature walks and hiking. Today, most water agencies allow some public access. The San Francisco Water Department allows access to trails around the eastern edge of the lakes that fill the earthquake valley in San Mateo County and access to routes on the western edge of the watershed to groups led by trained docents.

The Role of Private Nonprofit Groups

Private nonprofit organizations, such as the Trust for Public Land, Peninsula Open Space Trust (POST), Greenbelt Alliance, and Sempervirens Fund, have worked for many years to preserve and protect open space lands for eventual public use. Through gifts, purchases, and easements, these organizations can make choice lands available to public agencies. An outstanding example is POST's 4262-acre purchase of choice coastal land at Rancho Corral de Tierra in San Mateo County, adjacent to existing federal, state, and county parks, as well as San Francisco Watershed lands. In 2006 the Golden Gate National Recreation Area purchased this land for public open space. Cooperation among agencies, citizens, large donors, and the federal government brought about this remarkable acquisition. A connector trail through this land will someday reach the Bay Area Ridge Trail on the crest of the Santa Cruz Mountains.

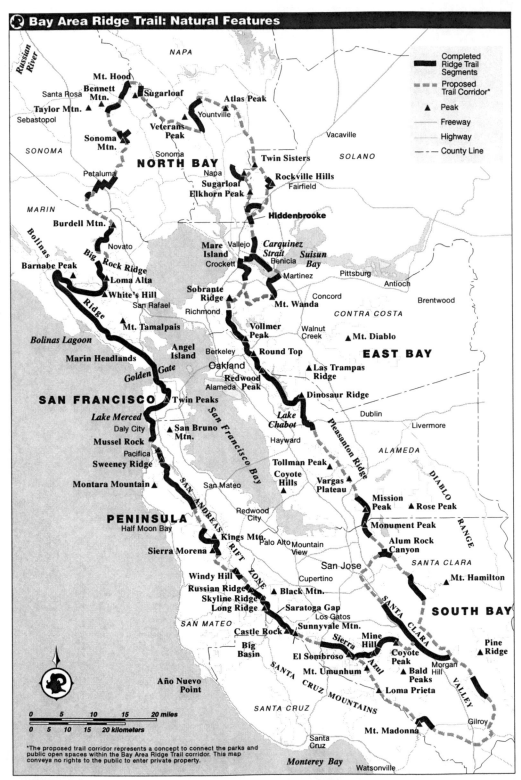

Legend

Completed Ridge Trail Segments

Proposed Trail Corridor*

▲ Peak

Freeway

Highway

County Line

NAPA

Russian River

Mt. Hood

Bennett Mtn.

Santa Rosa

Sugarloaf

Atlas Peak

Taylor Mtn. ▲

Sebastopol

Yountville

Veterans Peak

Vacaville

Sonoma Mtn.

SONOMA

Sonoma

SOLANO

Twin Sisters

NORTH BAY

Napa

Rockville Hills

Petaluma

Sugarloaf

Fairfield

Elkhorn Peak

MARIN

Hiddenbrooke

Burdell Mtn.

Novato

Mare Island

Vallejo

Carquinez Strait

Suisun Bay

Bolinas

Big Rock Ridge

Crockett

Benicia

Barnabe Peak

Loma Alta

Martinez

Pittsburg

Antioch

White's Hill

San Rafael

Sobrante Ridge

Concord

Brentwood

Richmond

Mt. Wanda

CONTRA COSTA

Ridge

Mt. Tamalpais

Vollmer Peak

Walnut Creek

▲ Mt. Diablo

Bolinas Lagoon

Angel Island

Berkeley

Round Top

EAST BAY

Marin Headlands

Oakland

▲ Las Trampas Ridge

Golden Gate

Redwood Peak

Alameda

▲ Dinosaur Ridge

SAN FRANCISCO

Twin Peaks

Dublin

Lake Merced

Lake Chabot

Livermore

Daly City

San Bruno Mtn.

Hayward

Pleasanton Ridge

ALAMEDA

Mussel Rock

Pacifica

Sweeney Ridge

Tollman Peak

DIABLO

Montara Mountain ▲

San Mateo

Coyote Hills

Vargas Plateau

RANGE

Redwood City

Mission Peak

▲ Rose Peak

PENINSULA

Half Moon Bay

Monument Peak

Kings Mtn.

Palo Alto

Mountain View

Alum Rock Canyon

Sierra Morena

RIFT ZONE

San Jose

SANTA CLARA

▲ Mt. Hamilton

Windy Hill

Cupertino

Russian Ridge

▲ Black Mtn.

Skyline Ridge

Long Ridge

Saratoga Gap

SOUTH BAY

SAN MATEO

Los Gatos

Sunnyvale Mtn.

Pine Ridge

Castle Rock

Sierra Azul

Mine Hill

Big Basin

El Sombroso

Coyote Peak

Morgan Hill

Año Nuevo Point

Mt. Umunhum

Bald Peaks

SANTA CRUZ MOUNTAINS

Loma Prieta

VALLEY

SANTA CRUZ

Mt. Madonna

Gilroy

Santa Cruz

Monterey Bay

Watsonville

0   5   10   15   20 miles

0   5   10   15   20 kilometers

*The proposed trail corridor represents a concept to connect the parks and public open spaces within the Bay Area Ridge Trail corridor. This map conveys no rights to the public to enter private property.

6

Introducing the Bay Area Ridge Trail

A combination of unique characteristics primed the Bay Area for the establishment of the Bay Area Ridge Trail: a glorious physical setting; a long history of outdoor recreation; a growing greenbelt; a conservation ethic; and a population of avid outdoor enthusiasts, conservationists, and educated and willing volunteers. Designed as a multiuse ridgeline route, this proposed 550-plus-mile trail will connect public parklands and watersheds of the Bay Area greenbelt that circles San Francisco Bay. It will eventually link more than 75 parks and public lands and provide magnificent views, visits to important historic sites, glimpses of the area's cultural heritage, and firsthand experience of the Bay Area's diverse ecosystems.

On a network of paths that traverses a broad corridor along the ridgelands, the Bay Area Ridge Trail provides recreational opportunities for hikers, mountain and road bikers, and equestrians. Many segments of the trail are accessible to wheelchair users. At least one segment of the Ridge Trail lies less than a half-hour's drive or bus ride from any Bay Area community. The scenic trail links communities along the ridgeline and will connect to bayside population centers and the San Francisco Bay Trail via feeder trails through existing city, county, regional, and federal parks.

The Beginnings

When William Penn Mott, Jr. was general manager of the East Bay Regional Park District in the 1960s, he proposed that a trail be established around the entire ridge of the Bay Area. His vision also included a trail around the bay, close to the water, and connector trails to the Sierra Nevada. Mott went on to serve as director of the California State Parks and later of the National Park Service. In the late 1980s, he lent his strong support and encouragement to achieving his vision of a ridgeline trail around the bay.

In 1986, during the review of the Land Use Element of the San Francisco General Plan, language was inserted that promoted public access to the watershed lands of the City and County of San Francisco. People for Open Space (POS), the predecessors of Greenbelt Alliance, began an effort to acquaint the city with the public-access policies of the region's other water departments. POS brought together the managers of water departments; county, regional, state, and federal parks departments; trail activists; and leaders of environmental organizations at a meeting in 1987, intending to demonstrate to San Francisco that other Bay Area watersheds' less restrictive public-access policies did not harm water quality. As an important outgrowth of that meeting, these groups recognized that watershed lands, parks, and preserves that surround the bay could be linked with a regional trail.

A coalition of activists, spurred by the energy and commitment of William Penn Mott, Jr. (then director of the National Park Service), set up the Bay Area Trails Council in September 1987, renamed the Bay Area Ridge Trail Council in late 1987. Brian O'Neill, superintendent of the Golden Gate National Recreation Area (GGNRA), was the first chairman. The Bay Area Ridge Trail Council was established as a project of POS/Greenbelt Alliance, which provided office space and administrative support in the early years. The National Park Service provided first-year funding, and GGNRA contributed staffing. The outpouring of support for the Bay Area Ridge Trail led the informal council to incorporate in 1992 as a private nonprofit organization. Today, the council

The Bay Area Ridge Trail Council's Mission

A coalition of volunteers and agencies, the Bay Area Ridge Trail Council plans, promotes, builds, acquires, and maintains the 550-mile Bay Area Ridge Trail, a multiuse trail that, when complete, will connect more than 75 parks and open spaces on the ridgeline surrounding the San Francisco Bay. Recognizing the growing recreational needs of the Bay Area's diverse populations, along with the desire of individuals to connect with their communities and the outdoor environment, the council creates links between parks, people, and communities, fulfilling the pioneering vision of William Penn Mott, Jr.

has a membership of 3500, two regional field coordinators, and a dedicated corps of grassroots volunteers.

Bay Area Ridge Trail Accomplishments

As of December 2007, approximately 310 miles of the Ridge Trail have been completed and are dedicated, signed, and in use. Many additional miles of trail are being planned or are under construction for dedication in the near future. The total Ridge Trail mileage is primarily calculated along the main route on a single alignment and does not include alternate routes, connector trails to the main route, or side trips. There is at least one Ridge Trail segment in each of the Bay Area counties. Most of the developed trail traverses public parklands around the Bay Area—with two exceptions, one a 4.5-mile trail in Skyline Wilderness Park, is on land leased from the State of California and operated as a park by a private group that offers its use to the public for a nominal fee. A second trail, the Lucas Valley Trail, crosses Lucasfilm private lands in Marin County.

This treasury of public lands unites the nine Bay Area counties that touch San Francisco Bay. The Bay Area Ridge Trail is a composite necklace of trails, made up of diverse jewels, for a variety of users, from hikers, equestrians, mountain bikers, and wheelchair users, to all who appreciate the beauty of this land. The public spaces it threads offer magnificent views of the Bay Area and places to sit, contemplate, relax, test endurance, build stamina, and restore the spirit.

Along these paths, an observant user can see many of the area's animal species, countless birds, and hundreds of different wildflowers in season. The parks through which the Bay Area Ridge Trail runs offer a wide variety of experiences depending on each trail's terrain and exposure to sun, rain, and wind. The presence of animal and plant life will vary according to such exposure, past usage, and present management. You will enjoy a unique experience on each segment of the Ridge Trail.

The Next Step: Closing the Gaps

Since 1987, the Bay Area Ridge Trail Council has been particularly successful in completing Ridge Trail segments on public lands. Going forward, about 44 percent of the total miles to be completed are in existing public parks and open spaces along the route. About 53 percent of the miles are on privately held lands, and 3 percent are on lands held by nongovernmental organizations. The Bay Area Ridge Trail Council actively reaches out to private landowners, works to build sound public policies that support the Ridge Trail, and assists community partners in fundraising and trail maintenance efforts—critical components in the completion of the remaining Ridge Trail miles.

Closing these gaps in the Bay Area Ridge Trail presents an immediate and immense challenge that will take years to fulfill. However, the council's long-range strategic target is to complete 400 miles of the Ridge Trail by 2012. Success in this effort relies on the council's leadership and the ongoing involvement and commitment of its members, volunteers, and public agency partners.

Volunteers play a key role in the programs and projects of the council. From an active corps who serve on the Board of Directors, to those who build trails and plan and carry out Ridge Trail events, and others who raise needed funds, the volunteers are the heart of the Bay Area Ridge Trail Council. Two outstanding volunteers, Dinesh Desai and Bob Cowell, hiked the entire Ridge Trail route in the summer of 1999. Newspaper, magazine, and TV coverage of this event raised public awareness and financial support of the trail. Several hiking and bicycling groups have challenged themselves to hike or ride a large number of Ridge Trail segments over an extended period. A Santa Clara County group, for instance, hiked 18 segments over a year-long period. Volunteers in the North Bay water trees along a newly landscaped segment of the trail.

Young people, too, can contribute to the Ridge Trail mission. The High Adventure Team of the Santa Clara County Council of the Boy Scouts of America created a patch for youths who hike or bike one segment in any of the four Bay Area sections of the Ridge Trail. Completing a trip in each of the four sections earns the participant all four patches for the full 424-inch Bay Area Ridge Trail "map." The program is open to Brownies and Cub Scouts, Girl and Boy Scouts, and other youth and school groups. Trail maintenance or construction of the trail under supervision of the public land agency is an alternate way to earn a patch. A pamphlet is available through the Boy Scout office (408-280-5088) or South Bay Scout Shop (408-279-2086).

Other Regional Trails in the Bay Area

After World War II, Californians' enthusiasm for an around-the-state, border-to-border loop trail surged, and easements were secured and rights of way developed for the California Riding and Hiking Trail. However, due to rapid building activity along the route and to lack of legal rights to the trails, most trail segments fell into disrepair and were subsequently closed. Today, the Bay Area Ridge Trail follows some segments of this early trail in Contra Costa and San Mateo counties in the East Bay and on the Peninsula.

The Anza Trail, a National Historic Trail, follows Captain Juan Bautista de Anza's attempt to find a land route from Mexico to San Francisco. In the Bay Area, the Anza Trail runs through Santa Clara, San Mateo, and San Francisco counties.

The statewide Coastal Trail hugs the shoreline through San Mateo, San Francisco, Marin, Santa Cruz, and Sonoma counties. In Marin, San Francisco, and San Mateo counties, the Ridge Trail and Coastal Trail share the same alignment.

The San Francisco Bay Trail proposes to circle the shoreline of the entire bay, following a plan originally developed and funded by legislation introduced by Senator Bill Lockyer. The Association of Bay Area Governments, the Metropolitan Transportation Commission, and the nonprofit San Francisco Bay Trail Project are now implementing plans for the Bay Trail, and as of 2007, more than 290 miles are completed.

The Skyline-to-the-Sea Trail connects Castle Rock State Park, on the crest of the Santa Cruz Mountains, with Big Basin State Park, on the Pacific Coast at the mouth

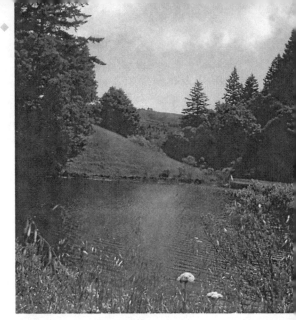

Horseshoe Lake, Skyline Ridge Open Space Preserve

of Waddell Creek. Since the inception of this 26-mile trail in 1969, hundreds of volunteers have built and maintained it during California Trail Days, with support and sponsorship from Sempervirens Fund, the State of California Department of Parks and Recreation, and presently, the California Trails and Greenways Foundation. The Skyline-to-the-Sea Trail also serves as a connector from the coast to the Bay Area Ridge Trail at Saratoga Gap in Santa Clara County.

Three Bay Area trails have been granted national trail status: The Anza Trail is a National Historic Trail; and both the Skyline Trail, which traverses six regional parks on the ridges above East Bay cities, and the Creek Trail, which follows Penitencia Creek in Alum Rock Park, are designated National Recreation Trails. The Bay Area Ridge Trail follows the Skyline and Creek trails and parts of the Anza Trail.

The Bay Area Ridge Trail Council seeks to connect neighboring communities by linking the Ridge Trail to other regional trails and to local trail networks. The connecting trails offer many local residents the opportunity to reach the long regional trails without ever starting a car. These links bind the communities together like the spokes of a bike wheel.

Other Long Trails

Long-distance trails connecting several sites, cities, and/or regions are a challenge to distance hikers and a source of volunteer action and pride in the areas they traverse. The oldest of these trails in the U.S. is the Appalachian Trail, which stretches from Springer Mountain in Georgia to Mt. Katahdin in Maine. Other well-known trails include the Long Trail in New England, the John Muir Trail in California's Sierra Nevada, the aforementioned Anza Trail, and the Pacific Crest and Coastal trails from Mexico to Canada. Around Lake Tahoe, the Tahoe Rim Trail traverses ridgetop lands, and in Southern California, the Santa Ana River Trail offers paved paths on both sides of the river leading to Huntington Beach. Other communities and regions are taking up the long trail idea.

The State of California's Recreational Trails Committee coordinates California's statewide effort to build trails that link communities and promote stewardship of and appreciation for the wealth of public land at our doorsteps. Along with the California Trails and Greenways Foundation, it conducts an annual conference for trail advocates and sponsors the annual spring California Trail Days to help build and maintain trails throughout the state. A National Trails Day event is held on the first Saturday of June in a different location around the country each year.

How to Use This Book

In late 1989, Tioga Press publisher Karen Nilsson and I submitted a proposal to the Bay Area Ridge Trail Council to produce a small guide for each completed Ridge Trail segment. Eventually, these guides were to be assembled in a book. The council accepted the proposal and agreed to make the maps and print the guides. Frances Spangle, with whom I coauthored other guidebooks, wrote the first four Marin County trips and one in San Mateo County. The Bay Area Ridge Trail Council eventually produced 18 guides, printed in two colors on a folded 11-inch x 17-inch sheet and offered for a small fee. After Karen Nilsson's untimely death, Thomas Winnett, publisher of Wilderness Press, a premier national guidebook press, graciously took over the project. The first edition of this book, dedicated to Karen, was the outgrowth of that proposal. This third edition incorporates and updates the early guides and the two previous editions, as well as including all the segments that have been completed in the intervening years—a total of 58 trips, totaling 300-plus miles as of press time.

The trail descriptions here are arranged in clockwise order around San Francisco Bay, begin in San Francisco on the Golden Gate Bridge, followed by Marin County, Sonoma County, then Napa County, and so on around the bay. Hence, the Marin County descriptions start at the south end and finish at the north end of each segment. As the route heads across the interior valleys of the North Bay, trail descriptions begin at the west end and finish at the east end. The East Bay descriptions start in the north and end in the south, and across the Santa Clara Valley the trips go from east to west. Heading up the Peninsula and into San Francisco, the route is described from south to north.

Trip Descriptions

Summary Information

The summary information for each trip lists the mileage of that particular Ridge Trail segment, the different types of users who may access it, the managing agencies, the most important of the regulations visitors must observe, and any nearby facilities, such as water and restrooms.

The agency and regulations sections list the name of each public or private agency responsible for the area, its hours of operation for the park or preserve, dog and bike rules, and fees. Rules regarding dogs range from parks that do not allow dogs on any trail to those that only require them to be under voice control. In general, dogs must be on a six-foot leash. Some trails pass through the jurisdictions of more than one agency, each with different dog regulations, all of which are noted.

Many parks charge an entrance fee, although some only require it on weekends, and group fees may be lower. There is usually a fee for amenities such as camping, horse rental, and swimming. Fees change every few years, so the exact charge is not given in this book. Call the agency that manages the park or special facility, or check its website for current fees.

Biking rules vary depending on the managing agency. Some allow mountain bikers on fire or service roads; a few allow them on narrow trails. Biking access is included in the introductory material for each trip; bikers will find Ridge Trail routes on the maps in this guide as well as on agency maps and on the icons on trailhead signs. See Appendix

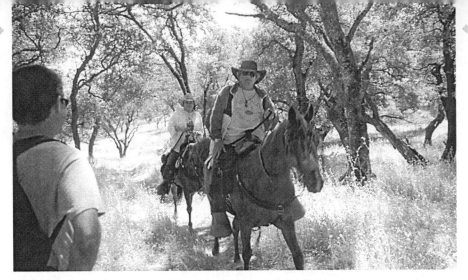

The River-to-Ridge Trail is open to hikers, equestrians, and bicyclists.

3 for a complete list of agency addresses, phone numbers, and websites. The Bay Area Ridge Trail Council website (www.ridgetrail.org) also supplies this information.

Getting There

For every trip in each of the five main book sections, this section gives directions to the trailhead from the nearest major road for each end of the trip. In a few instances, the trailhead differs for each class of user. Driving directions for each of the trailheads are provided in this section. If public transportation is available, general information about service is listed as well. For more information about public transit access to various portions of the Ridge Trail, please see Appendix 4.

On the Trail

This section describes the route, gives directions for trail junctions, tells you what you may see along the way, mentions animal and plant life, and sketches some geologic, historic, and cultural features that add to the interest of the trip. Since I scouted these trips at different times of the year and the appearance of flowers, shrubs, and trees and the presence of animal life varies seasonally, some aspects of the trail's surroundings may differ from what you see.

Maps

Each section begins with an overview map of the Ridge Trail route through the region that particular section covers; the Ridge Trail segments are shown as bold black lines. A separate map for each trip marks the Ridge Trail segment, as well as other trails, park trailheads, and major landmarks. Different thicknesses and dash patterns indicate the trails and their user groups at a glance. The combination of user-group symbols on the map, the accessibility information at the beginning of each trip, and the material in the text clarify the Ridge Trail route and appropriate users within each park or preserve. Additional information on the maps includes trailhead parking areas, major roads, and nearby landmarks, which when combined with the text, will direct you to the park.

Map Legend

TRAIL USES

Bay Area Ridge Trail

Connector Trails (gray)

Multiuse Trail

Hiking/Biking

Equestrian/Hiking

Hiking only

Other Trails (uses not specified)

Name Trail or Road Used by Bay Area Ridge Trail

Name Other Trail or Road Name

Regional Trails

Bay Area Ridge Trail

San Francisco Bay Trail

Juan Bautista de Anza National Historic Trail

American Discovery Trail

East Bay Regional Park District Regional Trails

Skyline-to-the-Sea Trail

(70) Interstate Highway

(34) U.S. Highway

(14) State Highway

Freeway

Major Road

Road

Unpaved Road

Rail Transit and Station (BART, MUNI, Caltrain, VTA, & Amtrak)

Other railroad (freight only)

TRAIL MAP SYMBOLS

P Trailhead Parking

EP Equestrian Parking

LP Limited Parking

T Transit Stop

Infrequent Transit Stop

Picnic Area

Campground

Group Campground

Ranger Station

Visitor Center or Museum

Restroom

Point of Interest

1250' Peak (elevation in feet)

Gate

Redwood Tree or Grove

Start/**End** Start and End of Trip

End/Start Multiple Trips per Map

Parks and Open Space Preserves along Bay Area Ridge Trail

Adjacent Public Lands and Watersheds

Private Property

Elevation Contours (200-foot intervals)

Stream

Body of Water

Marsh or Wetland

Overview Map Symbols

Completed Ridge Trail Segments

Proposed Ridge Trail Corridor (see note on overview maps)

Trail Corridor in Adjacent Counties (existing and proposed)

Freeway

Local Highway

County Line

North Arrow

The maps are generally based on the 7.5-minute series of U.S. Geological Survey (USGS) topographic maps, which are available from some sporting goods and outdoor stores and from the USGS online at http://store.usgs.gov or by writing to 345 Middlefield Road, Menlo Park, CA 94025.

Some additional trails in each park are shown on the maps, but user groups are not distinguished for these areas. For complete information, consult another Bay Area guidebook or request a park map from the managing agency. There are maps at some trailheads, but they may not be available when you visit. Some excellent guidebooks include *Peninsula Trails* and *South Bay Trails,* both coauthored by Jean Rusmore, Betsy Crowder, Frances Spangle, and Sue LaTourrette; and *North Bay Trails* and *East Bay Trails* by David Weintraub, all published by Wilderness Press.

Sharing the Trails

Hikers, mountain bikers, and equestrians share many segments of the Bay Area Ridge Trail. Wherever possible, the Ridge Trail tries to accommodate all users on a single route. If this is not possible, Bay Area Ridge Trail policy states that ". . . due to policy or regulation restrictions, environmental concerns, safety or physical terrain, the Bay Area Ridge Trail Council works cooperatively to secure an additional route that offers an equivalent trail experience."

Variations in speed, height, and power of each type of user require that there be some trail etiquette rules. Some general rules are:

- Observe trail-use signs.
- Be responsible, safe, and considerate.
- Stay on the trail.
- Respect private property.
- Minimize your impact.
- Protect plants and wildlife.
- Hikers and mountain bikers yield to equestrians—stop and remain quiet while an equestrian is passing.
- Mountain bikers yield to hikers—dismount and allow a hiker to pass.

A number of agencies have adopted additional rules for bikers. Maximum speed is 15 miles per hour; slow down to 5 miles per hour when passing or when sight distance is limited, and helmets are a standard requirement of most agencies. Some agencies use radar systems to increase awareness of park speed limits and to help bikers know their speed.

Some Hazards for Trail Users

Poison oak is ubiquitous in the Bay Area. It takes different forms, most often as a trailside shrub but mature plants climb trees and occasionally become small trees themselves. It has three-lobed leaves that are shiny green in spring and turn beautiful shades of red and orange in the fall, and it is extremely harmful to those allergic to it. Just to touch its leaves, berries, or leafless twigs can cause an itchy, blistery rash that takes several weeks to heal. Learn to recognize it and carefully avoid it.

Rattlesnakes are indigenous to the Bay Area, but far less widespread than poison oak. They have triangular-shaped heads, diamond markings on their backs, and rattles

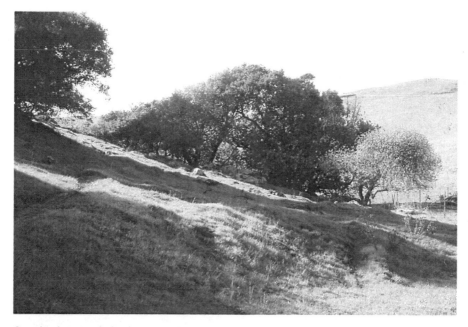

Grasslands in Lynch Canyon Open Space

or segmented sections on their tails. They generally try to avoid contact with humans. However, it's advisable to look down on warm spring days as you hike for rattlesnakes that may be sunning themselves on the trail. Also be sure to look where you put your hands when climbing on rocks.

Lyme disease is a potentially serious disease caused by the bite of the western black-legged tick. In their active months, between December and June, these tiny ticks can brush off trailside grasses and bushes onto your clothes. Wear light-colored clothing so you can see the ticks, keep your arms and legs covered, and tuck your pant legs into your socks.

Mountain lions are shy, native residents of wild lands in the Bay Area. Sightings of these creatures have become more frequent in recent years due to increased human use of their habitat. A mountain lion is about the size of a small German shepherd with a furry tail as long as its body. Trail users should stand facing any mountain lion they en-counter and make loud noises while waving their arms; do not run away because that may cause a mountain lion to see you as prey.

Feral pigs have spread over many acres of wild lands since they were introduced as hunting animals in the 19th century. While generally not dangerous to humans, they can be fierce when cornered. Do not approach any that you may see.

What to Wear and Take Along

Some basic rules for all trail users are to carry plenty of water, food, and snacks; have the appropriate equipment for your mode of travel; take an extra sweater or fleece and a windbreaker; wear a hat; and carry sunscreen. A small packet of band-aids can also be useful. All these items can easily fit in a light daypack.

Specialized equipment for trail users is readily available but not required. Many hikers prefer to wear boots; others find that sturdy shoes with good tread and adequate support are appropriate for most Bay Area trails. Some bikers prefer special mountain biking shoes that clip into their pedals, and many equestrians prefer to wear a protective helmet.

Where to Stay

Many Bay Area Ridge Trail travelers hike or ride one or two segments of the trail on day trips from their Bay Area homes. For those who want to take a longer trip, a weekend

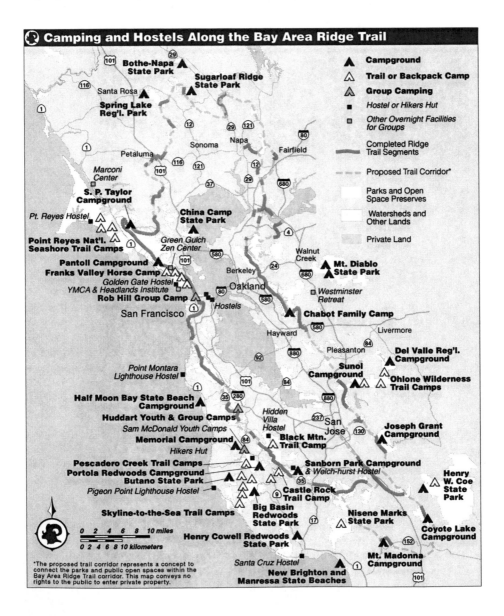

or more, there are many miles of continuous Ridge Trail through Marin, Contra Costa, Alameda, Santa Clara, and San Mateo counties. A Ridge Trail hike through the city of San Francisco would fill two days.

Hostels, primitive camps, and public park campgrounds, located within 2 to 6 miles of the trail, are generally the least expensive places to stay overnight. Charming bed and breakfast inns, comfortable motels, and luxurious hotels in towns and tourist areas near the trailheads are listed in local telephone books or with travel agencies.

As the public discovers the outstanding scenic and recreational qualities of the Bay Area Ridge Trail, local and national outing companies will undoubtedly offer hiking and riding trips on it with transportation to the trailheads and overnight accommodations.

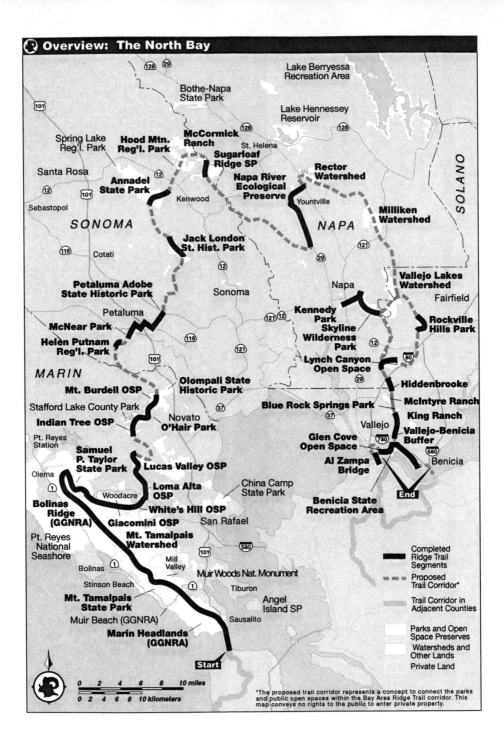

Lake Berryessa
Recreation Area

Bothe-Napa
State Park

Lake Hennessey
Reservoir

Spring Lake
Reg'l. Park

Hood Mtn.
Reg'l. Park

McCormick
Ranch

St. Helena

Santa Rosa

Annadel
State Park

Sugarloaf
Ridge SP

Napa River
Ecological
Preserve

Rector
Watershed

Yountville

Milliken
Watershed

Sebastopol

SONOMA

Kenwood

NAPA

SOLANO

Cotati

Jack London
St. Hist. Park

Sonoma

Napa

Vallejo Lakes
Watershed

Fairfield

Petaluma Adobe
State Historic Park

Petaluma

Kennedy
Park
Skyline
Wilderness
Park

Rockville
Hills Park

McNear Park

Helen Putnam
Reg'l. Park

Lynch Canyon
Open Space

MARIN

Olompali State
Historic Park

Hiddenbrooke

Mt. Burdell OSP

Blue Rock Springs Park

McIntyre Ranch

Stafford Lake County Park

Novato
O'Hair Park

Vallejo

King Ranch

Indian Tree OSP

Glen Cove
Open Space

Vallejo-Benicia
Buffer

Pt. Reyes
Station

Samuel
P. Taylor
State Park

Lucas Valley OSP

Al Zampa
Bridge

Benicia

Olema

China Camp
State Park

Loma Alta
OSP

Woodacre

Benicia State
Recreation Area

End

Bolinas
Ridge
(GGNRA)

White's Hill OSP

Giacomini OSP

San Rafael

Pt. Reyes
National
Seashore

Mt. Tamalpais
Watershed

Bolinas

Mill
Valley

Muir Woods Nat. Monument

Stinson Beach

Tiburon

Mt. Tamalpais
State Park

Angel
Island SP

Muir Beach (GGNRA)

Sausalito

Marin Headlands
(GGNRA)

Start

Completed
Ridge Trail
Segments

Proposed
Trail Corridor*

Trail Corridor in
Adjacent Counties

Parks and Open
Space Preserves

Watersheds and
Other Lands

Private Land

0   2   4   6   8   10 miles
0   2   4   6   8   10 kilometers

*The proposed trail corridor represents a concept to connect the parks
and public open spaces within the Bay Area Ridge Trail corridor. This
map conveys no rights to the public to enter private property.

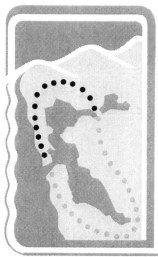

THE NORTH BAY

The Golden Gate Bridge 21

Marin Headlands from the Golden Gate Bridge to
Tennessee Valley. 25

Marin Headlands from Tennessee Valley to Shoreline Highway 31

Mount Tamalpais State Park 35

Mount Tamalpais State Park and Golden Gate
National Recreation Area 39

Golden Gate National Recreation Area and
Samuel P. Taylor State Park. 43

Samuel P. Taylor State Park to Loma Alta Open Space Preserve 49

Loma Alta Open Space Preserve to Lucas Valley
Open Space Preserve. 53

Lucas Valley Open Space Preserve 56

Indian Tree Open Space Preserve to O'Hair Park 59

Mount Burdell Open Space Preserve. 63

Helen Putnam Regional Park and McNear Park to
Petaluma Adobe State Historic Park 69

Jack London State Historic Park 73

Annadel State Park 79

Hood Mountain Regional Park and Open Space Preserve 83

Sugarloaf Ridge State Park. 86

Yountville Cross Road 91

River-to-Ridge Trail. 93

Skyline Wilderness Park and Napa Solano Ridge Trail 95

Rockville Hills Regional Park. 99

Lynch Canyon Open Space 103

Hiddenbrooke Trail. 106

Vallejo-Benicia Buffer. 109

Vallejo-Benicia Waterfront 113

The Golden Gate Bridge

Length 1.7 miles from South Vista Point to North Vista Point

Accessibility Hikers, bicyclists, and wheelchair users. Bridge can be windy or foggy, so wear layers.

Agency Golden Gate Bridge, Highway, and Transportation District

Regulations Hikers and wheelchair users are permitted on east sidewalk during daylight hours only. Bicyclists have 24-hour daily usage on sidewalks (the side determined on a daily basis); after daylight hours bike use is subject to a remotely controlled security check at gates on both ends of east sidewalk. Motorized bikes must be manually pedaled.

Facilities Viewing deck, small visitors center, and gift shops at San Francisco end of bridge, and water and restrooms at both ends of the bridge

This famous span, begun in 1933 and dedicated in 1937, was built to carry automobiles and pedestrians between South and North Bay communities and is one of the world's most spectacular and visited sites. Today, a trip by foot, bike, or wheelchair offers visitors a good opportunity to understand Bay Area geography and the route of the Bay Area Ridge Trail.

Getting There

SOUTH SIDE PARKING AREA: Take Highway 1 or 101 to parking just southeast of the toll gates, and follow the arrows directing you to the bridge walkway. (Returning from the north the route takes you under the span to the parking area.) Follow the signs that direct you to the wide path that leads under the bridge and up to the busy visitor plaza and the bridge's east walkway. Additional parking is available on the north side of Lincoln Boulevard on the east side of the bridge.

NORTH SIDE PARKING AT VISTA POINT: Take Highway 101 or 1 south, follow signs to turnoff for North Vista Point, and then take the pedestrian and wheelchair route on east sidewalk or bike route on sidewalk as signed.

On the Trail

On March 28, 1937, President Franklin Delano Roosevelt pressed a telegraph key in the White House that signaled the opening of the Golden Gate Bridge. Since that ceremonial event, this iconic San Francisco structure has been in continual daily use. More than 100,000 commuters cross it every day, 1 million tourists cross it every month, and 40 million drivers cross it every year. During its 70 years of operation, the bridge has been closed only three times, twice for extremely high winds and once when thousands of pedestrians crowded the decks to celebrate the 50th anniversary of its opening.

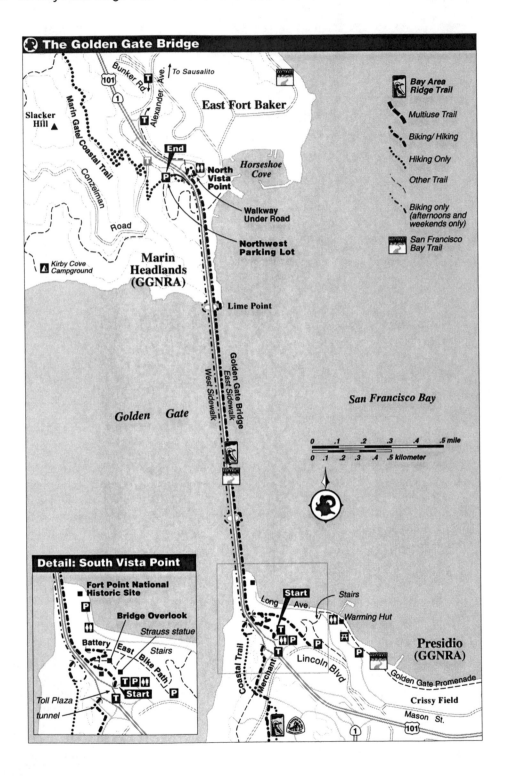

The Golden Gate Bridge

To Sausalito

Bunker Rd.

Slacker Hill ▲

Marin Gate Coastal Trail

Conzelman

Road

East Fort Baker

Alexander Ave.

End

North Vista Point

Horseshoe Cove

Walkway Under Road

Northwest Parking Lot

Marin Headlands (GGNRA)

Kirby Cove Campground

Lime Point

Golden   Gate

Golden Gate Bridge
East Sidewalk
West Sidewalk

San Francisco Bay

0   .1   .2   .3   .4   .5 mile
0 .1 .2 .3 .4 .5 kilometer

Legend
- Bay Area Ridge Trail
- Multiuse Trail
- Biking/ Hiking
- Hiking Only
- Other Trail
- Biking only (afternoons and weekends only)
- San Francisco Bay Trail

Detail: South Vista Point

Fort Point National Historic Site

Bridge Overlook

Strauss statue

Battery   East   Stairs

East Bike Path

Toll Plaza

tunnel

Start

Coastal Trail

Long   Ave.

Start

Merchant

Stairs

Warming Hut

Lincoln Blvd

Presidio (GGNRA)

Golden Gate Promenade

Crissy Field

Mason St.

On May 27, 1937, just a few months after its official dedication, the bridge was closed to traffic and opened to pedestrians only from 6 AM to 6 PM. Schoolchildren were bussed to the bridge and given flowers to toss over the side. More than 200,000 people came, passing through turnstiles that counted them. To this day, those who participated remember the thrill of that opening event.

Today, from the Vista Point adjacent to the south parking area you can see north across the Bay and southeast to the Golden Gate National Recreation Area beach along the Bay's waters. This long strand can be windy and foggy, but it is very popular with runners, joggers, dog walkers, sunbathers, windsurfers, and casual strollers. From the west end of this beach a trail reaches the bridge walkway.

At this Vista Point be sure to note the statue of Joseph Strauss, the chief engineer of the Golden Gate Bridge, and the man who insisted upon strict safety guidelines—helmets for all workers and supervisors and the installation of safety nets for the bridge workers. To read more about the "Halfway to Hell" workers, see the Al Zampa Bridge trip on page 121.

Leave the Vista Point and follow the arrows directing you to the bridge's east walkway. (If you avoid commute hours, your trip will be quieter.) As you look out to sea, think of the first explorers happening onto this slot in the coastline. Imagine those stalwart, adventurous men who risked foul weather, wild storms, lack of food and water, and uncharted ocean to sail north along this coast.

It is said that Sir Francis Drake was the first to land here and his name adorns many public and private places. A bay in Point Reyes National Seashore and north of the Golden Gate named for Drake is considered his more probable landing site. Records from the Spanish explorers tell us that Juan Manuel de Ayala and his subordinate, José Cañizares, were the first white men to sail into San Francisco Bay, in the historic ship *San Carlos*. Latecomer Captain John C. Frémont named the strait *Chrysopylae* (Greek for "golden gate"), before the discovery of gold in California, in his *Geographical Memoir upon Upper California, in Illustration of His Map of Oregon and California*, which was published in 1848.

If you walk across the bridge on a clear day, you can see northwest to the light station at Point Bonita and southwest to Mile Rock and Land's End, sentinels over the Bay's entrance. Alcatraz and Angel islands, both open to public tours, lie to the east. Farther inland, two other bridges, the Richmond-San Rafael and Oakland Bay Bridge, cross the bay's waters.

At midspan, you are 220 feet above the mean high-water mark, and the top of the tower is 500 feet above you. From the walkway you can see an international parade of ships with origins from exotic places: sleek naval vessels, elegant ocean liners, Bay harbor cruise boats, sturdy tugs, and sailboats of all sizes. You can get a sense of the volume and speed of the tide by watching the water as it passes the bridge columns.

As you approach the north end, look left at the rugged cliffs towering above a small beach. You can visit this beach via a trail under the bridge and then another trail that leads to North Bay Ridge Trail trips in the Marin Headlands. And on the east side of the bridge watch for the remains of a proposed fort on rocky Lime Point. Just beyond in a beautiful cove you can see Fort Baker, now refurbished and open for public visits.

When you see the North Vista Point exit, take the stairs that lead to a viewing area where you will have spectacular Bay and ocean views from a different perspective. Or, turn around and retrace your way to the south Vista Point with the City of San Francisco, its shoreline, high rise buildings and acres of public parks and open space laid out before you and the end of your round trip of 3.4 miles.

◆ ◆ ◆

The next leg of the Bay Area Ridge Trail begins on the west side of the bridge in the Marin Headlands from the Golden Gate Bridge to Tennessee Valley trip.

Marin Headlands from the Golden Gate Bridge to Tennessee Valley

Length 4.6 miles

Accessibility Hikers, equestrians, and mountain bikers

Agency Golden Gate National Recreation Area

Regulations Dogs are not permitted on the Ridge Trail and must be on-leash on some other Marin Headlands trails.

Facilities Water, restrooms, and telephone at Marin Headlands visitor center; restrooms and telephone at Tennessee Valley; backcountry camping at Hawk Camp or Haypress campgrounds

This dramatic trip takes you from the landmark Golden Gate Bridge into the hills of the Marin Headlands—you climb through open grassland and coastal chaparral to the ridge above Sausalito and descend into the wide ravine of Tennessee Valley. You'll have spectacular views of San Francisco Bay, the Marin Headlands, and the Pacific Ocean. On narrow paths and wide service roads, you'll climb and descend 600 feet; come prepared for wind and fog.

Getting There

By Car

SOUTH TRAILHEAD, GOLDEN GATE BRIDGE NORTHWEST PARKING (HIKER TRAILHEAD): Going north on Highway 101, take the Alexander Avenue exit and turn left (west) at the stop sign. Go west to Conzelman Road. Make an immediate right uphill and then an immediate left downhill to the parking lot.

Going south on Highway 101, take the Sausalito exit, go left at the stop sign, go right on Conzelman Road, and then immediately turn left onto the road to the parking lot.

BUNKER ROAD TRAILHEAD (MOUNTAIN BIKER/EQUESTRIAN TRAILHEAD): Going north on Highway 101, take the Alexander Avenue exit, downhill toward Sausalito, and pass a stop sign. Take the first left turn (west) into the Fort Baker-Fort Barry Tunnel. Signals regulate one-way auto traffic through the tunnel. Traveling south on Highway 101, take the Sausalito exit (before the Golden Gate Bridge), turn left at the stop sign and go immediately right under the highway toward Sausalito. Turn left at the second stop sign; the tunnel entrance is on your left. There is bike traffic in both directions, so watch for flashing yellow lights. Follow Bunker Road about 1.25 miles beyond tunnel to the trailhead on your right, which has parking for horse trailers and all trail users.

Additional parking for all trail users is available at the Miwok Trailhead at the east end of Rodeo Lagoon near the Headlands Institute. Limited parking for all trail users is available at the junction of Conzelman and McCullough roads with access to the Coastal Trail.

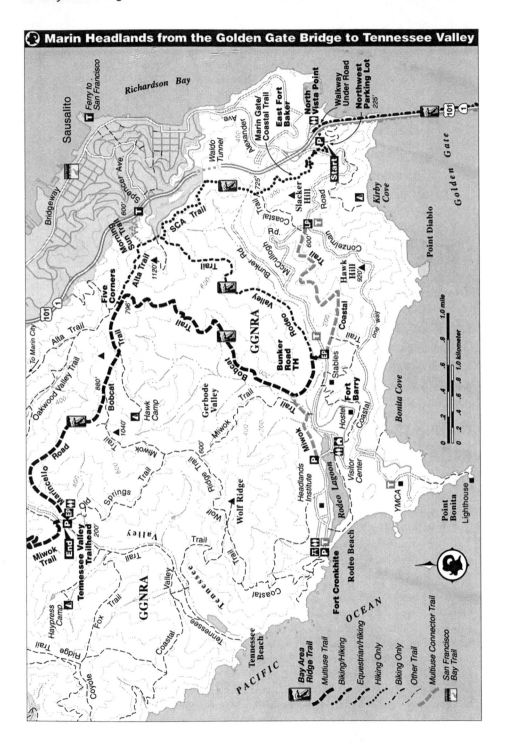

Marin Headlands from the Golden Gate Bridge to Tennessee Valley

Richardson Bay

Sausalito

Ferry to San Francisco

Bridgeway

Spencer Ave.

Alexander Ave.

Waldo Tunnel

Marin Gate/ Coastal Trail

East Fort Baker

North Vista Point

Walkway Under Road

Northwest Parking Lot

Golden Gate

Kirby Cove

Start

Slacker Hill

Road

Conzelman

McCullough

Point Diablo

Bunker Rd.

Hawk Hill

SCA Trail

Morning Sun Trail

Five Corners

Alta Trail

Coastal Trail

Rodeo Valley

GGNRA

Bonita Cove

To Marin City

Alta Trail

Oakwood Valley Trail

Bobcat Trail

Hawk Camp

Gerbode Valley

Miwok Trail

Bunker Road TH

Stables

Fort Barry

Coastal Trail

one way

Miwok Trail

Springs Trail

Wolf Ridge Trail

Wolf Ridge

Headlands Institute

Hostel

Visitor Center

YMCA

Point Bonita Lighthouse

Martinello Road

Old

Miwok Trail

End

Tennessee Valley Trailhead

Rodeo Lagoon

Rodeo Beach

Haypress Camp

GGNRA

Trail

Valley

Tennessee

Fox Trail

Coastal Trail

Tennessee

Fort Cronkhite

OCEAN

Ridge Trail

Coyote

Tennessee Valley

Tennessee Beach

PACIFIC

Bay Area Ridge Trail

Multiuse Trail

Biking/Hiking

Equestrian/Hiking

Hiking Only

Biking Only

Other Trail

Multiuse Connector Trail

San Francisco Bay Trail

1.0 mile

1.0 kilometer

NORTH TRAILHEAD, TENNESSEE VALLEY: From Highway 101 near Mill Valley take the Stinson Beach/Mt. Tamalpais exit and go west on Highway 1 (Shoreline Highway) for about 0.4 mile. Turn left (south) on Tennessee Valley Road, and continue to the parking lot at the end of the road.

By Bus

Several Golden Gate Transit buses stop at Spencer Avenue on Highway 101 daily for access to the Morning Sun Connector Trail. A MUNI bus runs from San Francisco to the Marin Headlands on Sundays only.

On the Trail

Hikers, equestrians, and **mountain bikers** take different trails to reach the Bay Area Ridge Trail route, and then they travel the same route from a junction often called Five Corners. Each user's route to this junction is described separately below in this order: hikers, equestrians, and mountain bikers. Trails in Marin County have a long history, and some trails retain their historic names. This narrative and the maps use the long-established names, although some of these do not appear on trail signs. However, the Ridge Trail route is clearly marked on signposts with the blue, white, and red logo.

Hikers start at the trailhead parking near the northwest portal of the Golden Gate Bridge. From the northwest corner of the parking lot, cross the road and pick up the Bay Area Ridge Trail, also the Coastal Trail, which starts in a Monterey cypress forest and climbs 0.2 mile to Conzelman Road. Cross Conzelman Road to railroad-tie steps, and begin a 600-foot climb up the open hillside. You zigzag along this narrow trail through coastal scrub that seems nondescript, but as the signs warn, it is habitat for the endangered Mission Blue butterfly.

Pause partway up the hill to look back at Lime Point. Juan Ayala, the first European to enter San Francisco Bay, called Lime Point a "white island rock" and anchored his ship, the *San Carlos*, nearby. The rock was later named for its covering of bird lime. Beyond the point lie the waters of the Golden Gate. The Golden Gate Bridge, begun in 1933 and dedicated in 1937, spans the narrow entrance to the bay that Ayala navigated more than two centuries ago, in 1775.

The trail climbs steeply northwest above Highway 101; traffic sounds fade and the view northeast widens to include Richardson Bay and the Belvedere Peninsula. At your feet, a bright variety of yellow daisies, blue lupine, pearly everlastings, and brilliant red Indian paintbrush grow amid bracken fern and the ubiquitous poison oak.

A small footbridge crosses seeping springs where moisture-loving yellow mimulus thrive. Turn around here to enjoy magnificent views of San Francisco's skyline, Alcatraz and Angel islands, and the East Bay hills beyond. Below you to the northeast, you can see the red-tiled roofs of East Fort Baker's historic buildings in Horseshoe Cove. This old fort, part of the Golden Gate National Recreation Area, is home to the Bay Area Discovery Museum, which offers imaginative activities for young people. Beyond Horseshoe Cove, you can see the bay, enlivened by the sight of yachts heeling over in the brisk winds coming through the gate.

At the ridgecrest, you come to a trail junction; to stay on the Ridge Trail route, go right (northwest) on the 0.8-mile SCA Trail, named for and built by the Student Conservation Association. The Coastal Trail goes left over Slacker Hill and then descends west to Rodeo Lagoon. If the day is clear, the views around the compass from this hill are dramatic; you'll have your first views west to the Pacific Ocean and northwest over the GGNRA's 12,000-acre Marin Headlands.

Continue northwest on the SCA Trail. After climbing up a slope where rattlesnake grass and oats blow in the wind, you come to a sign that states HIKERS, PRIVATE PROPERTY—turn west here. The single-track Ridge Trail heads west here at the head of Rodeo Valley; it follows the contour of the hillside below a row of houses. From this trail you can look 600 feet down into Rodeo Valley and see the west entrance of the tunnel beneath the ridge you have just walked along.

The narrow trail climbs gently along a grassy slope, accented by jagged outcrops of white rock and flowery in spring. You pass through a small eucalyptus grove and continue for a half mile before climbing to the ridgetop high above Sausalito. On the ridge, you meet the Rodeo Valley Trail, the Bay Area Ridge Trail equestrian route, which has climbed northeast from the Bunker Road Trailhead.

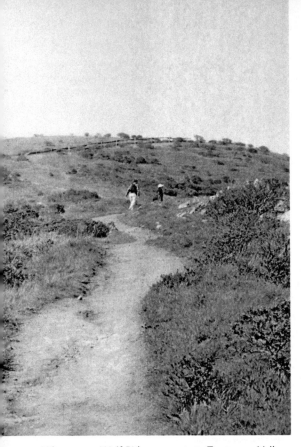
Hikers cross Wolf Ridge en route to Tennessee Valley.

Equestrians begin at the Rodeo Valley Trailhead off Bunker Road at the junction of the Coastal and Rodeo Valley trails in the Marin Headlands. Cross the wooden bridge, signed RIDGE TRAIL, over willow-bordered Rodeo Creek, and head north along the lower slope of the hill between Rodeo and Gerbode valleys. In spring, the field above the creek is bright with yellow mustard, and the air is filled with the calls of red-winged blackbirds.

Head east on the Rodeo Valley Trail for about 1 mile along the edge of the valley and past interesting rock outcrops. The trail winds toward the ridgetop for another mile, over steep pitches and gentle grades. At the ridgetop, it meets the north end of the SCA Trail, where equestrians join hikers to continue to Five Corners.

Now **hikers** and **equestrians** continue past a private road on the right and go left around a white, metal fire-protection gate onto the Alta Trail. Then you round the east side of a wooded, antenna-crowned hill, where you pass the 0.5-mile Morning Sun Trail, a 300-foot connector trail of railroad-tie steps from the Highway 101 Spencer Avenue exit in Sausalito. At this trailhead, you'll find parking, a telephone, and Golden Gate Transit bus connections.

Hikers and **equestrians** on the Bay Area Ridge Trail continue northwest from the Morning Sun Trail intersection along an oak-shaded hillside. Occasional views of the bay and patches of apricot-colored sticky monkeyflowers grace the trail. Look west to the Clyde Wahrhaftig Memorial Bench dedicated in 1998 to honor the memory of this renowned geologist who contributed greatly to the understanding of Marin Headlands' geology.

In about a half mile, you reach the convergence of five trails, known as "Five Corners" to Marin Headlands regulars, although no sign identifies it as such. Watch carefully for this junction—on foggy days it may be hard to see. Jog left (west) about 30 feet to meet the Bobcat Trail and turn right (northwest) on it. This is where **mountain bikers** coming up from Gerbode Valley meet **hikers** and **equestrians**.

Mountain bikers begin at the same trailhead as equestrians on Bunker Road (you can also park at the Miwok Trailhead at the east end of Rodeo Lagoon near the Headlands Institute). Cross the wooden bridge signed RIDGE TRAIL, and turn left (west) on the Rodeo Valley Trail (multiuse going west only). Turn right (northeast) at the Bobcat Trail junction, and begin your 2-mile trip up Gerbode Valley. Look for blue bush lupine blooming by the trailside in spring. Ahead is the site of the former Sam Silva dairy, one of the many Portuguese dairies along this coast in the mid-1800s. All that remains today are the groves of eucalyptus and Monterey cypress and a few persistent fruit trees and rose bushes. You can make out the cistern that supplied water to the site, high on the hill above.

Past the dairy, the trail begins its climb up a hillside, and you look out over the floor of the valley. In the 1960s, developers planned the city of Marincello in this valley. Martha Gerbode and other staunch conservationists succeeded in preventing the development plans by buying the land and turning it over to The Nature Conservancy; the headlands then became part of the Golden Gate National Recreation Area. The Bobcat Trail winds up the valley to the ridge and Five Corners junction.

From Rancho Sausalito to Golden Gate National Recreation Area

The open hills before you—from the Marin Headlands to Stinson Beach—were once part of the vast Rancho Sausalito. In 1822, enterprising Englishman William Richardson left his ship in San Francisco; two years later he married Mario Antonio Martinez, the daughter of Ignacio Martinez, the Mexican commandante of the Presidio. In 1841, Mexican governor of California Juan Bautista Alvarado granted him the 20,000-acre Rancho Sausalito. Failing ventures forced Richardson into debt, and he had to sell his land to Samuel Throckmorton in 1860. The land was subdivided, and many ranches were bought for use as dairies by Portuguese immigrants from the Azores. Hay to feed the dairy cows did not thrive along this foggy coast, however, and by the mid-1890s the Portuguese had abandoned their dairies.

The U.S. Army also occupied land in the headlands. The Army bought the tract that now serves the north end of the Golden Gate Bridge in 1855, and in 1873, it began installing fortifications there, the last of which was a Nike missile site, dismantled in 1974.

Today, most of the original Rancho Sausalito is part of the Golden Gate National Recreation Area. The grizzlies and elk that vaqueros and early settlers hunted are long gone, but bobcats, deer, foxes, and an occasional mountain lion still range over these hills.

From Five Corners, **all trail users** follow the Bobcat Trail due west up a slight incline to a spectacular view: Mt. Tamalpais to the northwest, Richardson Bay to the east, and the Pacific Ocean to the west. At the top of the incline you pass a little meadow fenced for "Resource Protection" against footsteps, hoof prints, and wheel tracks; in spring you will see buttercups, poppies, brodiaea, and scarlet Indian paintbrush—notice the native grasses waving in the breeze.

After a small dip and rise, you pass the trail that goes southwest a half mile downhill to primitive Hawk Camp. Pause here to look back for a last glimpse of San Francisco's skyline and the tip of the Golden Gate Bridge tower. Hawks soar above, watching for field mice and voles in open grasslands and for wary rabbits hurrying across the road to the cover of chaparral. Bear right to continue past the camp on the rocky, rutted Bobcat Trail.

In less than a quarter mile you reach the junction of Marincello and Bobcat trails, where you veer right again on the wide, 1.7-mile Marincello Trail, and the Bay Area Ridge Trail route to Tennessee Valley. (The Bobcat Trail veers left, uphill.) You follow the road laid out in the 1960s to the proposed Marincello development. Modest stands of Monterey pines, cypresses, and a few eucalyptus planted by the would-be developers of this city now crown the steep road banks. Clumps of willows and tall woodwardia ferns watered by seeping springs dot the roadside.

The hillside falls off steeply to the east into Oakwood Valley, beyond which lie Richardson Bay and Belvedere. The trail makes a wide curve west as you near the trailhead in Tennessee Valley, and the Miwok stables and corrals, part of an old dairy ranch, come into view. At the Tennessee Valley Trailhead you will find pleasant picnic tables under a grove of pines. For an easy 3.4-mile side trip from Tennessee Valley, follow a trail that leads to the coast at Tennessee Cove.

◆ ◆ ◆

The next segment of the Ridge Trail route continues north from here on the Miwok Trail to Shoreline Highway and Mount Tamalpais State Park beyond.

Marin Headlands from Tennessee Valley to Shoreline Highway

Length 3.8 miles

Accessibility Hikers, equestrians, and mountain bikers

Agency Golden Gate National Recreation Area

Regulations Dogs on leash are permitted on the Ridge Trail but are not allowed on other trails.

Facilities Restrooms and telephone at Tennessee Valley

The trailhead in Tennessee Valley lies at a low divide between Coyote and Wolf ridges, from which creeks flow east to Richardson Bay and west to the ocean. The Bay Area Ridge Trail route climbs northwest along the Miwok Trail, a narrow and sometimes steep trail that ascends 800 feet toward Coyote Ridge; you'll have sweeping views of San Francisco Bay, see bountiful spring wildflowers, and catch cool ocean breezes. Fog and wind will often accompany you over these coastal hillsides. You reach Highway 1 on a gentle descent along a wide service road.

A network of trails extends south into Gerbode and Rodeo valleys and north to Muir Beach and Green Gulch. These trails are popular and very busy on weekends. One trail leads 2 miles west to Tennessee Cove, well-known for its powerful surf. It was here in 1853 that the three-masted sidewheel steamship Tennessee ran aground in fog on a voyage from Panama. All aboard were saved.

Getting There

SOUTH TRAILHEAD, TENNESSEE VALLEY: From Highway 101 near Mill Valley take the Stinson Beach/Mt. Tamalpais exit and go west on Highway 1 (Shoreline Highway) for about 0.4 mile. Turn left (south) on Tennessee Valley Road and continue to the parking lot at the end of the road.

NORTH TRAILHEAD, SHORELINE HIGHWAY: From Highway 101 in Mill Valley take the Stinson Beach/Mt. Tamalpais exit and go 2.7 miles west on Highway 1 (Shoreline Highway). Continue 0.4 mile beyond Panoramic Highway turnoff north to roadside parking. There is space for four cars on the north side of the highway and for six cars on the south side. Do not block the fire road gate.

On the Trail

To begin this trip to Shoreline Highway, **hikers, equestrians,** and **mountain bikers** find the Bay Area Ridge Trail/Miwok Trail sign on the north side of the parking area at the east end of Tennessee Valley Road. Cross a bridge over a small creek, and

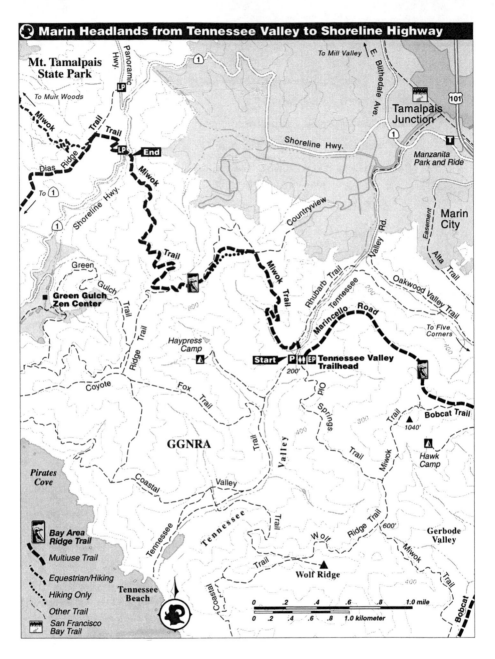

Marin Headlands from Tennessee Valley to Shoreline Highway

Mt. Tamalpais State Park

Panoramic Hwy.

To Mill Valley

Blithedale Ave.

101

To Muir Woods

Miwok Trail

Trail

LP

Tamalpais Junction

Shoreline Hwy.

Manzanita Park and Ride

LP End

Miwok

Dias Ridge

To 1

Countryview

Marin City

Shoreline Hwy.

Easement

Alta Trail

Trail

Miwok Trail

Oakwood Valley Trail

Green

Rhubarb Trail

Tennessee

Gulch

Marincello Road

To Five Corners

Green Gulch Zen Center

Ridge Trail

Haypress Camp

Start P EP Tennessee Valley Trailhead

200'

Old Springs

Bobcat Trail

1040'

GGNRA

Coyote

Fox Trail

Valley

Trail

Miwok Trail

Hawk Camp

Pirates Cove

Coastal

Valley

Tennessee

Wolf Ridge Trail

600'

Gerbode Valley

Miwok

Bay Area Ridge Trail

Multiuse Trail

Equestrian/Hiking

Hiking Only

Other Trail

San Francisco Bay Trail

Tennessee Beach

Trail

Coastal

Wolf Ridge

Bobcat

0   .2   .4   .6   .8   1.0 mile
0   .2   .4   .6   .8   1.0 kilometer

follow its course upstream through a grove of native scrub oaks and nonnative eucalyptus, commonly imported and planted as windbreaks for dairy ranches along the coast.

After 0.25 mile, the Ridge Trail/Miwok Trail begins to climb out of the canyon on switchbacks. Across the stream, you see a scattering of oaks and madrones on the grassy hillside and apricot-colored blossoms of sticky monkeyflower grow along the trail. In spring, open grasslands are bright with flowers—pink mallow, blue brodiaea, golden poppy, and blue ground iris.

You climb several flights of innovative hard rubber water bars—alternatives to railroad ties designed to prevent erosion and to allow both mountain bikers and equestrians to maneuver—the trail rises quickly toward the ridge ahead. Look west to see the Pacific Ocean through a notch in the hills at the end of Tennessee Valley. Soon you see east across Richardson Bay to Belvedere and Angel Island and beyond to the East Bay. Such vistas are surely what were envisioned for the Bay Area Ridge Trail.

Amid chaparral and rock outcrops, pink mallow, silver-leafed lupine, and blue-eyed grass bloom in open grassy patches. Silver-leafed lupine is an important host plant for the endangered Mission Blue butterfly; in order to protect the plants, the park service rerouted the trail on this steep grade.

Above your trail to the north, you see a grove of tall eucalyptus crowning the hill ahead. The Miwok Trail circles east of the grove. As you approach the grove, a narrow path marked for hikers only turns left (west) on a shortcut to Coyote Ridge ahead. Detour along this steep, grassy hillside in spring to see an extravagant display of wildflowers.

The Bay Area Ridge Trail route continues north on the Miwok Trail and then west beside a sheltered, shady forest where wood ferns carpet the ground. As you round the hilltop, you'll see the Miwok Trail extending north from Coyote Ridge. Near the ridgetop, you meet the Coyote Ridge Trail. You turn right on the Miwok Trail and wind in and out of deep canyons and cross chaparral-covered hills as you drop steeply into Tamalpais Valley. The Coyote Ridge Trail continues southwest to meet the Green Gulch and Fox trails and then meets the Coastal Trail.

The Miwok Trail/Bay Area Ridge Trail continues into Tamalpais Valley, with views of houses nestled on the hills. As you near the highway, you pass through woods of eucalyptus and oak, where ferns line the trail and toyon and elderberry flourish.

Just before the highway, a short section of trail buttressed with railroad ties and flanked by posts directs you to a point where **hikers, equestrians,** and **mountain bikers** have enough sight distance to safely cross Shoreline Highway. To the west you can see Muir Beach and the Pacific Ocean.

◆ ◆ ◆

Across the road, the Bay Area Ridge Trail route continues on the Miwok Trail over Dias Ridge, through Mount Tamalpais State Park. Find the trail in a small parking area on the far side of the highway.

Mount Tamalpais State Park: From Shoreline Highway to Pantoll Ranger Station

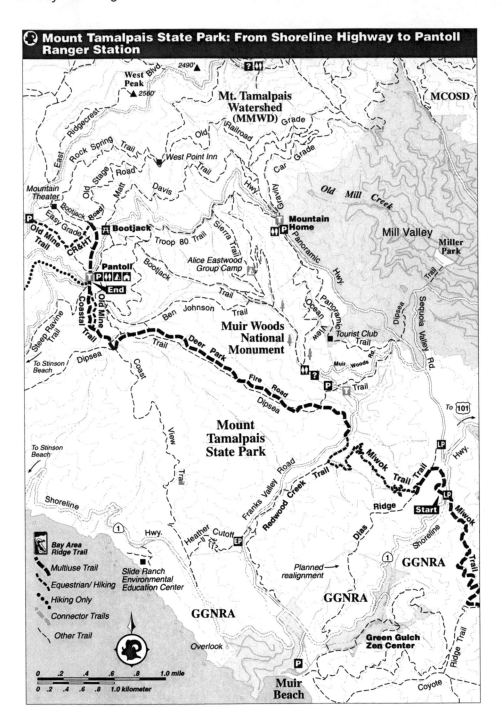

West Peak 2490'

West Peak 2560'

Mt. Tamalpais Watershed (MMWD)

MCOSD

Ridgecrest

East

Rock Spring Trail

Old Stage Road

Old Grade

Railroad Grade

Car Grade

West Point Inn

Matt Davis Trail

Mountain Theater

Old Mill Creek

Mill Valley

Miller Park

Easy Grade

Bootjack Road

CR&HT

Old Mine Trail

Bootjack

Troop 80 Trail

Sierra Trail

Gravity Car Grade

Hwy.

Mountain Home

Panoramic

Pantoll

End

Bootjack

Alice Eastwood Group Camp

Trail

Ben Johnson Trail

Ocean View

Panoramic

Tourist Club Trail

Dipsea

Sequoia Valley Rd.

Steep Ravine Trail

Coastal Trail

Old Mine

Deer Park Trail

Muir Woods National Monument

Muir Woods Rd.

To Stinson Beach

Dipsea

Coast Trail

Fire Road

Trail

To 101

Dipsea

View Trail

Mount Tamalpais State Park

Franks Valley Road

Redwood Creek Trail

Miwok Trail

Trail

Hwy.

To Stinson Beach

Ridge

Start

Miwok

LP

Shoreline

Heather Cutoff

EP

Dias

GGNRA

Bay Area Ridge Trail

Multiuse Trail

Equestrian/ Hiking

Hiking Only

Connector Trails

Other Trail

Slide Ranch Environmental Education Center

Planned realignment

GGNRA

GGNRA

Green Gulch Zen Center

Ridge Trail

Overlook

Coyote

0   .2   .4   .6   .8   1.0 mile

0 .2 .4 .6 .9 1.0 kilometer

Muir Beach

Mount Tamalpais State Park

From Shoreline Highway to Pantoll Ranger Station

Length	5.4 miles
Accessibility	Hikers, equestrians, and mountain bikers
Agency	Mount Tamalpais State Park
Regulations	Park is open from 7 AM to approximately sunset, dogs are prohibited, and bikes are limited to fire roads.
Facilities	Water, restrooms, walk-in campsites, and telephone at Pantoll Ranger Station; Franks Valley Horse Camp on Muir Woods Road

Watch raptors soar above open grassy slopes, take in views of the Pacific Ocean, follow a moist creekbed, and cross shaded oak woodlands and Douglas-fir forests; this trek through Mount Tamalpais State Park crosses the northwest corner of Muir Woods. You begin with a 500-foot elevation loss on the gentle, 2.1-mile Miwok Trail and then gain 1400 feet on a steady climb to Pantoll Ranger Station.

Getting There

By Car

SOUTH TRAILHEAD, SHORELINE HIGHWAY: From Highway 101 in Mill Valley, take the Stinson Beach/Mt. Tamalpais exit, and go 2.7 miles west on Highway 1 (Shoreline Highway). Continue 0.4 mile beyond the Panoramic Highway turnoff north to roadside parking. There is space for four cars on the north side of the highway and for six cars on the south side. Do not block the fire road gate.

ALTERNATE TRAILHEAD ON PANORAMIC HIGHWAY: Follow directions above, but turn north on Panoramic Highway, continuing north around the first sharp bend to roadside parking. Pass through gate on west side of road to Dias Ridge Fire Trail, and continue south a third of a mile to the Miwok Trail.

NORTH TRAILHEAD, PANTOLL RANGER STATION: From Highway 101 in Mill Valley follow the directions above, but turn north on Panoramic Highway and continue approximately 6 miles northwest to parking at ranger station, which charges a parking fee. Additional parking is available at the Bootjack Picnic Area, 0.2 mile before Pantoll, if Pantoll is full (a group parking fee applies).

Equestrians

Horse trailer parking on the road shoulder alongside Franks Valley Road provides access to the Redwood Creek Trail and the Deer Park Fire Road to Mt. Tamalpais.

By Bike

Mountain bikers can access the trail from Deer Park Fire Road off Franks Valley Road and Muir Woods Road.

By Bus

The West Marin Stagecoach stops at Pantoll Ranger Station a couple times each day.

On the Trail

This Bay Area Ridge Trail trip runs from the Golden Gate National Recreation Area through the southeast corner of 6000-acre Mount Tamalpais State Park. **Hikers, equestrians,** and **mountain bikers** begin on the Miwok Trail from Shoreline Highway and climb switchbacks on a gentle grade. In spring, purple iris and lavender bush lupine enliven the greasewood-covered hillside. At the ridgetop, you turn left (southwest) on the Dias Ridge Fire Road. On clear days, you'll have far-reaching views from broad, grassy Dias Ridge: west to San Francisco; east to Richardson Bay, Belvedere, Angel Island, and across to the East Bay. Mt. Tamalpais rises before you to the north. The Miwok Trail branches right (northwest) after 0.2 mile on the Dias Ridge Trail.

Mountain bikers continue west on the soon-to-be-restored Dias Ridge Trail to Highway 1, where you go north 0.25 mile and then turn right (north) on Franks Valley and Muir Woods roads and join hikers and equestrians on Deer Park Fire Road.

Hikers and **equestrians** turn on the Miwok Trail and descend into Franks Valley. The trail loses 500 feet on a comfortable grade; switchbacks pass through grassy clearings and oak groves, with views into the valley and of the ridge you will follow on Deer Park Fire Road. A meadowside bench halfway down the trail offers a good place to pause. You follow a tributary to Redwood Creek and arrive at a junction with the Redwood Creek Trail. A handsomely turned signpost notes that the Miwok Trail was built by the Youth Conservation Corps in 1981. The Miwok Trail ends here and you go upstream on the Redwood Creek Trail.

Redwood Creek begins high in the canyons above Muir Woods and flows into the ocean at Muir Beach. In fall and winter, you may see fish swimming in the creek (fishing is prohibited). The trail follows the creek as it bends around a jumble of rocks where giant bay laurels spread a wide canopy. A pool reflects the sky and overhanging branches of alders, making this an inviting place to stop for a snack before the long climb to Pantoll. Continuing upstream, you cross a footbridge and then head north to Muir Woods Road. The main entrance to Muir Woods National Monument is 0.75 mile up the road. However, you pick up the gated, signed Deer Park Fire Road directly across the road. Here, **bikers** join **hikers** and **equestrians** on this broad, unpaved fire road, which swings up through scanty chaparral into oak woodland. For 2.8 miles you climb steadily up the ridge to the Pantoll Ranger Station, a gain of 1400 feet. In about a half mile, the fire trail crosses the Dipsea Trail, the route of the 7-mile foot race from Mill Valley to Stinson Beach, held every June since 1905. The Dipsea Trail affords an alternate route for hikers; it more or less parallels the fire trail, crossing it several times as they climb to the ridge. In another half mile, the fire trail emerges on a stretch of meadow from which you can see the domes of a military installation on Mt. Tamalpais's west peak.

In spring, these grassy hillsides are bright with flowers. Red-tailed hawks and turkey vultures with wingspreads of nearly 6 feet often circle above the meadows, scanning

The Sleeping Lady

The 2571-foot East Peak of Mt. Tamalpais towers over the Bay Area; it has been upthrust by fault movement over millions of years. The mountain was revered by Coast Miwoks, who settled by its streams and along its coast and bay waters more than 7000 years ago. According to legend the long flank of the mountain when viewed from the south is a beautiful maiden sleeping with her head to the east and her feet facing the sea. New arrivals to this area were drawn to its peaks and slopes, and by the late 1800s, thousands of hikers thronged its trails on weekends. In 1896, the Mt. Tamalpais Railroad was extended to the summit. The Tamalpais Conservation Club, formed in the early 1900s, and other hiking clubs helped construct and maintain trails. In 1928, Mt. Tamalpais State Park was created.

them for hapless field mice or carrion. You may not see any black-tailed deer, but you can be sure they are nearby from their tracks along the trail.

The trail enters the forest again, where the shade is welcome on sunny days. Tall redwoods remind you that you are on the edge of Muir Woods National Monument, which you pass through farther up the trail, in a Douglas-fir forest. The trail steepens, veering left to emerge onto broad grasslands below Pantoll. To the west, you have a view of the Pacific Ocean, or as is often the case, the fog bank covering it. South and east are the bay and San Francisco's skyline. You join the Coastal Fire Road and head due north, passing the Dipsea Trail as it veers west on its way to Stinson Beach. Shortly you pass the Lone Tree Fire Road and continue north for about 0.7 mile to the Pantoll Ranger Station.

Hikers and **equestrians** can follow the Old Mine Trail to Pantoll through a Douglas-fir forest; the trail begins just beyond the Lone Tree Trail junction and runs adjacent to the Coastal Fire Road. Mountain bikers stay on the Coastal Fire Road to Pantoll. If you are not continuing north, you could arrange to meet friends at the Pantoll Ranger Station and have lunch at nearby Rock Spring or Bootjack picnic areas.

◆ ◆ ◆

From Pantoll, **hikers** can continue north on the Matt Davis Trail, which begins the next segment of the Bay Area Ridge Trail. The trailhead is just across Panoramic Highway from Pantoll. **Bikers** do not have a designated Ridge Trail route north from Pantoll to the Bolinas-Fairfax Road; **equestrians** take the Old Stage Road to enjoy the next trail segment.

Mount Tamalpais State Park and Golden Gate National Recreation Area: From Pantoll Ranger Station to Bolinas-Fairfax Road

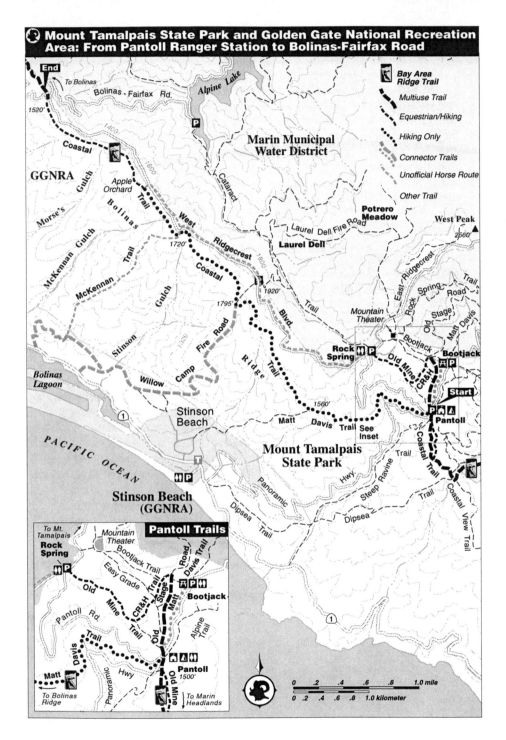

Bay Area Ridge Trail

Multiuse Trail

Equestrian/Hiking

Hiking Only

Connector Trails

Unofficial Horse Route

Other Trail

End

To Bolinas

Bolinas - Fairfax Rd.

Alpine Lake

1520'

1400

Coastal

Trail

Marin Municipal
Water District

GGNRA

Bolinas

Gulch

Apple
Orchard

Morse's

McKennan Gulch

McKennan Trail

West

Ridgecrest

1720'

1600

Coastal

Potrero
Meadow

West Peak
2560'

Laurel Dell Fire Road

Laurel Dell

East Ridgecrest Trail

Rock Spring Road

Stage

Old Matt Davis

Mountain
Theater

1800

1795'

1920'

Stinson Gulch

Fire Road

1300

Trail

Blvd.

Rock
Spring

Old Mine

Bootjack

Bootjack

CR&H

Start

Ridge

Trail

Willow

Camp

1560'

Pantoll

Bolinas
Lagoon

Stinson
Beach

Matt   Davis   Trail   See
Inset

Mount Tamalpais
State Park

PACIFIC OCEAN

Stinson Beach
(GGNRA)

Panoramic

Hwy.

Dipsea Trail

Trail

Steep Ravine

Trail

Coastal Trail

Coastal View Trail

Dipsea

Pantoll Trails

To Mt.
Tamalpais

Mountain
Theater

Rock
Spring

Bootjack Trail

Easy Grade

Old

Pantoll Rd.

Mine

Trail

CR&H Trail

Stage

Matt Davis Trail

Road

Bootjack

Alpine
Trail

Davis

Trail

Matt

Hwy.

Panoramic

Old Mine

Pantoll
1500'

To Bolinas
Ridge

To Marin
Headlands

0   .2   .4   .6   .8   1.0 mile

0   .2   .4   .6   .8   1.0 kilometer

Mount Tamalpais State Park and Golden Gate National Recreation Area

From Pantoll Ranger Station to Bolinas-Fairfax Road

Length 6.4 miles

Accessibility Hikers, equestrians, and mountain bikers

Agencies Golden Gate National Recreation Area and Mt. Tamalpais State Park

Regulations Pantoll Road and Ridgecrest Boulevard are open from 7 AM to sunset but may be closed in times of high fire danger or hazardous road conditions. Pantoll Ranger Station charges a parking fee. Mt. Tamalpais State Park is open from 7 AM to sunset and prohibits dogs. GGNRA and MMWD require that dogs be on a leash. Bikes are allowed on fire roads only.

Facilities Water, restrooms, and telephone at Pantoll Ranger Station; water and restrooms at Rock Spring; and water and restrooms at nearby Mountain Theater

High on the slopes of Mt. Tamalpais and along Bolinas Ridge, this route takes full advantage of the mountain's challenging trails, breathtaking views, forested glades, and flowery slopes. Coastal fog often obscures vistas in the morning and late afternoon. Choose a clear winter or spring day to appreciate views up and down the coast and the wildflowers that bloom along the trail. Hikers gain and loose several hundred feet in elevation.

Getting There

By Car

SOUTH TRAILHEAD, MOUNT TAMALPAIS PANTOLL RANGER STATION: From Highway 101 in Mill Valley, take the Stinson Beach/Mt. Tamalpais exit and go 2.7 miles west on Highway 1 (Shoreline Highway). Turn north on Panoramic Highway and continue approximately 6 miles northwest to parking at ranger station, where there is a parking fee. Additional parking is available at the Bootjack Picnic Area (which charges a group parking fee), 0.2 mile before Pantoll, if Pantoll is full.

NORTH TRAILHEAD, BOLINAS-FAIRFAX ROAD: From Pantoll Ranger Station in Mt. Tamalpais State Park, take Pantoll Road 1.3 miles to Ridgecrest Boulevard and Rock Spring. Turn left onto East Ridgecrest Boulevard and continue northwest to the Bolinas-Fairfax Road junction. Park on the south side of the road and cross the road to the trail entrance. Or take Bolinas-Fairfax Road west from Fairfax or east from Highway 1 to its junction with Ridgecrest Boulevard; parking on the south side of Ridgecrest Boulevard. Bolinas-Fairfax Road is subject to closure.

By Bus

A Golden Gate Transit bus runs from San Francisco to Pantoll on weekends and holidays only and continues to Stinson Beach. West Marin Stagecoach also stops at Pantoll a couple times each day.

On the Trail

Hikers, equestrians, and **mountain bikers** start this trip at Pantoll on different routes. Each route is described separately below.

Hikers begin on the Matt Davis Trail, at the stone steps across Panoramic Highway from the Pantoll parking lot. This well-kept old trail crosses the mountain and descends to Stinson Beach. A favorite of many hikers, it is named for the "dean of Mt. Tamalpais trail builders" and has been built and rebuilt over the years.

The trail curves to the left around a serpentine rock outcrop and for the next half mile contours through a forest of oaks and firs. Soon it enters a small ravine where a stream splashes over moss-covered rocks, and giant ferns stand 6 feet tall. Around the next bend, a grassy spot above the trail is blue with hound's tongue blossoms in March. Douglas irises bloom by the trail's edge in April.

Matt Davis Trail   *Elizabeth Byers*

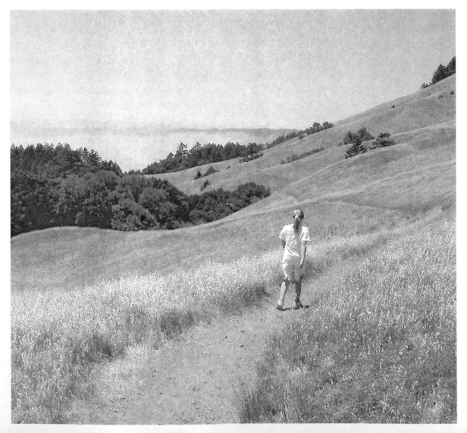

As the trail rounds a south-facing slope, it emerges from the woods to cross a steep, grassy hillside and climb over a saddle. From this vantage point, you see Bolinas Lagoon ahead (west) in the distance and, looking back (southeast), the San Francisco skyline. The trail winds in and out of a tree-filled gully, and—again on grassy slopes—reaches the junction with the Coastal Trail. You head north here, and the Matt Davis Trail continues down (left) to Stinson Beach.

Now a narrow path, the Coastal Trail (Bob Cook Memorial) turns upward to round a steep slope. From these heights you look down on the town of Stinson Beach, and on a still day you can hear the roar of the surf. As the trail enters a forested ravine, the sounds of surf fade in the presence of a splashing creek. From the far side of the ravine, you see the long curve of Stinson Beach, the Bolinas Lagoon, and the white line of waves breaking on Duxbury Reef beyond.

The trail continues across steep hillsides punctuated by great serpentine outcrops. Spreading bay trees, their roots buttressed by these rocks, cling to the hillside in gullies. Deer tracks crisscross open slopes above dark, forested ravines. At the forest's edge far below, grazing does and their fawns raise their heads as they sense intruders. In the sky, vultures with wingspans of 6 feet circle on strong updrafts that rise from the steep slopes. On fine days, bright-winged hang gliders share the skies, born aloft by the same updrafts. From launch sites near Ridgecrest Boulevard, they slowly wheel their way down to land on Stinson Beach. By March, buttercups and California poppies begin to appear in the grass, soon followed by a colorful array of spring wildflowers.

The Coastal Trail continues in and out of folds across the ever-steeper hillside, climbing toward a spur of Bolinas Ridge. Here you meet the Willow Camp Fire Road, which descends to Stinson Beach from Ridgecrest Boulevard; you continue on the Coastal Trail, across a small saddle, and enter a ravine. On the other side of the ravine, a stone bench beside the trail overlooks the sea. It honors Bob Cook, the Eagle Scout who conceived this trail and persisted in its completion by volunteers.

Around another open slope, the trail enters woods of bay trees where a lively creek rushes down Stinson Gulch. Across a bridge, ferns, mossy rocks, and a grove of moisture-seeking maples grow in damp contrast to the exposed hillsides. From the creek, the trail climbs up the hillside to Ridgecrest Boulevard, and you walk on the roadside around a bend for about 500 feet to the McKennan Gulch Trail gate. You have your first views of the Marin hills and mountain peaks to the northeast. On clear days, you can see Mt. St. Helena in the distance.

The Coastal Trail resumes beyond the McKennan Gulch Trail gate and drops into a tight gully. Railroad-tie steps lead to a rivulet where a Bay Area Ridge Trail sign marks the route. At this point you leave Mt. Tamalpais State Park and enter Golden Gate National Recreation Area lands for the last 2 miles of the trip.

You are above the woods of McKennan Gulch and below a small knoll. After crossing a little flat dotted with great boulders, where a fence keeps out feral pigs, the trail follows close to Ridgecrest Boulevard. Below you, an apple orchard in a green, spring-fed meadow marks the site of a mountain cabin. Here the unsigned equestrian trail from the east side of Ridgecrest Boulevard joins the Coastal Trail on the Bay Area Ridge Trail route.

Equestrians leave Pantoll Ranger Station, cautiously cross Panoramic Highway, and take the paved Old Stage Road past three left-branching hiking trails. You continue to the junction of the historic California Riding and Hiking Trail, marked by a water trough, and follow this shaded trail up steep slopes. From the open grasslands above, you have spectacular panoramic views of San Francisco, the ocean, and the multiple peaks of Mt. Tamalpais. After negotiating railroad-tie steps, you join the Old Mine Trail for a short stretch and then cross Ridgecrest Boulevard to Rock Spring parking lot.

There is no signed equestrian trail for the next 3 miles, northwest from Rock Spring to "Apple Orchard." Therefore, from the Rock Spring parking lot, riders head northwest on the California Riding and Hiking Trail, which follows the east shoulder of Ridgecrest Boulevard. You pass the Laurel Dell Fire Road (roadside parking available) and continue to the McKennan Gulch Trail gate (west side of Ridgecrest Boulevard) to join hikers on the Coastal Trail along Bolinas Ridge. Although an authorized equestrian route does not exist on the east side of Ridgecrest Boulevard, the Bay Area Ridge Trail Council continues to pursue viable alternatives. For current information regarding both the bike and equestrian alignments, please contact the Bay Area Ridge Trail Council.

Ahead, a tall fir forest extends over the ridgetop. The Bay Area Ridge Trail, accessible at this point to both **hikers** and **equestrians**, bears west under the trees to cross a broad chaparral-covered hillside. You then descend switchbacks through scrub oaks and cross a seasonally dry streambed before climbing steeply into a mixed woodland.

The trail levels off and 0.25 mile farther enters a ridgetop redwood forest. Trees in this forest, some as much as 50 feet in circumference, were heavily logged in the 1850s to build Gold Rush San Francisco. Today, a grove of stately second-growth redwoods shades the summit of Bolinas-Fairfax Road at the end of Ridgecrest Boulevard.

Bikers use Pantoll Road north from Pantoll Ranger Station to Rock Spring and then bear left on Ridgecrest Boulevard.

◆ ◆ ◆

At the junction of Bolinas-Fairfax Road and Ridgecrest Boulevard, the next leg of the Bay Area Ridge Trail begins on the Bolinas Ridge Trail, which is open to **hikers**, **equestrians**, and **bikers**.

Golden Gate National Recreation Area and Samuel P. Taylor State Park

From Bolinas-Fairfax Road to State Park Entrance

Length 12.8 miles to Samuel P. Taylor State Park; 12.2 miles to parking at Platform Bridge at Tocaloma; 11.1 miles to alternate trailhead at Olema Hill on Sir Francis Drake Boulevard

Accessibility Hikers, equestrians, and mountain bikers

Agencies Golden Gate National Recreation Area and California Department of Parks and Recreation

Regulations Bolinas Ridge Trail and Cross Marin Trail are open during daylight hours and subject to closure in times of high fire danger. Leashed dogs are permitted on Bolinas Ridge Trail. Leave gates to cattle-grazing lands as you find them. When in doubt, close the gate. Pantoll Road and Ridgecrest Boulevard are open from 7 AM to sunset but may be closed in times of high fire danger or hazardous road conditions.

Facilities Water and restrooms at Samuel P. Taylor State Park

From the heights of Bolinas Ridge you'll have magnificent views of the sparkling ocean, tree-covered ridges, deep canyons, oak-dotted hills, and distant peaks. You'll also glimpse Marin County history as you pass trails named for early landholders and tread the paths of Mexican ranchers, Anglo settlers, rugged loggers, and prosperous dairymen.

Getting There

By Car

SOUTH TRAILHEAD, BOLINAS-FAIRFAX ROAD AND RIDGECREST BOULEVARD JUNCTION: From Pantoll Ranger Station in Mt. Tamalpais State Park, take Pantoll Road 1.3 miles to Ridgecrest Boulevard and Rock Spring. Turn left onto Ridgecrest Boulevard, and continue northwest to Bolinas-Fairfax Road junction. Park on the south side of the road and cross the road to reach the trail entrance, or take Bolinas-Fairfax Road west from Fairfax or east from Highway 1 to the junction of Ridgecrest Boulevard and park on the south side of the road. Bolinas-Fairfax Road is subject to closure.

NORTH TRAILHEAD, JEWELL TRAIL: Take Sir Francis Drake Boulevard to Samuel P. Taylor State Park. Park at the main entrance, and go northwest 2.1 miles on Cross Marin Trail to junction with Jewell Trail. Off-road parking is prohibited, and there isn't a bridge across the creek at Jewell Trail. Limited additional parking is available at Tocaloma at the junction of Sir Francis Drake Boulevard and Platform Bridge Road, 3.5 miles north

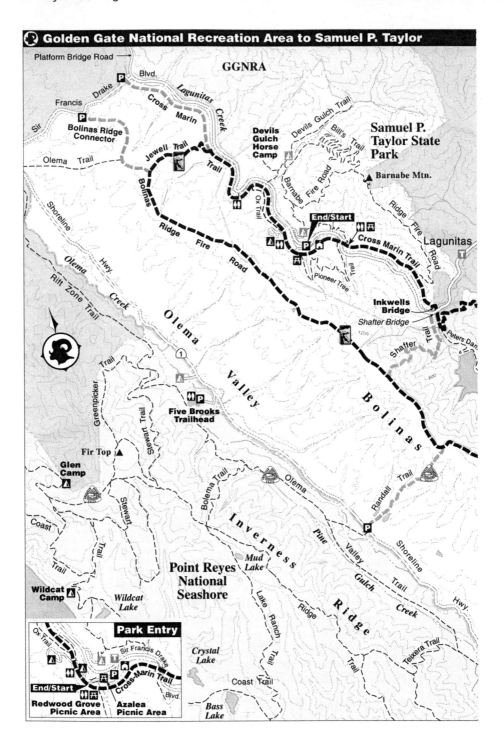

Golden Gate National Recreation Area to Samuel P. Taylor

Platform Bridge Road →

GGNRA

Blvd.

Drake

Francis

Cross

Marin

Lagunitas Creek

Sir

Bolinas Ridge
Connector

Devils
Gulch
Horse
Camp

Devils Gulch Trail

Bill's Trail

Samuel P.
Taylor State
Park

Olema Trail

Jewell Trail

Trail

Barnabe Fire Road

▲ Barnabe Mtn.

Bolinas

Ridge

Fire

Road

Ox Trail

Ridge Fire Road

End/Start

Cross Marin Trail

Lagunitas

Shoreline

Olema

Hwy.

Creek

Rift Zone Trail

Pioneer Tree

Trail

Olema

Valley

Inkwells
Bridge

Shafter Bridge

Shafter

Trail

Peters Dam

Bolinas

1

Greenpicker

Trail

Stewart Trail

Fir Top ▲

Glen
Camp

Five Brooks
Trailhead

Bolema Trail

Olema

Randall Trail

Coast

Stewart

Trail

Trail

Wildcat
Camp

Wildcat
Lake

Point Reyes
National
Seashore

Mud
Lake

Inverness

Pine

Valley

Gulch

Shoreline

Trail

Creek

Hwy.

Ridge

Lake Ranch Trail

Ridge Trail

Coast Trail

Teixera Trail

Park Entry

Ox Trail

Sir Francis Drake

Crystal
Lake

End/Start

Cross-Marin Trail

Blvd.

**Redwood Grove
Picnic Area**

**Azalea
Picnic Area**

Bass
Lake

State Park and Loma Alta Open Space Preserve

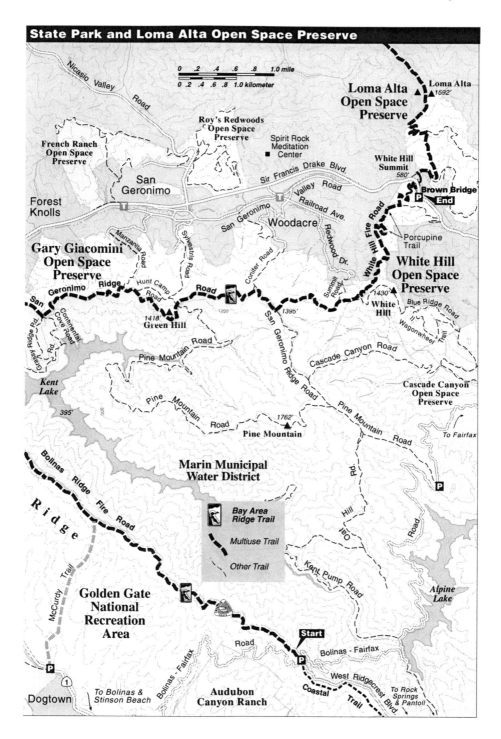

Loma Alta Open Space Preserve

Loma Alta ▲1592'

Nicasio Valley Road

Roy's Redwoods Open Space Preserve

Spirit Rock Meditation Center

White Hill Summit 580'

Brown Bridge **End** P

French Ranch Open Space Preserve

San Geronimo

Sir Francis Drake Blvd.

Valley Road

Railroad Ave.

Redwood Dr.

Porcupine Trail

Forest Knolls

Woodacre

White Hill Fire Road

White Hill Open Space Preserve

Gary Giacomini Open Space Preserve

Manzanita Road

Sylvestris Road

Conifer Road

San Geronimo Ridge

Hunt Camp Road

Road

Summit Road

1430' ▲

Blue Ridge Road

Green Hill 1418'

1200'

1395'

White Hill

Wagonwheel Trail

Continental Cove Road

Greasy Ridge Rd.

Pine Mountain Road

San Geronimo Ridge Road

Cascade Canyon Road

Kent Lake

395'

Pine Mountain Road

Pine Mountain ▲1762'

Pine Mountain Road

Cascade Canyon Open Space Preserve

To Fairfax

Marin Municipal Water District

Bolinas Ridge Fire Road

Ridge

Hill Rd.

Road

Oat

Bay Area Ridge Trail

Multiuse Trail

Other Trail

Golden Gate National Recreation Area

McCurdy Trail

Kent Pump Road

Alpine Lake

P

P

Dogtown

1

To Bolinas & Stinson Beach

Bolinas - Fairfax

Road

Audubon Canyon Ranch

Start P

Bolinas - Fairfax

West Ridgecrest Blvd.

Coastal Trail

To Rock Springs & Pantoll

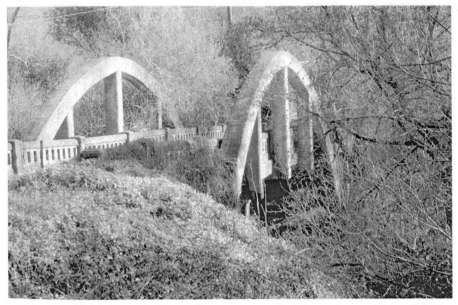

Platform Bridge at Tocaloma

of the main park entrance. Park along the road on Sir Francis Drake or off-road behind the bridge, which is accessible from Platform Road. Go south 1.5 miles on Cross Marin Trail to Jewell Trail junction.

EQUESTRIAN TRAILHEAD: Park on roadside at Devils Gulch Trailhead along Sir Francis Drake Boulevard.

ALTERNATE NORTH TRAILHEAD, NORTH TERMINUS OF BOLINAS RIDGE TRAIL AT OLEMA HILL: On Sir Francis Drake Boulevard go 4.1 miles northwest of Samuel P. Taylor State Park or 0.6 mile west of Tocaloma (Sir Frances Drake Boulevard/Platform Bridge Road junction) to the parking area on the south side of the road.

By Bus

A Golden Gate Transit bus runs from San Francisco to Samuel P. Taylor State Park on weekends and holidays.

On the Trail

A wide, unpaved road descends northwest along the crest of Bolinas Ridge, gradually losing 1300 feet in more than 12 miles. You'll travel through damp forests on soft and springy leaf duff; wind through tall chaparral on bare, rocky sandstone; and cross open, cattle-grazed grasslands. Weather and temperature vary as well: Long, exposed stretches of trail can be windy or hot, and summer fog often covers the open ridge. The Cross Marin Trail is paved from Platform Bridge south through Samuel P. Taylor State Park and is mostly in shade.

The San Andreas Fault runs through Olema Valley, just west of the trail; it made history in 1906 when it gave San Francisco and Marin County a violent shake. In the sheltering arm of Point Reyes, to the northwest, Drake's Bay is named for Sir Francis Drake, who is said to have anchored there in 1579.

To start your trip at the Bolinas-Fairfax Road summit, **hikers, equestrians,** and **mountain bikers** walk or ride into the cool, dark Douglas-fir and redwood forest. As you wind along the wide service road, you'll notice a low, wire-mesh fence on your left, designed to exclude feral pigs from Audubon Canyon Ranch, west of the ridge. Feral pigs were once imported for sport hunting but have proliferated and are now a menace to wild plants and animals; humans should avoid them because they can be aggressive if provoked.

Before long, you emerge from the conifer forest to pass into chaparral and coastal scrub, where dense vegetation makes a low, prickly border on both sides of the trail. From occasional openings in the chaparral you can see to the coast and even hear breakers crashing on Duxbury Reef. Look south behind you to see Mt. Tamalpais, Marin County's most prominent landmark.

After 3.4 miles, you pass the McCurdy Trail, where it begins a 1.7-mile descent west. It reaches Highway 1 at Woodville (also known as Dogtown), which boasted a number of flourishing lumber mills during the logging period. You stay on the Ridge Trail and continue through a luxuriant second-growth forest. In 2 miles, you reach the Randall Trail, which also descends 1.7 miles to Highway 1 in Olema Valley. The widowed Sarah Seaver Randall, a pioneer in the valley, had a ranch here where she operated a successful dairy and raised a large family. Her home, awaiting historic designation still stands nearby.

Along the ridge beyond the Randall Trail, the forest thins and pastures edge the trail. Turkey vultures wheel through the skies, and a cacophony of bird song comes from the trees. The cows that graze here may remind you of pictures of Mexican ranchers who raised cattle for their hides and hunted the once-numerous elk. When the Anglos arrived, their dairy herds grazed in these fields and supplied milk to dairies that became famous for their products. The cows you see today are mostly beef cattle.

You pass the Shafter Trail, named for the Shafter brothers, astute lawyers from Vermont who became rich landowners in Marin County. James Macmillan Shafter's house, known as "The Oaks," still stands on private property near the Bear Valley Trail in Point Reyes National Seashore; it now functions as a retreat center for the Vedanta Society. According to legend, one of the Shafter cows fell into a large fissure created by the 1906 earthquake.

Redwood Logging on Bolinas Ridge

Like much of this area, this part of the ridge and surrounding slopes were once clothed with a majestic redwood forest. The demand for lumber during the Gold Rush obliterated the forest within a few years. Oxen dragged cut logs down to Bolinas Bay, which was deep enough for ships at that time, before erosion-born silt filled it. The devastation of the redwoods was so great that even some loggers expressed dismay. Today, some second-growth trees have attained splendid heights, and salal, Oregon grape, and huckleberry form a shiny undergrowth.

Although the Shafter Trail (open to **hikers, equestrians,** and **mountain bikers**) descends east to the Shafter Bridge over Lagunitas Creek on Sir Francis Drake Boulevard, the Ridge Trail route continues north on the Bolinas Ridge Trail. Beyond the Shafter Trail junction, the Bay Area Ridge Trail route along the Bolinas Ridge Trail is completely out in the open; it drops into little ravines and then climbs up rounded knolls to take in views west to wooded Inverness Ridge and north to Tomales Bay. On clear days, the blue waters of Tomales Bay shimmer in the sunshine, carrying your eye to the bay's outlet on the coast. The San Andreas Fault continues north through this long finger of water into the Pacific Ocean.

Beside a spring-fed pond you come upon evidence of past habitation—a depression for house foundations and five eucalyptus trees planted in a tight row. The Longley family occupied a house here until 1888, where Thomas Longley reportedly operated a roadhouse. The house was later moved several miles downhill and eventually destroyed. Today the eucalyptus trees, called "The Five Sisters," can be seen from Tomales Bay. Nothing else remains to tell the settler's tale, but cows still come to drink from the pond.

You continue through this pastoral scene for 4 miles beyond the Shafter Trail turnoff. Open grasslands extend up to the forested ridgeline and down to the barns nestled in Olema Valley. The Bolinas Ridge Trail curves east around cattle chutes and corrals, and you reach a junction with the Jewell Trail. From here, the Bay Area Ridge Trail route follows the Jewell Trail 0.9 mile east to the Cross Marin Trail; the Bolinas Ridge Trail goes 1.3 miles north to Sir Francis Drake Boulevard.

You descend on the Jewell Trail, following the ridgecrest through steep grasslands punctuated by white, lichen-covered outcrops. Clumps of wind-sculpted oaks frame dramatic views of Barnabe Mountain in the east and Pine Mountain farther south. In spring, many-hued wildflowers brighten this spare landscape. Rounding a curve at the former Omar Jewell ranch homesite, you pass another line of eucalyptus and a few fruit trees.

Now you drop down rapidly to a gate at the Cross Marin Trail on the edge of Lagunitas Creek. Samuel P. Taylor's mill on this stream, formerly called Papermill Creek, once produced paper bags and newsprint for San Francisco. The Bay Area Ridge Trail route continues on the Jewell/Cross Marin trails to 2700-acre Samuel P. Taylor State Park. It follows Lagunitas Creek on the historic North Pacific Coast Railroad (later the North Shore and then the Northwestern Pacific Railroad) right-of-way. The railroad, bankrolled by the Shafter brothers and other financiers in the 1870s, extended from Sausalito to Samuel P. Taylor's mill and continued on to logging camps in Cazadero.

To reach park headquarters, go right (south) for 2.1 miles on the Cross Marin Trail. If you parked at Platform Bridge or have a shuttle car waiting there, however, go left (northwest) 1.5 miles on the Cross Marin Trail.

Equestrians heading to Devils Gulch Camp and trails east can follow the Cross Marin Trail south to the old horse corral, ford Lagunitas Creek, and then cross Sir Francis Drake Boulevard to the camp's entrance road.

◆ ◆ ◆

The next leg of the Bay Area Ridge Trail continues southeast.

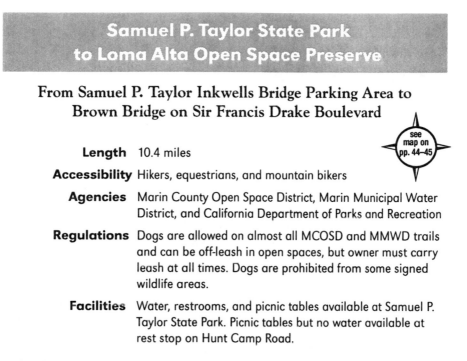

Samuel P. Taylor State Park to Loma Alta Open Space Preserve

From Samuel P. Taylor Inkwells Bridge Parking Area to Brown Bridge on Sir Francis Drake Boulevard

see map on pp. 44–45

Length	10.4 miles
Accessibility	Hikers, equestrians, and mountain bikers
Agencies	Marin County Open Space District, Marin Municipal Water District, and California Department of Parks and Recreation
Regulations	Dogs are allowed on almost all MCOSD and MMWD trails and can be off-leash in open spaces, but owner must carry leash at all times. Dogs are prohibited from some signed wildlife areas.
Facilities	Water, restrooms, and picnic tables available at Samuel P. Taylor State Park. Picnic tables but no water available at rest stop on Hunt Camp Road.

Make a long, undulating, ever-upward trip to 360-degree views of the North Bay, its deep canyons and wooded ridges crowned by Mt. Tamalpais, and then descend on the Porcupine Trail to Brown Bridge in White Hill Open Space Preserve.

Getting There

By Car

WEST TRAILHEAD, INKWELLS BRIDGE, SAMUEL P. TAYLOR STATE PARK: All modes leave the park's main entrance on Sir Francis Drake Boulevard about 10 miles west of Highway 101 in Marin County. If you're coming from the south, in the vicinity of Greenbrae take Sir Francis Drake Boulevard going northwest; pass through the towns of San Anselmo, Ross, and Fairfax; and look for the park entrance on your left. If you're coming from the north on Highway 101, take the Lincoln Avenue exit; go south; turn west on 4th Avenue (which becomes Red Hill Avenue); and after 1.4 miles (in the vicinity of Creekside Park) join Sir Francis Drake Boulevard going northwest; pass through the towns of San Anselmo, Ross, and Fairfax; and look for the park entrance on your left. Roadside parking, especially at Inkwells Bridge, is limited.

EAST TRAILHEAD, BROWN BRIDGE, LOMA ALTA OPEN SPACE PRESERVE: Follow directions above for Samuel P. Taylor State Park but about 2 miles past Fairfax, look for roadside parking for the White Hill Underpass Trail alongside Brown Bridge. Trail entrances are on both sides of the bridge.

EQUESTRIAN PARKING: Limited horse trailer parking is available at Baywood Equestrian Center. Call ahead (415-460-1480) to ensure that there's space. A spur trail leads up to the Ridge Trail.

By Bus

West Marin Stagecoach is available on weekdays. You may request that the bus stop at White Hill or Inkwells/Shafter Bridge.

On the Trail

Leave Samuel P. Taylor State Park's parking lot and picnic areas, and join the Cross Marin Trail going east. In intermittent shade on this wide, unpaved service road you follow the course of Lagunitas Creek and parallel Sir Francis Drake Boulevard for about 1.5 miles. When you reach the Inkwells Bridge, also known as the Marie Dhority Bridge, you cross the creek as it flows through the canyon below. In fall, the creek does look dark, like black ink, as it flows quietly around huge rocks on its way to San Geronimo Valley and Kent Lake. In winter it can be a raging torrent as it makes its way to Tomales Bay. During early winter, after the first rains, you may glimpse coho salmon moving upstream to spawn.

Carefully cross Sir Francis Drake Boulevard (traffic can be heavy) and continue up the service road on the left side of the creek. On the right side of the creek, the Shafter Trail connects to the Bolinas Ridge Trail.

In less than a quarter mile your route, the San Geronimo Ridge Road, turns uphill into the Gary Giacomini Open Space Preserve. The trail, a wide, often rutted, and almost always rocky, fire road, becomes a series of uphill segments followed by brief, somewhat level sections. The first half mile is in full sun, but after rounding a high bluff you enter a forest of tall conifers and bigleaf maples.

After about a mile, you may see a road going off right, but it is closed. Another goes left, downhill, but do not take it. The Bay Area Ridge Trail route is marked by signs on waist-high posts, sometimes set back from the road a little, but clearly visible. When you come to a second fire road going left, the Hunt Camp Road, you can descend on it to a modest opening in the Douglas-fir forest where there are a couple of venerable picnic

---

Watching for Coho Salmon

Lagunitas Creek was for decades a nationally famous coho salmon and steelhead fishery. Loss of spawning habitat in the latter half of the 20th century, however, led to a drastic decline in the creek's spawning population. By the mid-1980s there were only about 100 salmon returning annually. In the early 1980s volunteers with Trout Unlimited, a national salmon, trout, and steelhead conservation organization, worked to protect the fish and the creek. With the restoration of degraded habitat and the artificial spawning of many fish, the population was gradually restored. Lagunitas Creek has an annual run of about 500 fish. To look for salmon spawning in the winter, visit the Leo Cronin Coho Salmon viewing site on the west side of Sir Francis Drake Boulevard (parking is limited).

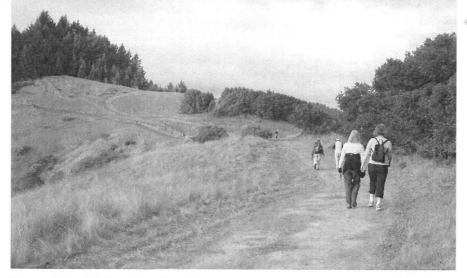

Hikers in White Hill Open Space Preserve   *Elizabeth Byers*

tables. When I scouted this trail with some friends, we ate our lunch here before climb-ing uphill to rejoin the main trail.

Now you continue eastward through chaparral—waist-high manzanita, ceanothus, and occasional small liveoak trees. Here, you will also see "pygmy" cypress trees, a natu-ral phenomenon due to the serpentine rock habitat. Less than a mile after rejoining the main trail you reach the trail's highest point at 1410 feet rising above steep, wooded can-yons topped by successive ridges dominated by Mt. Tamalpais towering in the south.

Traversing high grasslands and going past more rounded hills you reach a low, rocky mound and a Ridge Trail sign pointing left. After passing a road to a private residence, you begin a gradual downhill trend. Following this trail, which narrows briefly, you wind downhill through open country. Then you pass below a steep hillside where part of the trail slid out after a heavy winter rain in 2005. To your right and downhill is Camp Tam-arancho, property of the Boy Scouts who granted an easement over the land for this seg-ment of the Ridge Trail.

The last mile or two of this lengthy trip follows a zigzag course downhill through oak and madrone forest, welcome shade on a hot day. Eventually the trail is on the for-mer route of Sir Francis Drake Boulevard, and patches of old pavement are visible un-derfoot. When you come out of the forest and round the last turn, ahead of and below you is Brown Bridge. This structure, the largest single-span structure west of the Missis-sippi River, is a 380-foot steel bridge near the crest of White Hill. The span, which is partially brown in color, is named in honor of Marin County Supervisor Hal Brown. It was built over a hillside that continually slid out during heavy winter rains, taking the road with it. Now, the hill can slide under the bridge, which is well anchored on the hillside. The trail parallels the bridge, then goes under it, crosses a wooden bridge, and shortly ends just below White Hill Summit. You will find the parking area nearby where you may have left a car for the drive back to the beginning of the trail at Samuel P. Tay-lor State Park.

◆ ◆ ◆

The next leg of the Ridge Trail begins across Sir Francis Drake Boulevard in Loma Alta Open Space Preserve.

Loma Alta Open Space Preserve to Big Rock Ridge

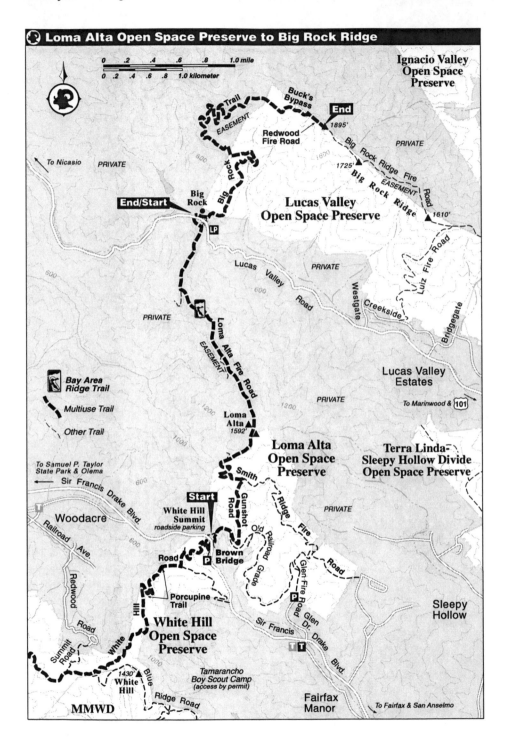

0 .2 .4 .6 .8 1.0 mile
0 .2 .4 .6 .8 1.0 kilometer

Ignacio Valley
Open Space
Preserve

Buck's
Bypass

Trail

End
1895'

EASEMENT

Redwood
Fire Road

1800

PRIVATE

To Nicasio   PRIVATE

Big Rock

800

Big Rock Ridge Fire Road

1725'   EASEMENT

Big Rock Ridge

End/Start   Big
Rock

1610'

LP

Lucas Valley
Open Space Preserve

Lucas Valley Road

600

PRIVATE

Westgate   Creekside

Luiz Fire Road

Bridgegate

600

PRIVATE

Loma Alta Fire Road

EASEMENT

Lucas Valley
Estates

To Marinwood & 101

**Bay Area
Ridge Trail**

Multiuse Trail

Other Trail

1200   1200

PRIVATE

1000

Loma
Alta
1592'

Loma Alta
Open Space
Preserve

Terra Linda-
Sleepy Hollow Divide
Open Space Preserve

To Samuel P. Taylor
State Park & Olema

Sir Francis Drake Blvd.

600

Smith   Road

PRIVATE

Woodacre

Railroad   Ave.

Gunshot Road

Start
White Hill
Summit
roadside parking

Old Railroad Grade

Ridge Fire Road

Sleepy
Hollow

Redwood

Road

600

Road

**Brown
Bridge**   P

Porcupine
Trail

Glen Fire Road   Glen Dr.

Sir Francis Drake

P

Hill

**White Hill
Open Space
Preserve**

Summit Road

White

1430'
White
Hill

Blue

Ridge Road

Tamarancho
Boy Scout Camp
(access by permit)

1000

Blvd.

T

Fairfax
Manor

To Fairfax & San Anselmo

MMWD

Loma Alta Open Space Preserve to Lucas Valley Open Space Preserve

From Sir Francis Drake Boulevard to Lucas Valley Road

Length	3.7 miles
Accessibility	Hikers, equestrians, and mountain bikers
Agencies	Lucasfilm Ltd. and Marin County Open Space District
Regulations	Trail is open from dawn to dusk. Dogs on leash are permitted on Lucasfilm lands, and they must be under voice control on MCOSD fire road.
Facilities	None

Cross open grasslands on old ranch roads with around-the-compass views. This steep trip climbs the hill that separates San Geronimo and Lucas valleys (with an elevation gain of 1092 feet and a loss of 1052 feet) on a wide, rocky, and exposed trail. It is best taken on cool mornings in summer or bright sunny days in winter.

Getting There

SOUTH TRAILHEAD: From Highway 101 take the San Anselmo exit (4th Street), and cross over the freeway. After 2 miles bear right on Sir Francis Drake Boulevard, and continue 4 miles to parking on the east side of the road. Carefully cross Sir Francis Drake Boulevard to the trail entrance under the east side of the bridge.

NORTH TRAILHEAD: From Highway 101 take the Lucas Valley Road exit, and go west on Lucas Valley Road. After about 6 miles, you reach the summit and the landmark Big Rock, where there is roadside parking.

On the Trail

Hikers, equestrians, and **mountain bikers** begin on the wide ranch road laid out on a segment of the old narrow-gauge North Pacific Coast Railroad bed. After a short descent through a small glen (one of two shaded stretches on the trip), you reach a wooden gate with the familiar MCOSD logo. Continue to the left beyond the gate, where another trail branches right (downhill). You soon make a sharp turn north to mount open grasslands with wide views on your 1.6-mile ascent to Loma Alta.

To the south, Mt. Tamalpais looms over the entire North Bay, while San Pedro Mountain and its long, lower line of hills stretches east to the edge of the bay. At your feet grow orange poppies, blue-eyed grass, and other spring wildflowers. By summer, most flowers have disappeared, but clumps of native bunchgrasses, nibbled by wildlife, still line the road. Ever higher you climb, and after turning due north, your views expand to include the Richmond-San Rafael Bridge and all of San Francisco and San Pablo bays.

At about 800 feet, you enter a shaded corridor where a cluster of oak trees flourishes, nourished by a spring on the hill to your left. It is a pleasant place to pause to take a drink and read your map. A little rivulet, fed by runoff from the spring and by winter rains, splashes its way south through the narrow ravine below the trail to join Fairfax Creek.

Beyond the tree canopy, the vegetation on this south-facing ridge reverts to sun-loving plants—sage, sticky monkeyflower, and ubiquitous poison oak. Perky stalks of pearly everlasting topped by creamy white flower tufts stand tall above the grasses. The trail continues unwaveringly straight up this ridge, aptly matching its name, Gunshot Fire Road. Off to the left (northwest), you may notice a huge rock outcrop, its surface weathered to a dull gray. Although unnamed, it is probably twice the width of and taller than Big Rock, which marks the end of this trail. These and other outcrops in this area are known as "knockers" and are probably composed of Franciscan mélange.

After a short, almost level stretch, you climb another steep pitch to reach a junction. Turn left (west) here, on the Smith Ridge Fire Road (now 0.75 mile from the trailhead); a right turn here would take you about 4 miles southeast to the preserve boundary. Pause at this junction to take in splendid views south—of Angel Island, the Bay Bridge, and the San Francisco skyline.

The trail now heads due west on a gentler route. Scattered clumps of young bay trees grow along the edges, and wildflowers flourish in the roadside drainage ditches. When the sun warms the air, you may detect the turpentine scent of yellow tarweed; Indians ground the seeds of this sticky-leafed plant into edible dry cakes. The blue-gray rocks underfoot appear to contain serpentine, the California state rock.

Fine views of sometimes fog-shrouded Bolinas Ridge and Pine Mountain open up before you, and on clear days, you'll see all the high peaks of West Marin, from Mt. Tamalpais in the south to Black Mountain in the north. Much of this land is public open space, including White Hill, Gary Giacomini, and Roys Redwoods open space preserves, in the nearer view. What a treasure trove to enjoy and support!

Now you climb steadily, winding up the ridge. A few small and mostly unused trails branch right (east), but you stay on the wide Ridge Trail. After less than a mile on the Smith Fire Road, you enter the Lucasfilm Limited property on an easement trail.

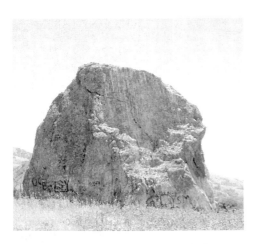

This easement, graciously offered to MCOSD users, crosses George Lucas's Loma Alta and McGuire ranches and includes just the trail itself. Watch carefully to stay on the trail; you will pass several junctions with trails that are not open to the public.

From the entrance into the Lucasfilm property (a working cattle ranch) turn right (east) and ascend beside the fenced property line. Tight clusters of redwood and bay trees fill the canyon below you, where moisture assures their growth. In late spring, the sun glances off the shiny surfaces of dry oatgrass. The wide, steep Ridge Trail route soon reaches a junction, where you veer left

Big Rock marks the end of this Ridge Trail segment.

toward the summit of Loma Alta—only 0.4 mile farther; the right-branching trail enters public property.

Continue upward on a brief but steep climb. At the broad, rounded summit (1592 feet), the trail levels off a little and you look down on the other side of the mountain. Savor the views over lunch or a snack: grassy ridges indented by tree-filled canyons, distant mountains traversed by other Ridge Trail routes, and valleys cut by rushing streams. Big Rock Ridge lies to the north—a long flank of mountain above Lucas Valley with two communication towers on its 1895-foot summit. The next leg of the Ridge Trail route climbs up this ridge to its summit.

The rocky road meanders down the east- and north-facing hills of the Lucasfilm ranches; your descent is gentle and undulating at first but steepens farther along. You can see houses nestled in Lucas Valley and the Luiz Fire Road zigzagging up Big Rock Ridge through the Lucas Valley Open Space Preserve.

Huge rocks are scattered among the grasslands; some shelter emerging oaks from sun and wind damage. After passing a farm road on the left and going under a single-strand power line, you see two corrals—one built of shiny new wire, the next a venerable, well-used wooden structure. An unnamed ridge creased by canyons filled with oak and bay trees rises to your left.

As you descend close to the fence line on your right, you look into a wooded canyon (private property) and a hill beyond scarred by a vertical barren patch. The trail makes a wide swing left (west) and winds down the north side of an open hillside. Your view now takes in grassy Shroyer Ridge straight ahead, topped by a patchy forest of redwoods that extends into its indented south side.

At 2.65 miles, you pass a ranch road heading left, downhill, and you see a semicircular fenced area in a quiet glen of the former McGuire Ranch. Here, in the protection of the enclosing hills, the air is filled with birdsong and the soft hush of wind in the trees. Losing elevation at every step (foot or hoof) or turn of the bike wheel, look left at a spring above the road. It is probably responsible for the muddy trail and lush growth on the right hillside—bay trees, bracken ferns, and, of course, poison oak. A nasty thistle, known as knapweed, thrives along this road, its tangled web of small branches armed with sharp barbs and light purple flowers.

The east-facing ridge above you is topped by windblown trees, pruned high by cattle. The steep slope is strewn with serpentine boulders and rocky rubble. As you drop farther downhill, fractured, almost dusty serpentine rock extends out onto the trail. Around the next curve you can see east down Lucas Valley to the bay, with Mt. Diablo looming beyond. You lose a few hundred more feet in elevation, pass another wooden corral, and reach Lucas Valley Road.

◆ ◆ ◆

Big Rock lies on the other side, marking the end of this 3.7-mile Ridge Trail segment and the beginning of the next—on the north side of Lucas Valley Road at the base of Big Rock.

Lucas Valley Open Space Preserve

Big Rock Trail from Lucas Valley Road to Buck's Bypass

see map on p.52

Length	3.7 miles one-way
Accessibility	Hikers, equestrians, and mountain bikers
Agency	Marin County Open Space District
Regulations	Preserve is open from dawn to dusk daily, and dogs on leash are permitted.
Facilities	None

Climb to high points where Marin County's mountains and valleys are laid out before you and San Francisco and the Golden Gate Bridge loom in the south on this out-and-back hike, which has some steep sections.

Getting There

From Highway 101 take the Lucas Valley Road exit, and go west on Lucas Valley Road. After about 6 miles, you reach the road's summit and the landmark Big Rock, where there is roadside parking.

On the Trail

From a fenced trail entrance at the foot of Big Rock at the summit of Lucas Valley Road take the Big Rock Trail. On this well-laid-out trail constructed by the Marin County Open Space District for the Bay Area Ridge Trail Council, you cross little bridges over rivulets and drain pipes, where sword fern and printer's fern thrive in shady nooks, and climb to a high viewpoint.

At first you contour around the south side of a 1000-foot hill. Then, heading north on this pleasant, 3-foot- to 4-foot-wide trail, you rise gently on the east side of the hill. Below you on the right, one branch of Miller Creek flows through a beautiful, wooded canyon—predominately live oak and bigleaf maple with an occasional buckeye.

After about a mile your trail crosses a bridge over the western arm of Miller Creek and then doubles back to cross the creek again. It heads due west and crosses into the private property of the Lucasfilm Company, which granted an easement to the MCOSD for this trail. Trail users must stay on the trail.

The trail climbs steadily through grasslands accented by splendid live oaks clinging with great tenacity to the steep hillside and offering welcome shade on hot summer days. At one of the larger creeks, over which a fine bridge crosses, there is a trailside garden supporting beautiful spring wildflowers—lupines, poppies, trillium, and farewell-to-spring—set against a backdrop of immense stony outcrops.

When I hiked this trail with a friend, a herd of cattle was grazing below the trail, quite oblivious to our passing. (It is always wise to give cattle a wide berth if they should be near the trail and allow them time to move away.)

The trail zigzags uphill through high grasslands on wide sweeps, north, then south, and again north, then south, each time gaining elevation. You can see its track above you. After the last zigzag, the trail trends east, makes a last steep pitch, and comes out at a relatively flat area. Here, a gate and a hiker's stile lead into the upper reaches of the Lucas Valley Open Space Preserve. MCOSD signs remind you to stay on the trail. Continue about a half mile to Buck's Bypass where the Ridge Trail route terminates at an elevation of 1800 feet, the high point on this ridge.

If you look north from these lofty hilltops, you can see Mt. Burdell, where another leg of the Ridge Trail climbs to its 1588-foot summit. Someday this segment of the Ridge Trail will connect with other Ridge Trail segments in Marin County that reach Mt. Burdell.

For now, turn around for views west and south—the familiar sites of White Hill and Mt. Tamalpais—often rising above the ground fog on a winter day—and the route of other Ridge Trail segments. Go back through the gate to find some relatively level grasslands on the ridge where you can spread out your backpack lunch and enjoy these views. Until the next leg of the Ridge Trail is completed, you must retrace your way downhill on this trail. Or, you could follow this trail, the Big Rock Ridge Trail, east to Novato on Highway 101.

◆ ◆ ◆

In the meantime, the next completed leg of the Bay Area Ridge Trail begins in Indian Tree Open Space Preserve, 6 or 7 miles as the crow flies, but about 14 miles longer via West Marin roads to the trailhead on Vineyard Road in Novato.

Children, too, enjoy these well-graded trails.   *Elizabeth Byers*

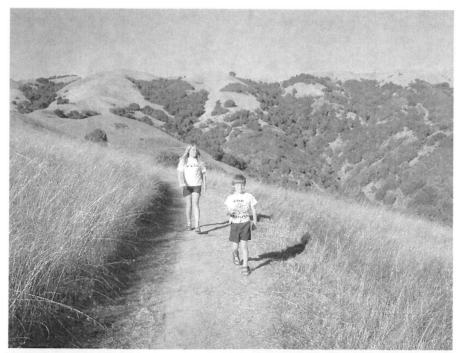

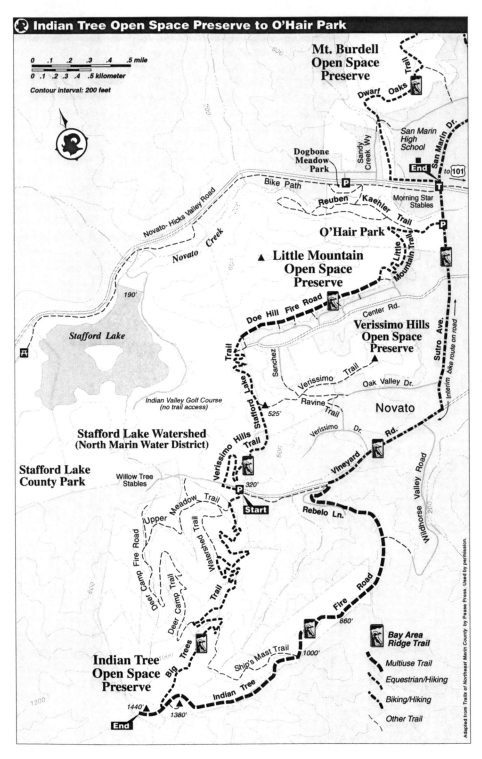

Indian Tree Open Space Preserve to O'Hair Park

0 .1 .2 .3 .4 .5 mile

0 .1 .2 .3 .4 .5 kilometer

Contour interval: 200 feet

Mt. Burdell
Open Space
Preserve

Dwarf Oaks Trail

San Marin
High
School

San Marin Dr.

Dogbone
Meadow
Park

Sandy Creek Wy

End

to 101

Bike Path

Novato-Hicks Valley Road

Reuben

Kaehler Trail

Morning Star
Stables

O'Hair Park

Novato Creek

▲ Little Mountain
Open Space
Preserve

Little Mountain Trail

Doe Hill Fire Road

Center Rd.

Verissimo Hills
Open Space
Preserve

190'

Stafford Lake

Sanchez

Verissimo Trail

Oak Valley Dr.

Stafford Lake Trail

Indian Valley Golf Course
(no trail access)

Ravine Trail

525'

Novato

Verissimo Dr. Rd.

Sutro Ave.

Interim bike route on road

Stafford Lake Watershed
(North Marin Water District)

Verissimo Hills Trail

Vineyard

Wildhorse Valley Road

Stafford Lake
County Park

Willow Tree
Stables

320'

Start

Rebelo Ln.

Upper Meadow Trail

Watershed Trail

Deer Camp Fire Road

Deer Camp Trail

Fire Road

860'

Bay Area
Ridge Trail

Ship's Mast Trail

1000'

Multiuse Trail

Indian Tree
Open Space
Preserve

Big Trees

Equestrian/Hiking

Biking/Hiking

Indian Tree

Other Trail

1200

1440'

1380'

End

Adapted from Trails of Northeast Marin County by Pease Press. Used by permission.

Indian Tree Open Space Preserve to O'Hair Park

From Vineyard Road to Indian Tree and through Verissimo Hills and Little Mountain Preserves to O'Hair Park

Length	9 miles (includes 6 miles round-trip to Indian Tree and 3 miles to O'Hair Park)
Accessibility	Hikers, equestrians, and mountain bikers
Agency	Marin County Open Space District
Regulations	Bikes are allowed on Doe Hill Fire Road, which is accessible from Center Road, but must turn off after about a half mile when the wide trail ends. They are prohibited on Indian Tree, Verissimo Hills, Stafford Lake, and Little Mountain Open Space Preserve trails.
Facilities	None

Explore Indian Tree's redwood and Douglas-fir forests on a shady and well-graded out-and-back trip (with an elevation gain and loss of 720 feet). Then head north over grassy hillsides above Stafford Lake, around Little Mountain, and through forest to O'Hair Park. The Little Mountain Trail starts on a fire protection road; otherwise, narrow, well-graded, and shaded trails cross these preserves, with minor elevation change.

Getting There

By Car

NORTHERN TRAILHEAD: From Highway 101 in Novato, turn west on San Marin Drive. Cross Novato Boulevard onto Sutro Avenue, and go over the Novato Creek bridge to roadside parking at O'Hair Park.

SOUTHERN TRAILHEAD: Follow the directions above but continue south on Sutro Avenue past O'Hair Park to Vineyard Road. Turn right (west), follow Vineyard Road for a little over a mile, and park on the south side of the street, immediately after the last house, in an unpaved area.

By Bike

Follow directions above on Novato city streets marked INTERIM BIKE ROUTE to Vineyard Road, go about three quarters of a mile, turn left (south) on Rebelo Lane, and then turn uphill on Marin County Open Space District Indian Tree Fire Road. Each trailhead is marked with a Ridge Trail logo, as well as the distinctive MCOSD sign.

On the Trail

There is not yet a trailhead at the south end of Indian Tree Open Space Preserve, so this segment of the Ridge Trail first visits Indian Tree on a 6-mile out-and-back trip, before continuing northwest through Verissimo Hills and Little Mountain open space preserves.

Indian Tree Open Space Preserve

Hikers and **equestrians** descend gently from the trailhead on Vineyard Road along a fenced trail into a small meadow, lusciously green in springtime and sprinkled with shiny yellow buttercups. Shortly you pass a green gate and turn left. You ascend switchbacks through oaks and sparse redwoods. The open understory allows a riot of springtime wildflowers to flourish—magenta shooting stars, white and light pink milk-maids, deep red Indian warriors, and later, blue hound's tongue.

In a small clearing, notice a huge rock slab seemingly teetering on a narrow point. Moisture-loving bay laurel trees are scattered among the oaks, Douglas firs, and red-woods. You'll recognize the bay tree by its aromatic leaves, similar to those of the Greek bay tree, but somewhat stronger. (Some people call them "spaghetti" leaves.) After about 0.75 mile you reach a clearing that offers splendid views east to the bay and north to the bare, 1440-foot peak of Mt. Burdell (the destination of the next Ridge Trail segment).

The trail makes a wide swing west and continues uphill, passing a trail that goes right, into the Stafford Lake Watershed. Where the forest is dense, especially on north- and east-facing slopes, moss grows on older oak tree trunks and shade-loving plants thrive—maidenhair and printer's ferns, chocolate-colored mission bells, creamy white globe lilies, and white coral bells.

On a narrow ridge between two canyons, you stroll under a canopy of tall redwoods, Douglas firs, and a few madrones that stretch for sunlight. Fine-leafed huckleberry bush-es fill the understory; deer and birds favor their small, blue-black berries. Soon you pass the Deer Camp Trail and curve left along a split-rail fence to continue on the Big Trees Trail. After about 0.25 mile, you emerge from the forest into chaparral on the edge of a deep canyon. A pause here will reward you with views east to the Novato baylands, the former Hamilton Air Base, and Mt. Diablo in the distance. The Indian Tree Fire Road, the bike route to the Indian Tree Preserve Summit, snakes up the opposite ridge. On a chilly day this southwest-facing stretch feels good; on a hot day, you will hurry by.

Back in the cool forest, you soon arrive at a junction with the Ship's Mast Trail, which was probably named for the very tall, perfectly straight redwoods growing here. You continue directly ahead on the Big Trees Trail, while the Ship's Mast Trail contours around the head of the deep canyon you looked into from the chaparral area; it eventu-ally connects to the Indian Tree Fire Road.

You climb steadily on the last leg of the Big Trees Trail, and then level off a little and emerge in a wide meadow. Join a dirt road that runs through the meadow, and follow this road through a gentle swale. Veer right uphill on a narrow footpath that leads to a lush meadow bursting with spring wildflowers of every hue—cream-colored iris, purple lupine, and yellow buttercups. Ahead are the big trees—a solitary clump of immense redwoods. From the footpath between them, take a few steps left (be careful!) to stand at the edge of an abrupt drop-off above the deep canyon you saw from the trail. Now the whole North Bay spreads before you.

When you have savored the flowers, trees, and views, return on the dirt road through the meadow, and bear right on the footpath into the forest to start your downhill trip. Return to Vineyard Road and turn left (west).

Mountain bikers are not allowed on the Big Trees Trail, so you begin the out-and-back Indian Tree segment by following Vineyard Road to Rebelo Lane and picking up the Indian Tree Fire Road there. Take the fire road to the top of the preserve. Return the same way and go right on Vineyard Road to Sutro Avenue. Turn left and continue to O'Hair Park.

Verissimo Hills and Little Mountain Open Space Preserves to O'Hair Park

Hikers and **equestrians** go west on unpaved Vineyard Road for less than 0.25 mile to the Verissimo Hills Trail entrance. The trail begins on the north side of the road at a stile and green MCOSD gate. Go through the gate, making sure to close it behind you (and the cows).

Start up the trail in a tight canyon, and soon cross a little bridge over an intermittent creek that nourishes an immense bay tree with an almost-hollow trunk. Making a switchback to the right, you begin a serious ascent of the east side of this canyon. At an overlook with a bench, you can see the densely forested hillside you just traversed in the Indian Tree Preserve.

You ascend several switchbacks under the intermittent shade of live oaks and bays. On a quiet spring morning I heard only birdsong and the rustle of leaves in a gentle breeze. After reaching the top of the first hill the trail follows the contour of the shady north-facing hillside and then turns sharply north. A sign on a gate in an open expanse announces that you are now on the Stafford Lake Trail. The narrow trail undulates up and down small hills, just below the eastern ridgeline boundary of the Stafford Lake

Catch a glimpse of Stafford Lake from the trail.

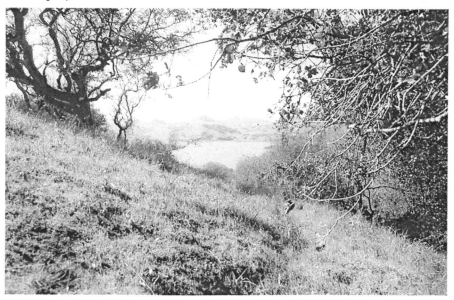

Watershed. Small openings through the trees allow quick views of Stafford Lake, with its little island and the dairy farms surrounding it. As hawks and turkey vultures quietly ride the winds above you, the distant sound of lawnmowing tractors reminds you that the intense green meadows below are the Indian Valley Golf Course.

Soon you leave the hilltop and descend a north-facing hillside through a deciduous oak forest. When the young, yellow-green leaves unfurl in spring against the dark brown limbs, these trees are uniquely beautiful. After a cold snap in fall, their leaves turn a rich tawny, golden-brown. Rounding several switchbacks you reach the end of this trail in a damp meadow in the Verissimo Hills Open Space Preserve. Cross the meadow and go through the stile in the fence that surrounds a cluster of homes at the end of Center Street.

Bear right on the Doe Hill Fire Road in the Little Mountain Open Space Preserve. Signs ask all users to avoid the trail after heavy rains. You skirt the base of Little Mountain on this wide trail; the south-facing exposure can be hot in summer. Tree-filled canyons indent the grassy hillside, collecting rain and spring water. You cross several streams on sturdy wooden bridges built over small dams made of rock-filled gabions. Stands of live oaks beside the trail provide shade for you and refuge for the many birds you may see or hear, especially in early morning or late afternoon.

Mountain bikers are allowed on the short, wide Doe Hill Fire Road, accessible from Center Road, but must turn off after about a half mile, when the wide trail ends.

Hikers and **equestrians** veer left on the narrower Little Mountain Trail at the base of a steep creek canyon. In May, early-blooming blue brodiaea wave above drying grasses, and clusters of orange poppies cover the sloping hillside. You enter a cool woods of bay and oak trees and, after a couple of zigzags, descend gradually along the east side of Little Mountain. Crossing little streams that tumble down the mountainside, this well-graded trail takes you through dense woods of tall, rather spindly trees reaching high for light. After a long traverse beside a handsome split-rail fence, the trail turns to the right and descends quickly to a junction. Make a sharp left turn on the trail that crosses Novato Creek and ends on Novato Boulevard.

◆ ◆ ◆

If you are going on to Mt. Burdell Open Space Preserve, **hikers** and **equestrians** cross Novato Boulevard opposite the west entrance of San Marin High School to the Dwarf Oaks Trail. **Equestrians** ride alongside Morning Star Farms and to the Brookside Trail entrance gate. **Bikers** follow the signed INTERIM BAY AREA RIDGE TRAIL biking route along San Marin Drive, turn left onto San Andreas Drive, and soon reach the preserve gate on the San Andreas Fire Road.

Mount Burdell Open Space Preserve

From O'Hair Park or San Andreas Fire Road
to the West Entrance of Olompali State Historic Park

Length 7.1 miles (includes 1.9 miles between O'Hair Park and San Andreas Fire Road and 5.2 miles round-trip to Mt. Burdell)

Accessibility Hikers, equestrians, and mountain bikers

Agency Marin County Open Space District

Regulations Dogs on leash are generally permitted, but both dogs and bikers are prohibited from the Dwarf Oaks Trail.

Facilities None

Climb through grasslands dotted with ancient oaks to spectacular vistas of North Bay ridges from the 1558-foot peak of Mt. Burdell. The largest of Marin County Open Space District's holdings, these nearly 1600 acres of oak savanna and grasslands are interspersed with dense woodlands. Hikers and equestrians can begin from O'Hair Park and cross a Sensitive Wildlife Area on the Dwarf Oaks Trail. Mountain bikers join them at San Andreas Fire Road, and all users follow wide fire roads to the peak; the trails are steep and rocky, with little shade. Summers are hot here, so be sure to get an early start and come prepared.

Getting There

By Car

O'HAIR PARK TRAILHEAD: From Highway 101 in Novato, turn west on San Marin Drive. Cross Novato Boulevard onto Sutro Avenue, and go over the Novato Creek bridge to roadside parking at O'Hair Park.

SAN ANDREAS FIRE ROAD TRAILHEAD: From Highway 101 in Novato, turn west on San Marin Drive. At San Andreas Drive, turn right and continue about a half mile to the preserve entrance, marked by a green gate and Marin County Open Space District sign. Park on the street, being careful not to block any driveways.

By Bike

From Highway 101 in Novato mountain bikers take San Marin Drive southwest to San Andreas Drive, turn right (northwest), and go to parking at the preserve gate on San Andreas Fire Road in Mt. Burdell Open Space Preserve.

By Bus

A few Golden Gate Transit buses stop at the intersection of San Marin Drive and Novato Boulevard.

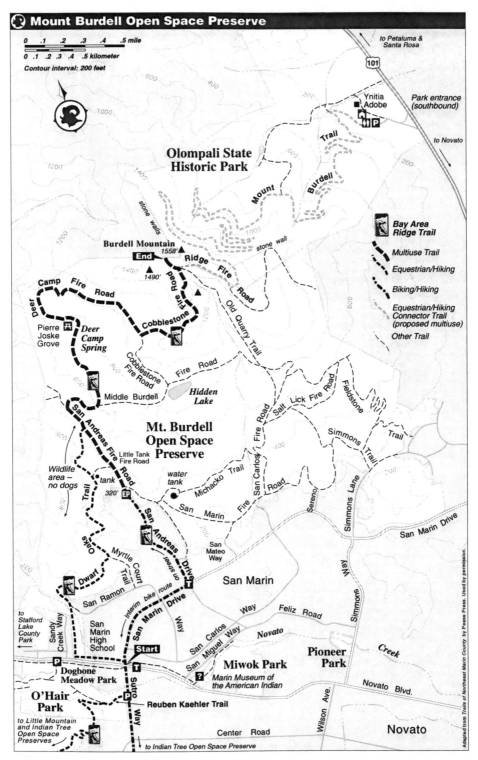

Mount Burdell Open Space Preserve

0   .1   .2   .3   .4   .5 mile
0   .1   .2   .3   .4   .5 kilometer

Contour interval: 200 feet

to Petaluma &
Santa Rosa

101

Ynitia
Adobe

Park entrance
(southbound)

to Novato

Olompali State
Historic Park

Mount Burdell Trail

stone walls

**Bay Area
Ridge Trail**

Multiuse Trail

Equestrian/Hiking

Biking/Hiking

Equestrian/Hiking
Connector Trail
(proposed multiuse)

Other Trail

Burdell Mountain
End 1558'
Ridge Fire Road
1490'

stone wall

Old Quarry Trail

Camp Fire Road
Deer

Cobblestone Fire Road

Pierre
Joske
Grove

Deer
Camp
Spring

Cobblestone
Fire Road

Middle Burdell

Fire Road

Hidden
Lake

Mt. Burdell
Open Space
Preserve

San Andreas Fire Road

Little Tank
Fire Road

Wildlife
area –
no dogs

tank
320'
EP

water
tank

Michacko Trail

San Carlos Fire Road

Salt Lick Fire Road

Fieldstone Trail

Simmons Trail

Sereno

Fire Road

San Marin

Simmons Lane

San Marin Drive

Oaks
Trail

San Andreas Drive

Myrtle Court
Trail

San Mateo
Way

Dwarf

Interim bike route

San Ramon

San Marin Drive

San Marin
High
School

Start

Feliz Road
Way

San Carlos Way

San Miguel Way

Novato
Way

San Marin

Pioneer
Park

Creek

to
Stafford
Lake
County
Park

Sandy Creek Way

Dogbone
Meadow
Park

Miwok Park

Marin Museum of
the American Indian

Novato Blvd.

Wilson Ave.

Simmons Way

O'Hair
Park

to Little Mountain
and Indian Tree
Open Space
Preserves

Sutro Way

Reuben Kaehler Trail

Center Road

to Indian Tree Open Space Preserve

Novato

Adapted from Trails of Northeast Marin County by Pease Press. Used by permission.

On the Trail

From O'Hair Park to San Andreas Fire Road

Hikers and **equestrians** can begin this trip across Novato Boulevard from the last leg of the Indian Tree to O'Hair Park segment. From roadside parking on Sutro Avenue, go northeast across Novato Boulevard. Cross it and go left (west) on the sidewalk in front of San Marin High School. Continue to the signed entrance (Dwarf Oaks Trail) into Mt. Burdell Open Space Preserve. The short, shady 0.6-mile trail dedicated in October 2001 traverses an easement between the school fence and the enclosed gardens of the Brookside subdivision. Cross the rust-colored steel bridge over a tributary of Novato Creek and soon enter Mt. Burdell's 6-acre southwest meadow. In spring, this meadow glows with bright orange California poppies and yellow suncups; by summer, golden oat grass covers the sloping fields. Red-tailed hawks soar overhead, and rusty-breasted bluebirds dart after insects.

Just past a sturdy vehicle bridge at the end of San Ramon Drive, you head northwest and climb grassy slopes on the Dwarf Oaks Trail. On this Ridge Trail segment, dedicated in 1990, you head east and traverse the hillside above a neighboring subdivision. Deciduous oaks crowd the banks of a tiny stream that courses through a fold in the hillside. Shortly, you enter an evergreen oak and bay forest, punctuated in fall by the golden leaves of a few Kellogg oaks. Little streams tumble over rocks in shady canyons in this sensitive wildlife area; white milkmaids and blue hound's tongue brighten the trailside. You leave the forest momentarily and reach a mossy rock garden and a mound with seemingly stunted oak trees growing from cracks in the rock—probably the trees that give their name to the Dwarf Oaks Trail.

When you leave the rock garden, you cross a grassy slope where several streamlets trickle down the hillside in spring. Head due north across a meadow filled with bright yellow buttercups in spring. Shortly, you come to the gate at San Andreas Fire Road and the beginning of the multiuse trip up Mt. Burdell to the boundary of Olompali State Historic Park.

From San Andreas Fire Road to the West Entrance of Olompali State Historic Park

The multiuse Ridge Trail route begins on the San Andreas Fire Road, a wide park patrol service road that heads north from the San Andreas gate. The trail hugs the wooded east side of the sensitive wildlife area and ascends gradually through a canyon to reach the preserve's central valley. Northwest across this valley, let your gaze stretch to the surrounding 1200-foot hills, fringed with dark tree silhouettes. To the east, Mt. Burdell rises 1558 feet; to the west is the low hill of the wildlife area. In the near foreground, a cattle pen beyond the preserve boundary sets a pastoral tone for the trip. If you are in this valley at sunset, you may be rewarded with a spectacular view of the northwest mountains outlined against a glowing, red-orange sky.

All trail users veer east from the valley on the Middle Burdell Fire Road through sloping grasslands to a grove of ancient, deciduous white oaks. One old giant's diameter measures close to 5 feet. In winter the gnarled, widespread limbs of these trees present striking, gaunt silhouettes against the greening fields. In their summer dress these oaks cast welcome shade for human visitors and seasonal bovine residents. (Huge fallen limbs serve as convenient resting places.) The Ridge Trail's Mt. Burdell segment was dedicated in this handsome grove in October 1990.

Just across from this majestic grove, the marked Ridge Trail route goes left on the Deer Camp Fire Road. You head due north through the grasslands and then climb to a broad, wooded plateau. Here, shady Deer Camp, a 25-acre picnic and camping site fenced against cattle intrusion, invites you to pause for a snack or lunch. Organized groups can get permission for overnight camping; they must carry their own water, and no fires are allowed. You'll find a portable toilet, hitch rails, and a circle of log benches situated under some fine Kellogg (black) oaks, large live oaks, and many bay trees.

Resuming your upward way, follow a long, steep curve around an isolated clump of buckeye trees on your right. The buckeyes' bare limbs shine silvery in winter but burst with new growth as early as February to herald spring. By May, the spikes of white flowers tinged with pink fill the air with a sweet fragrance. In dry years, the buckeye trees' leaves shrivel and drop in early summer to compensate for lack of water. As you ascend steadily for the next half mile, look for the preserve's biggest elderberry tree standing alone beside a curve in the trail: leafless in winter, covered with branchlets of fine leaves and clusters of cream-colored flowers in summer and heavy with blue-gray, edible berries in fall.

Shortly after the trail levels off beside a luxurious woods, you reach the Cobblestone Trail junction, where you turn left for the summit. As you start your climb, the relay tower near the west shoulder of Mt. Burdell appears above the forested ridgetop—but your destination is still 400 vertical feet and about 1 mile away. This trail takes its name from the basalt rock that was quarried here to pave San Francisco streets in the 1860s and 1870s. Basalt, a dark igneous stone, can be readily split, chipped and made into cobbles. From pits on the west side of Mt. Burdell, Chinese laborers dug out and chipped rectangular stone blocks (about 6 inches wide, 15 inches long, and 4 inches thick). The workers loaded the cobbles onto wooden sleds and slid them down the steep mountainside. Scars of the sleds' descent are still visible from this trail.

Continue uphill on the rocky trail, past lush clumps of California bay trees growing among boulders on north-facing slopes. It's said that the Olompali Miwok Indians used these boulders as hunting blinds, or perhaps set game traps near them. As you ap-

Mount Burdell's Early Residents

The Coast Miwoks lived in this area from the 1300s to the mid-19th century, subsisting on shellfish from the marshes and acorns and wild game from the oak-studded hills to the west. The Miwoks' last chief, Camilo Ynita, received a Spanish land grant in 1834 and named the village and surrounding lands Rancho Olompali. Ynita later sold part of the rancho to James Black, who passed some of the land to his daughter as a wedding present. Mary Black married Galen Burdell, the first San Francisco dentist and the man for whom the mountain was named. The Burdells built a fine house on the east side of the mountain and developed orchards and gardens on the site of the large Miwok village, Olompali. Today, it is the site of Olompali State Historic Park.

proach the summit of Mt. Burdell, on the left you see a private road to the relay tower, a telephone company repeater station. On the right, the Old Quarry Trail, for hikers and equestrians only, drops 800 feet in elevation down the steep canyon between Mt. Burdell and the ridge you just conquered.

With the summit just a few feet beyond the preserve boundary, you bear right onto the paved Burdell Mountain Ridge Road leading to the rock quarries. The main quarry is on your left, well worth a short walk to see the exposed, layered rock walls of the pits where cobbles were removed. Although small trees and shrubs have gained toeholds in the crevices and masked some of the walls, the size of the pit helps you empathize with the Chinese laborers who excavated it by hand. Just beyond the main pit are smaller diggings, even more overgrown.

An overlook on the other side of the road offers a hawk's-eye view of the preserve and the distant, high ridges that almost circle northern Marin County. If the day is bright, you can make out Hicks Mountain to the northwest, Mt. Tamalpais to the south, and the shoulder of Mt. Burdell curving around to the west; when fog lies in the valleys, the ridgetops seem like islands floating in a misty sea.

After enjoying the vistas and the red-tailed hawks and turkey vultures that may circle aloft, return past the quarries to a trail on your right. It leads to a very old rock wall, hand-built by Chinese laborers, that marks the boundary of Olompali State Historic Park. Step into a high meadow on the other side of the wall to see the Petaluma River flowing through flat marshlands toward San Francisco Bay.

Hikers and **equestrians** may take the 5-mile Mt. Burdell Trail to Olompali State Historic Park, which descends through white oak and madrone woodlands to the site of the largest Miwok village in Marin County and the Burdell home and gardens. (The Ridge Trail Council is working with its agency partners to determine a biking route through this park.)

To return to your trailhead, retrace your steps downhill on the Cobblestone Fire Road to the Deer Camp Fire Road junction. For different views, a slightly steeper route and a rainy-winter surprise, veer left on the Cobblestone Fire Road. The road curves south to enter a beautiful mature oak and bay woods. Soft duff under the great tree branches erupts with mushrooms in spring and nurtures ferns year-round; in early spring, white milkmaids and blue hound's tongue greet the observant eye.

Follow the trail southwest along a high, open, west-facing shoulder and a sparse, steep mountainside on your left. At the Middle Burdell Fire Road junction lies a great meadow nestled in a high valley, surprisingly inundated in wet winters by storm waters washed from the surrounding slopes. The fenced, flooded meadow is known as Hidden Lake, and is said to have been deep enough for swimming 40 years ago. Today, when dry, it provides seasonal cattle-grazing.

Bear right on the Middle Burdell Fire Road and go around the meadow/lake under a lush forest canopy to the crest of a west-facing, steep hillside. You descend rapidly, curving northwest through grasslands ablaze with brilliantly colored wildflowers in spring. Soon you reach the Deer Camp Fire Road junction in the grove of handsome white oaks. Continue 0.25 mile downhill on the Middle Burdell Fire Road to the preserve's central valley.

◆ ◆ ◆

The next segment of the Bay Area Ridge Trail begins in Petaluma's Helen Putnam Regional Park.

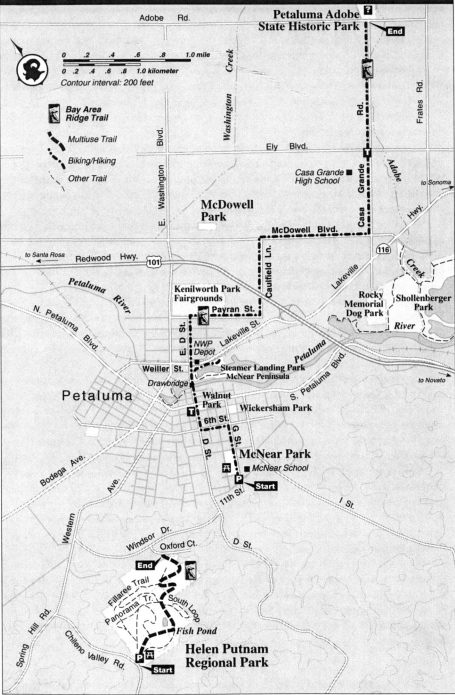

Helen Putnam Regional Park and McNear Park to Petaluma Adobe State Historic Park

Petaluma Adobe
State Historic Park

End

Adobe Rd.

0 .2 .4 .6 .8 1.0 mile
0 .2 .4 .6 .8 1.0 kilometer
Contour interval: 200 feet

Washington Creek

Adobe Rd.

Frates Rd.

Bay Area Ridge Trail

Multiuse Trail

Biking/Hiking

Other Trail

Ely Blvd.

Casa Grande High School

Casa Grande

Adobe Hwy.

to Sonoma

E. Washington Blvd.

McDowell Park

McDowell Blvd.

Caulfield Ln.

Lakeville

116

to Santa Rosa

Redwood Hwy.

101

Petaluma River

N. Petaluma Blvd.

Kenilworth Park
Fairgrounds

Payran St.

Lakeville St.

E. D St.

NWP Depot

Weiller St.

Drawbridge

Steamer Landing Park
McNear Peninsula

Petaluma Blvd.

Creek

Rocky Memorial Dog Park

Shollenberger Park

River

to Novato

Petaluma

Walnut Park

6th St.

D St.

G St.

Wickersham Park

S. Petaluma Blvd.

McNear Park

McNear School

Bodega Ave.

Ave.

Start

11th St.

I St.

Western

Windsor Dr.

Oxford Ct.

D St.

End

Fillaree Trail

Panorama Tr.

South Loop

Fish Pond

Spring Hill Rd.

Chileno Valley Rd.

Helen Putnam Regional Park

Start

Helen Putnam Regional Park and McNear Park to Petaluma Adobe State Historic Park

From Helen Putnam Park to Oxford Street and from 11th and G Streets to Casa Grande/Adobe Roads

Length	5.9 miles (includes 1.2 miles through Helen Putnam Regional Park and 4.7 miles from McNear Park to Petaluma Adobe State Historic Park)
Accessibility	Hikers and mountain bikers
Agency	Sonoma County
Regulations	Helen Putnam Regional, McNear, and Walnut parks are open during daylight hours. Petaluma Adobe State Historic Park is open from 8 AM to 5 PM and charges an entrance fee.
Facilities	Water and restrooms at Helen Putnam and McNear parks, water and restrooms at Petaluma Adobe State Historic Park

This pleasant stroll through a regional park and Petaluma's historic neighborhoods is rich in history. You'll pass restored Victorian houses around McNear and Walnut parks and cross the Petaluma River on a historic drawbridge to arrive at General Mariano Vallejo's ranch. The relatively level sidewalks and bike lanes are shaded until you reach city limits along Casa Grande Road, where trees are few; you'll follow the paved road shoulder to reach Petaluma Adobe State Historic Park, where a large eucalyptus grove awaits.

Getting There

By Car

WEST TRAILHEAD, HELEN PUTNAM REGIONAL PARK: From Highway 101 take the East Washington Boulevard exit. Continue on East Washington and cross the Petaluma River. Turn left on Petaluma Boulevard and right on Western Avenue. Go 2 miles and turn left (south) on Chileno Valley Road. Continue another mile to the parking area.

MCNEAR PARK: From Highway 101 take the East Washington Boulevard exit, go west on it to Payran Street, turn left (south), and then turn right (west) on East D Street. Turn left (south) on 6th Street and then right (west) on G Street to parking along this street or on 11th and F streets.

EAST TRAILHEAD, EUCALYPTUS GROVE, AT INTERSECTION OF ADOBE ROAD AND CASA GRANDE ROAD: From Highway 101 take the East Washington Boulevard exit, and go east on it to Adobe Road. Turn right (south), and proceed to off-road parking at edge of a large eucalyptus forest on the west side of the road.

By Bus

A Golden Gate Transit bus runs along 4th and C streets daily.

On the Trail

Helen Putnam Regional Park

In late fall 1995, the Bay Area Ridge Trail Council dedicated a trail in Helen Putnam Regional Park and the route from McNear Park to Petaluma Adobe State Historic Park as an official segment of the Bay Area Ridge Trail.

The paved 1.2-mile trail through Helen Putnam Regional Park begins at the southwest corner of the park near the playground and picnic area. It passes a cattail-lined fish pond and the creek that feeds it. The trail then heads northeast and rises 480 feet to the top of a pretty knoll that offers views of the surrounding hills and the town of Petaluma. The trail currently ends at Oxford Court, but it is hoped that someday the short gap between Helen Putnam and McNear parks will be closed.

McNear Park to Petaluma Adobe State Historic Park

The next Bay Area Ridge Trail route begins at McNear Park on the corner of 11th and G streets. A small grove of redwoods shades the picnic tables, benches, and horseshoe pits on lush green lawns. Nearby are tennis courts and brightly colored slides, swings, and climbing apparatus for young children, with plenty of benches from which parents can supervise the juvenile scene.

Hikers and **mountain bikers** leave the park, heading east along G Street. Opposite sides of the street offer sun or shade—take your pick depending on the day's weather. Turn left (north) on 6th Street and admire several large and handsome Victorian houses. Mature trees in well-kept gardens surrounded by picket fences cast shade over the sidewalk, which is welcome in summer.

At East D Street you go right (east) and pass more Victorians and the historic city post office. At the intersection of East D Street and South Petaluma Boulevard, a few black walnut trees in Walnut Park remain to give credence to the park's name. In yet another of this city's many parks, you will find green lawns, benches, and picnic tables.

Side Trip to McNear Building

An optional two-block detour to the historic McNear Building heads north along South Petaluma Boulevard from the east side of Walnut Park. Petaluma's downtown has 99 buildings recorded in the National Register of Historic Paces. The McNear Building's graceful iron front is typical of the sheet- or cast-iron façades popular here in the 1880s and 1890s; they were prefabricated in San Francisco and shipped here by boat along the Petaluma River. The Petaluma River was an important commerce route for other goods as well, beginning with the Gold Rush, when it was used to ship supplies for 49ers. Until 1950, grain and farm products were transported downriver to San Pablo Bay and San Francisco.

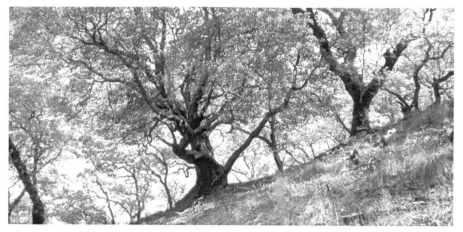

New leaves emerging on oak trees

From each of the park's four corners, a broad walkway leads to the charming, round bandstand in its center.

Continue along East D Street to the Petaluma River, just three blocks beyond Walnut Park. You cross the river on the historic D Street drawbridge, one of the oldest drawbridges still in use in California; its steel roadbed lifts for watercraft too tall to pass under it. Vacationing boaters from San Francisco Bay often use the mooring and landing facility upstream of the bridge. As you cross the river, look downstream to McNear Island, zoned for eventual park use by the town.

On the other side of the bridge there is a quarter-mile spur trail along the riverfront known as the Petaluma River Trail in an area known as Steamer Landing Park. It includes a spacious plaza paved with bricks upon which are engraved the names of donors or people honored by donor-friends. Several attractive benches with a central raised circular planter adorned with flowers offer a pleasant place to watch the activity along the Petaluma River. This small park also encompasses the western end of McNear Island.

In the next half mile, you go through a mixed commercial and residential neighborhood on East D Street. At the Sonoma-Marin Fairgrounds and Kenilworth Park on Payran Street, turn right (south) and continue for 0.5 mile to a shopping center on the corner of Caulfield Lane. Turn left (east) on Caulfield Lane, where you will find sidewalks on the north side of the street and bike lanes on both sides. New subdivisions fill the land on either side of the street, and tall fences and flowering plum trees line the sidewalks. Make a right turn (south) on McDowell Boulevard to find ranch-style housing, wide bike lanes, and only a little shade.

At Casa Grande Road you turn left, continuing east past even newer subdivisions and the playing fields and sprawling buildings of Casa Grande High School. A planted median strip and new trees along the sidewalks continue until Ely Boulevard. You are now about a mile from La Casa Grande, General Mariano Vallejo's partially restored adobe ranch headquarters and the end point of this segment. Since crossing the Petaluma River, you have traveled over what was once part of Vallejo's vast landholdings. The Sonoma Mountains to the northeast, the land east to Sonoma Creek, and thousands of acres from the shores of San Pablo Bay north to Glen Ellen were part of Vallejo's huge Rancho Petaluma. Vallejo grazed Mexican longhorn cattle on his extensive acreage,

Petaluma's "First Citizen"

Longtime Petaluma residents may remember McNear Park's benefactor, George P. McNear, who was born here in 1857. He donated the land for the park, as well as a handsome sum to maintain it. He also donated land for McNear School, just east of the park, and for a local golf course. McNear was prominent in many civic affairs and played an important part in the poultry industry here, which earned Petaluma the nickname "Egg Basket of the World." In 1937, when McNear was an active 80 years old, a historian declared him "the first citizen of Petaluma."

raised sheep and goats, and grew a variety of crops to supply the ranch's needs. Today, some of the land along Casa Grande Road remains in agricultural use.

Your route rises toward the foothills, where California oaks, sycamores, and bay laurel trees fill gentle folds in the hillsides. You reach the state-owned eucalyptus grove, on your left at the southwest corner of Adobe and Casa Grande roads, the end of this Bay Area Ridge Trail trip. You may have left a shuttle car here at off-road parking on Adobe Road. If you are returning to McNear Park, you might enjoy a visit to Petaluma's riverside shops and restaurants on 2nd Street, just two blocks north of the Ridge Trail route on D Street.

Across busy Adobe Road is Vallejo's adobe ranch headquarters, where you can visit some of its rooms and learn the story of food and meat production in the days of the Mexican ranchos. Several picnic tables under mature trees, a running stream, and a monument to Vallejo enhance the grounds outside the adobe. Although your Petaluma trip ends here, you will traverse other lands in Vallejo's holdings as you circumnavigate the Bay Area on its ridgelines in the Vallejo-Benicia Buffer and Benicia-Vallejo Waterfront trips (pages 109–117).

◆ ◆ ◆

The next leg of the Bay Area Ridge Trail starts in Jack London State Historic Park near Glen Ellen on the other side of the Sonoma Mountains. As yet, the route to this park has not been designated.

Jack London State Historic Park

From Sonoma Mountain Trail to Junction of Hayfields and Cowan Meadow Trails

Length 11.7 miles round-trip (includes 4.4 miles round-trip on connector trail, 4 miles round-trip on Sonoma Mountain Trail, and 3.3 miles round-trip to Hayfields/Cowan Meadow junction; additional 0.8 mile round-trip to park's northeast boundary)

Accessibility Hikers, equestrians, and mountain bikers

Agency California Department of Parks and Recreation

Regulations Park is open from 8 AM to dusk.

Facilities Water, restrooms, and telephone

Join this leg of the main Ridge Trail route—the Sonoma Mountain Trail—from a connector trail through redwood and oak forests. After an out-and-back trip on the Sonoma Mountain Trail segment, follow the Ridge Trail along lively streams, through dense forests, and across scattered grasslands on the eastern flank of Sonoma Mountain. You'll travel wide park service roads and new, well-designed, narrow trails to reach lofty heights: a gain of 608 feet in elevation on the Sonoma Mountain Trail and 1220 feet on the Hayfields Trail, where you'll have grand views of the Valley of the Moon.

Getting There

From Highway 101 in Sonoma County, take Highway 12 to Glen Ellen, and turn southwest on Arnold Drive. Turn left (west) on London Ranch Road to the park entrance on the left. Turn right to the western parking area just across London Ranch Road.

On the Trail

Since there is no trailhead at the southern extension of the main Bay Area Ridge Trail, the first 2 miles of this trip follow connector trails (the Lake and Mountain trails) to meet the Ridge Trail route, the Sonoma Mountain Trail. **Hikers** and **mountain bikers** begin on the Lake Trail, from the middle of the westernmost parking lot. **Equestrians** take the trail from the parking area's north corner and follow short paths through the trees to join the Lake Trail. Bear right on this park service road.

The multiuse Lake Trail skirts the north and west sides of a beautiful private vineyard, the vines of which add lovely shades of red and tawny gold to the fall scene. Once the prized vineyard of Jack London, who laid it out on stepped terraces, it still produces wine today. After 0.4 mile on the service road, **hikers** can cut right onto a narrow trail through redwood and fir woods and then rejoin **mountain bikers** and **equestrians** at the reed-rimmed lake, created by London for swimming, fishing, and poolside partying.

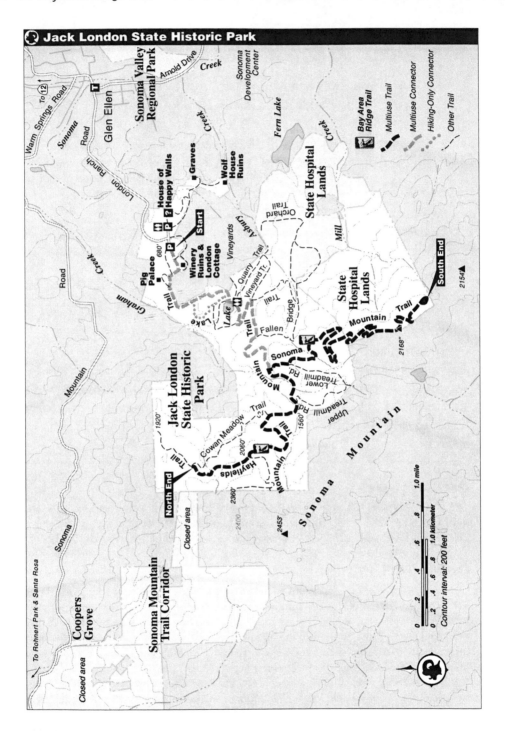

Jack London State Historic Park

To Rohnert Park & Santa Rosa

Warm Springs Road

To (12)

Sonoma Road

Glen Ellen

Arnold Drive

Sonoma Valley Regional/Park

Creek

Sonoma Development Center

Fern Lake

Creek

Bay Area Ridge Trail

Multiuse Trail
Multiuse Connector
Hiking-Only Connector
Other Trail

London Ranch Road

House of Happy Walls

Graves

Wolf House Ruins

State Hospital Lands

Mill Creek

Pig Palace

680'

Start

Winery Ruins & London Cottage

Vineyards

Asbury

Orchard Trail

State Hospital Lands

South End

2154'

Graham Creek

Quarry Trail

Vineyard Tr.

Lake

Lake Trail

Bridge Trail

Fallen

Mountain Trail

State Hospital Lands

2168"

Sonoma

Lower Treadmill Rd

Sonoma Mountain

Jack London State Historic Park

1920'

Cowan Meadow Trail

Mountain Trail

Upper Treadmill Rd

1560'

2060'

Hayfields

Mountain Trail

Sonoma Mountain

2360'

2400'

North End

Closed area

Sonoma

Coopers Grove

Closed area

Sonoma Mountain Trail Corridor

2453'

0   .2   .4   .6   .8   1.0 mile

0 .2 .4 .6 .8 1.0 kilometer

Contour interval: 200 feet

Today, the lake's curving stone dam offers park visitors a sunny place to rest on their trek up the mountain.

Beyond the lake all users turn right (due west) to join the Mountain Trail, which in 0.15 mile swings south through a cool, dark forest of redwoods and Douglas firs. In openings where large redwoods were cut long ago, tanoaks, madrones, and bigleaf maples now fill the void. After climbing steadily for 0.2 mile, you reach a junction with the Fallen Bridge Trail, which goes left toward Asbury Creek. Mays Clearing lies before you, a wide meadow with fine views south over the valley and east to the mountains that rise above it. In fall, look for the clear red berries that hang from long tendrils of the native honeysuckle vine; in winter, white snowberries attract deer and birds but are poisonous to humans.

Follow the Bay Area Ridge Trail sign that points the way right and uphill on the Mountain Trail. You climb through Woodcutters Meadow, where fallen tree limbs are strewn among scattered, moss-covered rocks, and clumps of California fescue and ferns wave in the breeze. As you pass the Upper Fallen Bridge Trail on the left, the trail swerves right to make a hairpin turn north and then south through lovely Pine Tree Meadows. Filled with many native flowers in spring, especially purple iris, pink checkerbloom, and shiny yellow buttercups, this meadow is a delight to behold.

Continue on the Mountain Trail as it swings right and climbs again through woods to reach the Sonoma Mountain Trail.

South Along the Sonoma Mountain Trail

Turn left to begin the out-and-back trip to the park's southern boundary on the southern segment of the Ridge Trail route. The trail heads generally south through a forest of Oregon white oak, California bay, and bigleaf maple, zigzagging on wide sweeps. Here and there, young Douglas firs spring up in openings created by fallen trees. You cross the deep trough of Asbury Creek, lined by ferns and large-leafed, creamy-blossomed aralia.

Beyond the creek, small, lacy-leafed hazelnut trees and California buckeyes grow under a high canopy of magnificent deciduous Oregon white oaks. In spring, large candles of buckeye blossoms, white to light pink, fill the air with their fragrance. Numerous specimens of hound's tongue, a tall, blue-blossomed cousin of forget-me-not (in the Borage family), grow along the trail. You may also see mission bells nodding their bell-shaped heads—deep purple and greenish spotted—a special springtime treat.

Low walls demarcate this carefully designed trail, constructed from rocks and downed tree logs that trail builders removed to smooth the trail surface. From a few clearings, you can see Fern Lake and the red-roofed buildings of the Sonoma Developmental Center in the valley below. A ring of mountains encloses this valley, and almost due north, Mt. St. Helena rises to 4344 feet. From another opening you can look back northwest to 2463-foot Sonoma Mountain, topped by its radio transmitter tower.

The trail sweeps widely to the west and then east; you then head due south through the forest and into the Developmental Center property. A sign announces the trail's name and its builders—crews of volunteers and California Conservation Corps members under the able direction of Toni McRorie.

Now on the second leg of the Sonoma Mountain Trail, at about 2000 feet, you follow several small switchbacks in and out of the forest. In spring, flowers bloom in small sunny meadows—deep blue lupine, purple-tufted brodiaea, and tiny pink linanthus. Bring your wildflower book to identify the glorious specimens. From a wide clearing, you can see the Napa River to the east, where it flows through the marshlands to San Pablo Bay. Mt. Diablo rises beyond, easily visible on a clear day.

Just after crossing the indistinct track of an old road on your left, you come to the south boundary of the Developmental Center. Beyond is private property—do not enter! Loop to the right on a short trail and retrace your route to the junction with the Mountain Trail, which you left some 2 miles back.

North to the Junction of Hayfields and Cowan Meadow Trails

At the junction of Sonoma Mountain and Mountain trails, turn left from the Sonoma Mountain Trail, or continue straight on the Mountain Trail if you skipped the Sonoma Mountain Trail round-trip. Shortly you cross South Graham Creek; in winter and spring it may overflow onto the road, but you can usually rock hop across. In the rainy season,

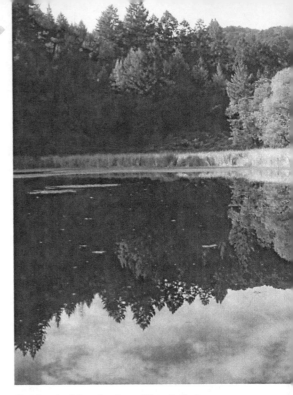

Pond at Jack London State Historic Park

rushing water cascades over rocks in a moist, fern-clad canyon upstream. Bear right at the junction with Upper Treadmill Road, continuing on the Mountain Trail for 0.1 mile to Middle Graham Creek. After crossing the creek, you come to a rest area with a picnic table. Ferns grace the trail banks beneath large redwoods, and hazelnut leaves glow golden against the dark redwood trunks in fall.

Just 0.2 mile beyond the rest area, and after a third Graham Creek crossing, you reach the junction of Mountain and Cowan Meadow trails. The multiuse Ridge Trail route stays on the Mountain Trail, swinging left and gaining more than 400 feet in elevation in 0.65 mile. You pass another vista point with views south to a tree-topped knoll and west toward the Sonoma Mountain summit. Bear right at the next junction, on the Hayfields Trail. After 0.2 mile, you begin to descend rapidly for another 0.2 mile, north toward the marshy confluence of three arms of North Graham Creek and the upper junc-

Jack London's Beauty Ranch

No trip to this park is complete without a visit to Beauty Ranch, Jack London's cherished estate. By 1876, London had already achieved international fame for his adventure stories *Call of the Wild* and *The Sea Wolf.* Jack and his wife, Charmian, then moved to Sonoma Valley to escape busy city life, and he began work on Beauty Ranch. Over the remaining years of his life, he embarked on continual projects to improve the land and repair or construct buildings.

tion with the Cowan Meadow Trail. The Ridge Trail ends here, as of this writing, but you can continue 0.4 mile northeast under the power lines to the park boundary at about 1920 feet. Your return descent is speedier than your ascent, and you soon reach the historic buildings of the former Jack London ranch.

The 0.5-mile Beauty Ranch Trail leads to the ranch buildings, the winery and distillery, and the House of Happy Walls, built by Charmian London after Jack's death. Charmian lived at the ranch until her death at the age of 84, after which the House of Happy Walls became a museum with artifacts of the London legend; today it is also the park visitor center. Jack London's gravesite is about a half mile by trail from the House of Happy Walls. Follow the park road about a quarter mile beyond to the handsome rock walls of Wolf House, all that remains of the Londons' dream house. In 1959 the state acquired some 40 acres of the original ranch; today, Jack London State Historic Park has expanded to more than 800 acres.

◆ ◆ ◆

In the future, proposed trails will connect this Bay Area Ridge Trail segment to segments in Petaluma to the south, and Annadel and Sugarloaf Ridge state parks to the north. For now, the next segment begins 7 miles north in Annadel State Park.

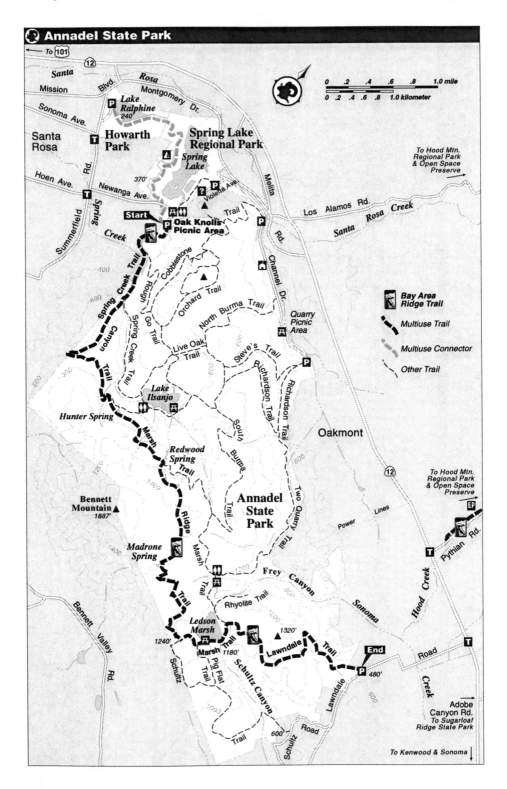

Annadel State Park

To 101

Santa
Rosa Blvd.
Mission
Sonoma Ave.
Santa
Rosa
Hoen Ave.
Summerfield Rd.

12
Montgomery Dr.
Lake Ralphine 240'
Howarth Park
Spring Lake Regional Park
Spring Lake 370'
Newanga Ave.
Spring Creek
Start
Oak Knolls Picnic Area

Violetta Ave.
Melita Rd.
Los Alamos Rd.
Santa Rosa Creek

To Hood Mtn. Regional Park & Open Space Preserve

0 .2 .4 .6 .8 1.0 mile
0 .2 .4 .6 .8 1.0 kilometer

Cobblestone
Orchard Trail
North Burma Trail
Channel Dr.
Quarry Picnic Area
Steve's Trail

Spring Creek Trail
Rough Go Trail
Live Oak Trail
Richardson Trail

Canyon Trail
400
600
600

Lake Ilsanjo
South Burma
Richardson Trail

Bay Area Ridge Trail
Multiuse Trail
Multiuse Connector
Other Trail

Hunter Spring
Redwood Spring Trail

Oakmont
600
12
To Hood Mtn. Regional Park & Open Space Preserve

Bennett Mountain 1887'
Marsh Trail
Ridge Trail
1200
1400

Annadel State Park
Two Quarry Trail
Power Lines
Sonoma
PY
Pythian Rd.
Hood Creek

Madrone Spring
Marsh Trail
1200
Frey Canyon
360

Bennett Valley Rd.
Rhyolite Trail
1200

Ledson Marsh
1240'
Marsh Trail 1180'
Schultz Canyon
Pig Flat Trail
Schultz Trail

1320'
Lawndale Trail
End 480'

Road
Creek

1000
600
Schultz Road
Trail

Adobe Canyon Rd.
To Sugarloaf Ridge State Park

To Kenwood & Sonoma

Annadel State Park

From Spring Lake Park to Annadel's East Gate at Lawndale Road

Length	8.6 miles
Accessibility	Hikers, equestrians, and mountain bikers (unsuitable for road bicyclists or inexperienced riders)
Agency	California Department of Parks and Recreation
Regulations	Spring Lake Park is open from 8 AM to sunset and charges an entrance fee. Annadel State Park is open from sunrise to sunset, does not permit dogs on trails, and requires that bikers observe state park rules.
Facilities	Water, restrooms, and telephone at Oak Knolls Picnic Area in Spring Lake Park; water and restrooms at Channel Drive parking lot; and restrooms at Lake Ilsanjo and at the intersection of Marsh and Two Quarry trails in Annadel State Park

Gradually climb over grassy hillsides and through oak woodlands and conifer forests on the west side of Bennett Mountain along wide, rocky service roads. You gain 1100 feet and then lose 1000 feet as you descend past spring-fed meadows on a well-graded trail to Annadel's east side. The west- and south-facing slopes can be hot in summer; north- and east-facing slopes are forested.

Getting There

WEST TRAILHEAD, SPRING LAKE PARK: From Highway 101 in Santa Rosa, take Highway 12 east. At Farmers Lane (marked Highway 12), continue straight onto Hoen Avenue and pass Summerfield Road. Turn onto the first street on the left (Newanga Avenue), and follow Newanga as it veers right after one block. Continue to the Spring Lake Park entrance, and go right to parking at Oak Knolls Picnic Area.

EAST TRAILHEAD, LAWNDALE ROAD: From Highway 101 in Santa Rosa, take Highway 12 east about 9 miles, turn right (south) on Lawndale Road, and continue about 1.5 miles to a small parking area on the right side of the road.

On the Trail

Two local parks are connected by trail to Annadel State Park—Howarth Park and Spring Lake Regional Park. This trip begins in Spring Lake Park at the Oak Knolls Picnic Area and follows a graveled road due south on the levee beside Spring Creek. In summer the creek is dry, but in winter water flows from the northwest side of Bennett Mountain through Annadel State Park to the flood-control basin of Spring Lake. The levee trail, much favored by local mountain bikers, hikers, and equestrians, runs along the base of a west-facing hillside, just outside Annadel State Park's boundary.

After a half mile, the trail crosses the creek and then continues another half mile to the Annadel State Park boundary. You cross a concrete weir for Spring Creek flood control and go straight ahead for 0.2 mile to enter an oak-and-buckeye woodland on the Canyon Trail in Annadel State Park's 5000 wilderness acres. The stone foundations on your right are all that remain of a cabin built by one Dr. Summerfield, a former owner of this land. Annadel State Park was once part of Rancho Los Guilicos, granted in 1839 to a Scottish sea captain, John Wilson. Wilson was married to Ramona Carrillo de Pacheco. Since he was away at sea most of the time, his nearly 19,000 acres remained relatively untouched.

You continue on the wide, rocky Canyon Trail and emerge from the shady forest into a gentle valley. Ahead you see the low, rounded ridge of Taylor Mountain with the large homes of a nearby subdivision in the foreground. After you make a hairpin turn to the left, your uphill way begins in earnest. From the open hillside you look north to Spring Lake and beyond to Rincon Valley. On clear days, Mt. St. Helena's long shoulder and its taller, prominent left hump, is visible in the distant north. Looking south from this trail at 1000 feet, you see Bennett Mountain's 1887-foot summit just outside the park. If you come here in late March or early April, you may find the rare white fritillary blooming in moist grasslands.

After 1.5 miles on the Canyon Trail, you reach a junction with the Marsh Trail. Make a sharp right turn, and continue climbing on the redesigned, narrower Marsh Trail. You'll see splendid examples of northern oak woodlands made up of Oregon white oaks, black oaks, buckeyes, and occasional manzanitas along this trail. Beautiful, lush stands of California fescue, a native gray-green bunchgrass with tall, graceful stalks and feathery flower heads, fill the spaces between rounded, moss-covered boulders on the forest floor. The Pomo people who used to live here collected fescue seeds for food.

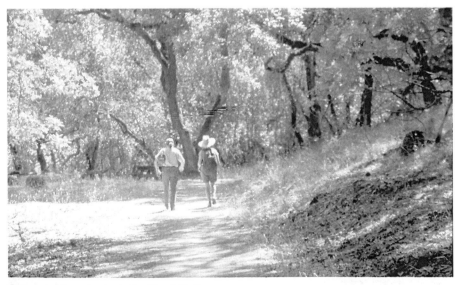

Oregon white oaks shade the Marsh Trail.

Land of the Bitakomtara

Native American tribes were the first inhabitants of the land this Bay Area Ridge Trail segment traverses. The Bitakomtara, a southern group of Pomos, occupied approximately 200 square miles in the Santa Rosa area, from Laguna de Santa Rosa east to Sonoma Creek, and south from Mark West Creek nearly to Cotati. Probably about 20 tribelets lived in the area, and each spoke a slightly different dialect.

The Bitakomtara lived well on this land, harvesting acorns from several species of oaks, fishing the creeks, and hunting or trapping game, especially deer, squirrels, and rabbits. Many years have passed, but little has changed this lands' meadows and woods since then. You will find a near wilderness here, especially on remote sections of the Bay Area Ridge Trail route. Oak trees stud the hillsides, their acorns litter the trails, springs feed bubbling creeks, and the bulbs, berries, seeds, and grains that Native Americans used to harvest grow in meadows and forests.

In the shade of redwoods and Douglas firs, with soft duff underfoot, you cross the headwaters of Spring Creek. Here, where ferns drape the road banks and redwoods tower overhead, a quiet serenity prevails. You proceed through the forest, and after 1.6 miles on the Marsh Trail, reach a junction with a well-designed segment of the Ridge Trail. Make a sharp right turn onto the 3.3-mile Ridge Trail, formerly Upper Steve's Trail, and head south on a gentle uphill grade. A high forest canopy arches over skeletons of huge manzanitas, and in moist places, spring blossoms of scarlet columbine stand between 1 and 3 feet tall.

You enter a woods of oak and buckeye and curve around the head of an intermittent stream, traveling due east. As you cross rivulets and streams on this trail, notice that the drainages are covered with large flat-topped rocks that replace former culverts. Known as armored drains, these wide, gently scooped-out aprons are easier to maintain and are more pleasant to cross in all seasons.

You emerge from the woods and skirt a sloping meadow southwest of Ledson Marsh; the meadow grasses are golden in summer and vivid green in winter and spring. Fine specimens of manzanita thrive here, and spring wildflowers and bunchgrasses fill the meadow after winter rains. Oregon white and California black oaks dot your route through the grasslands. Some of these trees are over 200 years old. Although they continue to set seed, an overabundance of rodents—mice, voles, and squirrels—that eat the acorns are preventing the oaks from regenerating in spite of the efforts of the rodents' natural predators: hawks, owls, and coyotes.

You cross a historic rock wall that marks a boundary established by early landowners. These rocks, and those strewn about the hillsides, are mostly basalt, an igneous rock of the Pliocene Age Sonoma Volcanics formation that is found throughout the Sonoma and Mayacmas Mountains.

From your vantage point at 1198 feet, look northeast across the meadows and Ledson Marsh to 2730-foot Hood Mountain, named in honor of William Hood, who owned Rancho Los Guilicos for almost 30 years. On October 21, 2006, a trail from the Oakmont area in the Valley of the Moon to Hood Mountain's summit was dedicated as a

5-mile segment of the Bay Area Ridge Trail. Northwest lies 2729-foot Bald Mountain (on the Bay Area Ridge Trail route through Sugarloaf Ridge State Park). Lower Red Mountain, immediately west of Sugarloaf Ridge State Park on private property, is easily recognized by its unusual color.

The Ridge Trail turns left (north) on the Marsh Trail toward Ledson Marsh. In 0.3 mile you reach a picnic table under a huge, double-trunked oak and flanked by three large manzanitas. This shady spot offers fine views of the reed-rimmed marsh and your route across the meadow above it. In fall, the reeds' gold and brown tones present a subdued contrast to the dark green woods.

When you feel refreshed, rejoin the Marsh Trail and pass the Pig Flat Trail junction. Continue 0.4 mile around the east side of the marsh, and cross a bridge over the outlet stream; a low dam contains winter runoff from the surrounding hillsides. When summer's heat prevails, the marsh dries up. Continue through a veritable coyote-bush forest (*baccharis*), accented by a few struggling live and blue oaks, to another junction on the north side of the marsh. Then swing right onto the Lawndale Trail, here a rocky road, heading for the park's east entrance.

In the next 0.3 mile, look for piles of dark basalt rock, remains of late 19th-century cobblestone quarrying. European immigrants chipped and shaped basalt rocks into paving stones and sent them by barge and train to San Francisco. Cobblestone quarrying was a thriving industry until modern automobile users began to prefer smoother rides.

On the final leg of this Ridge Trail trip, a 2.2-mile section of the well-designed Lawndale Trail, was built by state park employee Toni McRorie and volunteers. It ambles through a redwood-and-fir forest, following a gentle downhill slope. A study of fire ecology has left black scars on some redwoods, although the trees are still alive. Upon leaving the wooded area, you traverse a south-facing hillside in a grassy canyon and go through a gate at the Lawndale Road parking area.

After your trip, stop in at the park office to see an exhibit about how the Pomo people quarried and shaped obsidian into arrowheads, knives, scrapers, and spearheads. Since these artifacts are significant clues to the culture of the Native Americans who once inhabited this area, visitors are asked to leave them intact.

◆ ◆ ◆

The next leg of the Bay Area Ridge Trail begins in Hood Mountain Regional Park, about 4 miles northeast of this parking area.

Hood Mountain Regional Park and Open Space Preserve

Length	3.1 miles one-way
Accessibility	Hikers, equestrians, and mountain bikers
Agency	Sonoma County Regional Parks
Regulations	Preserve charges a small parking fee at entrance.
Facilities	Historic Hood Mansion; equestrian-trailer parking at Eliza Road; kiosk at trailhead with area maps; parking, water, and restroom at trailhead

A vigorous uphill trip follows Hood Creek through forests and meadows, passes several ponds, and then climbs to the top of Hood Mountain.

Getting There

From Highway 12 between Santa Rosa and Kenwood, turn north onto Pythian Road. **Hikers** and **mountain bikers** stay to the right when the road forks and go 0.75 mile on the Sonoma County Park District Road to the county's parking area. **Equestrians** veer left off Pythian Road onto Eliza Road to equestrian parking near the Hood Mansion.

On the Trail

From the kiosk at the parking area take the trail that follows the upper side of the fence around the parking area to the park district's sign where you read, among other tempting destinations, that Hood Mountain is 3.1 miles ahead. The Ridge Trail route follows the Lower Johnson Road Trail, which shortly becomes the park road. It goes up steeply and there is little shoulder, so listen for oncoming cars. Hood Creek flows far below in a narrow, wooded canyon; you can hear it on a calm day.

Bear right past a private home with a wide swath of green lawn, and then almost immediately go right again. On a wide trail you zigzag uphill passing three big water tanks and then go left beside a sturdy split-rail fence on the park boundary. As you progress ever upward, look for sword ferns on the trail banks and huge boulders lying beside the trail. There is downed wood scattered throughout the forest, probably left from some previous logging operation. (Current logging practices require slash to be left onsite.)

At the next junction you make a sharp right turn onto the Panorama Ranch Trail, which is edged by a low rock wall. After crossing three minor creek drainages, you then take a high-sided, fiberglass bridge over a larger creek in a heavily wooded canyon. At an unmarked trail junction I took the left trail that goes uphill when I scouted the trail; the right seemed to go down. The left-hand route goes through a wide meadow, bears left on a wide track, and goes steadily uphill to meet the Pond Trail. The right-hand trail, however, is the official Ridge Trail route and also reaches the Pond Trail junction.

Shortly you reach the junction of Pond and Valley View trails. The Valley View Trail is now marked as the Ridge Trail route. If you take the Valley View Trail, you will

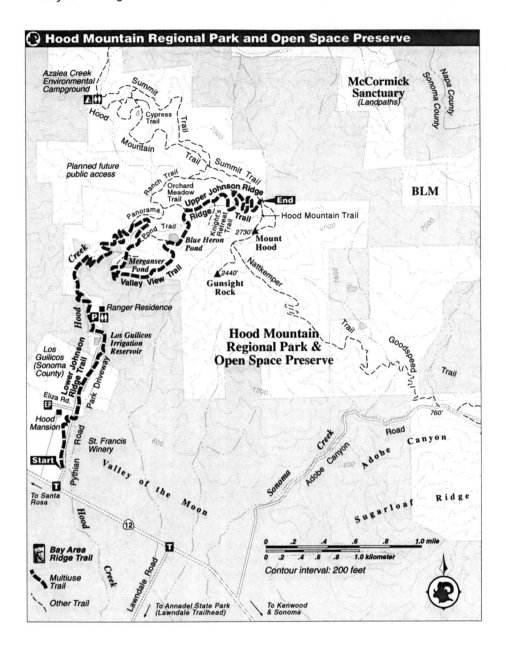

Hood Mountain Regional Park and Open Space Preserve

Azalea Creek Environmental Campground

Summit

Hood

Cypress Trail

Mountain

Trail

Trail

Summit Trail

Planned future public access

Ranch Trail

Orchard Meadow Trail

Upper Johnson Ridge

Panorama

Ridge Trail

Knight's Retreat Trail

Pond Trail

2730'

Blue Heron Pond

Mount Hood

Merganser Pond

Valley View Trail

Creek

Gunsight Rock

2440'

Nattkemper

End

Hood Mountain Trail

McCormick Sanctuary (Landpaths)

Napa County
Sonoma County

BLM

Ranger Residence

Los Guilicos Irrigation Reservoir

Los Guilicos (Sonoma County)

Lower Johnson Ridge Trail

Hood

Eliza Rd.

Hood Mansion

Park Driveway

St. Francis Winery

Start

Pythian Road

Valley of the Moon

To Santa Rosa

Hood

12

Bay Area Ridge Trail

Multiuse Trail

Other Trail

Creek

Lawndale Road

To Annadel State Park (Lawndale Trailhead)

Hood Mountain Regional Park & Open Space Preserve

Sonoma

Adobe Canyon Creek

Adobe

Canyon

Road

Sugarloaf

Ridge

760'

Goodspeed

Trail

Trail

600

800

1200

1600

2000

To Kenwood & Sonoma

0   .2   .4   .6   .8   1.0 mile
0 .2 .4 .6 .8 1.0 kilometer

Contour interval: 200 feet

head downhill, hearing and glimpsing Merganser Pond through the trees way below you. When you emerge from the forest, you arrive at a point where the view merits the name of the trail. You make a sharp turn left around the point and then head across the middle of the densely forested mountainside. After about a quarter mile this route veers left and climbs back uphill to join the Pond Trail, a total distance of 1.5 miles.

If you take the Pond Trail, you head east and soon pass the Blue Heron Pond, a small, circular body of water surrounded by tall trees and a cool site for a hot summer day picnic. In fact, not far beyond in a small clearing there is a picnic table. This route crosses many drainages lined with flat rocks, which are easily managed in summer and late fall. The going may be a little too wet after serious winter storms.

Rather abruptly you leave the forests and pass a sloping meadow surmounted by a row of widely-spaced, large deciduous trees. It may be an abandoned fruit orchard, as the name of a trail from here seems to imply—the Orchard Meadow Trail, which takes off left. However, just beyond here a Ridge Trail sign directs you to the right on the Upper Johnson Ridge Trail. You are in the forest again and heading uphill. Shortly on your left behind a fence you see a little cabin with a white door, known as the Hendrickson Historic Site. Another nearby cabin is in poor condition.

In these cool woods look for California fescue, a narrow, long-leaved, gray-green bunchgrass that drapes the banks and spills over the trail tread. The Pomo Indians valued this grass and collected its seeds for food.

Continuing on the Upper Johnson Ridge Trail you climb steadily through the forest over a series of humps and hollows on this steep, well-worn trail. It zigzags for more than a half mile before finally emerging in a wide, circular opening at Hood Mountain's 2730-foot summit. From this circular opening enclosed by tall manzanita shrubs you can take the trail southeast to 2440-foot Gunsight Rock for splendid views over the Sonoma Valley. On a clear day you can see two other summits on Ridge Trail routes—southeast across the canyon to the top of neighboring Bald Mountain in Sugarloaf Ridge State Park and almost due south to Sonoma Mountain in Jack London State Historic Park.

After enjoying the splendid views and the pleasure of reaching the summit, **equestrians** and **bikers** head downhill on the Upper Johnson Ridge Trail. **Hikers** can join them on this trail or zigzag down the narrow Summit Trail through the densely forested, steep hillside to rejoin the Upper Johnson Ridge Trail farther down the mountain and from there return to the parking areas.

◆ ◆ ◆

The next segment of the Ridge Trail lies southeast of Hood Mountain in Sugarloaf Ridge State Park.

Sugarloaf Ridge State Park

From Visitor Center to Bald Mountain Summit

Length   5.4 miles round-trip, 6.7 miles using hikers' alternate return

Accessibility   Hikers, equestrians, and mountain bikers

Agency   California Department of Parks and Recreation

Regulations   Park charges an entrance fee. Dogs are prohibited from trails.

Facilities   Phone at visitor center, water, and restrooms

A challenging 1550-foot climb from an enclosed, remote valley to the top of Bald Mountain, where you'll take in far-flung views of Northern California. Cross oak woodlands and chaparral slopes, and detour to a seasonal vernal pool on wide service roads with a short paved segment. These trails can be hot in summer.

Getting There

From Highway 12 east of Santa Rosa or northwest of Kenwood, turn north on Adobe Canyon Road, and continue to the end. The parking area is on the left after the park entrance kiosk and visitor center. People hauling horse trailers can park them just past the barn 0.5 mile beyond the kiosk.

On the Trail

Equestrians ride from the barn to the group campsite parking area to join the Lower Bald Mountain Trail. Go northwest, uphill, and meet the **hiker** and **mountain biker** route at the Bald Mountain Trail. Some riders and hikers may join you having taken the Goodspeed Trail downhill from Gunsight Rock in Hood Mountain Regional Park and Open Space Preserve.

Hikers and **mountain bikers** start this trip on the trail across the road from the kiosk. The wide, multiuse, Stern Trail starts from the visitor center east of the kiosk and heads uphill (northwest) through grasslands and past scattered clumps of scrub oak to join the Ridge View Trail for the trip up the mountain. You may be joined here by hikers and equestrians who have come over from Mount Hood on the Goodspeed Trail or from the park entrance on the Pony Gate or Canyon trails. In 1976 Mrs. Marjorie Stern dedicated 300 acres of her land in Kenwood to enlarge Sugarloaf Ridge State Park, and it is for her that the Stern Trail is named. She also helped to create Annadel State Park, another link in the Bay Area Ridge Trail.

After rounding several switchbacks, you pass the Lower Bald Mountain Trail coming up from the Group Campground. In less than a half mile, you reach the junction with the Lower Bald Mountain Trail, where equestrians join the main Ridge Trail route.

When you meet the Bald Mountain Trail, a paved road built for service vehicle access to the microwave station on Red Mountain, go around a metal gate across the road,

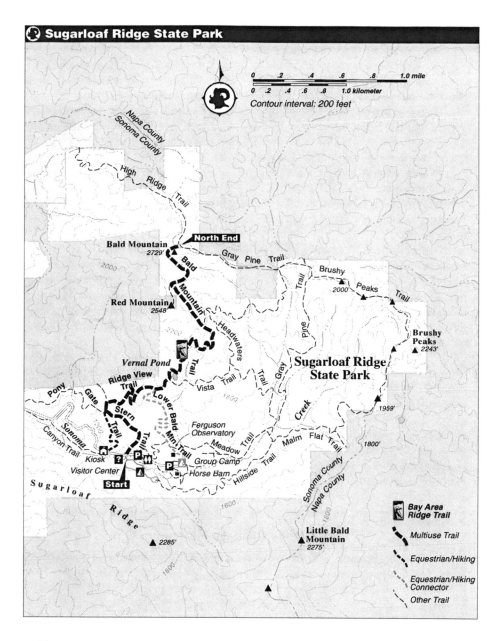

Sugarloaf Ridge State Park

Contour interval: 200 feet

Napa County / Sonoma County

High Ridge Trail

Bald Mountain
2729'

North End

Gray Pine Trail

Brushy

2000'

Peaks

Trail

Bald Mountain

Red Mountain
2548'

Headwaters

Trail

Brushy Peaks
▲ 2243'

Pony

Gate

Vernal Pond

Ridge View Trail

Vista Trail

1600

Gray

Pine

Trail

Creek

Sugarloaf Ridge State Park

▲ 1959'

Sonoma Canyon Trail

Stern Trail

Lower Bald Mtn. Trail

Ferguson Observatory

Meadow

Trail

Malm Flat Trail

▲ 1800'

Kiosk

Visitor Center

Group Camp

Horse Barn

Hillside Trail

Start

Sonoma County / Napa County

Sugarloaf

Ridge

1600

1600

▲ 2285'

1800

Little Bald Mountain
2275'

▲

Bay Area Ridge Trail

Multiuse Trail

Equestrian/Hiking

Equestrian/Hiking Connector

Other Trail

and begin your ascent in earnest. The road cuts reveal large veins of bluish-green serpentine, California's state rock and an indicator of fault zones. The St. John's Mountain Fault crosses this mountain.

Look west over the Sonoma Creek canyon to ridge after ridge of coastal mountains that stretch to the sea. When early morning fog lies in the interior valleys, the ridgetops peek out, giving the effect of islands rising from misty inland seas. Conical-shaped Hood Mountain rises to the northwest—at 2730 feet, it is the highest point in neighboring Hood Mountain Regional Park and the summit of the Ridge Trail route in that park. On clear days, you can see south to Mt. Tamalpais in Marin County. Below you are the park's meadows, barns, and visitor center.

Due south beyond the park's boundary is the rugged linear ridge from which Sugarloaf Ridge State Park takes its name. The bare rock columns on its north face are remnants of nearby Mt. St. Helena's volcanic activity some 7 million years ago.

High road banks and modest oak-fir-madrone woodlands along this trail offer much-needed shade on summer mornings. In spring, clumps of iris brighten the road with lavender or cream blossoms. Apricot-colored sticky monkeyflowers, purple asters, and the tawny, two-foot-tall stalks of native bunchgrass last into summer.

Hikers, equestrians, and **bikers** continue steadily uphill on the Bald Mountain Trail. You pass the Vista Trail, on which a short detour takes you to a lovely vernal pool. When winter rains fill this seasonal wetland, a unique community of plants blooms; as the water recedes, they die in concentric rings. Enjoy the pool from the trail and respect its fragile environment.

Return to the Bald Mountain Trail, where the vegetation alternates between woodland and chaparral, depending on soil and exposure. Chaparral covers the slopes on south-facing stretches of the trail. Farther uphill, oaks and madrones fill little ravines, often accompanied by bay trees. The oaks and madrones on these hillsides are old-growth trees, unlike the hardwood forest in the valley below, which was stripped by a settler in the 1880s. He burned the wood to make charcoal and sold it to heat homes and run steam engines in nearby communities.

Occasionally turn back to look over this steep, rugged terrain. There is little agricultural activity in these mountains, except for a large vineyard just outside the southern boundary of the park and a few large ranches to the west. Instead, many acres of this land are public open space, including this 2700-acre park—Sugarloaf Ridge State Park—and Hood Mountain Regional Park, just west of here.

Continue upward on the paved road, around bends that head into small ravines. At about 2200 feet, you pass the Red Mountain Trail and begin to see black oaks and bigleaf maple trees on the east-facing slopes that drain into Sonoma Creek's headwaters. Across a steep ravine to the northeast, you see the grass- and brush-covered slopes of

Sugarloaf Ridge History

There is evidence that Native Americans lived here as long ago as 5000 B.C. The most recent peoples were the Wappos, whose village was called Wilikos. Their firm resistance to the intruding Spaniards earned them the name *Wappo*, a derivative of the Spanish word *guapo* meaning "brave or handsome." Weakened by cholera and smallpox, the tribe's numbers diminished and they were eventually relocated to a Pomo reservation. The last full-blooded Wappo died in 1909.

The Spaniards ran cattle on these hills before the arrival of the first settlers in 1867. Farming was not successful here, and in 1920 the State of California purchased these lands for a reservoir, which never materialized. Later, Sonoma State Hospital built a swimming pool and cookhouse for a summer camp program. Finally, in 1964 this land became part of the California State Park System.

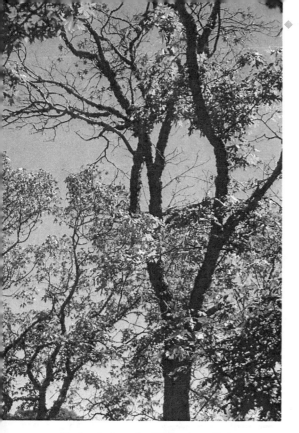

Black oak, Sugarloaf Ridge State Park

the park's northern ridge, along which the Gray Pine Trail extends to meet the Brushy Peaks Trail.

You leave the paved road where it turns sharply left and ascends private Red Mountain. Your route, still the Bald Mountain Trail, goes right and then immediately left. You descend a very steep dirt road and then traverse open, sloping grasslands dotted with bright wildflowers in spring and glowing, rosy-red buckwheat in fall.

About a half mile from the turnoff you round the north side of Bald Mountain's summit and reach the junction with the High Ridge and Gray Pine trails. The former heads downhill, a tempting direction after the last upward pitch, but you take the Gray Pine Trail right for about 100 yards and then go right again to reach the rounded, bare summit. An exhilarating 360-degree sweep around the compass greets you.

You will find two vista displays to help identify (clockwise from San Francisco): the towers of the Golden Gate Bridge, Mt. Tamalpais, the Sonoma hills, Mt. St. Helena, long Blue Ridge between Napa County and the Central Valley, Mt. Diablo, and then San Francisco. Even Snow Mountain to the north and the Sierra Nevada to the east are visible on a clear winter day.

With Northern California at your feet, this is a pleasant place for a picnic. Find a protected shelf just below the summit with a view north to Mt. St. Helena. The Bay Area Ridge Trail route between this park and the next completed segment in Napa County is Hood Mountain Regional Park. As of this writing, there is no completed segment from Sugarloaf's summit to the Hood Mountain summit, but the Goodspeed Trail from the park entrance will take you there.

When it's time to descend, you can return the way you came—the downhill trip is faster! However, **hikers** and **equestrians** can combine the Gray Pine and Meadow trails for an interesting and extended return trip.

◆ ◆ ◆

The next leg of the Ridge Trail starts on Solano Avenue in Napa.

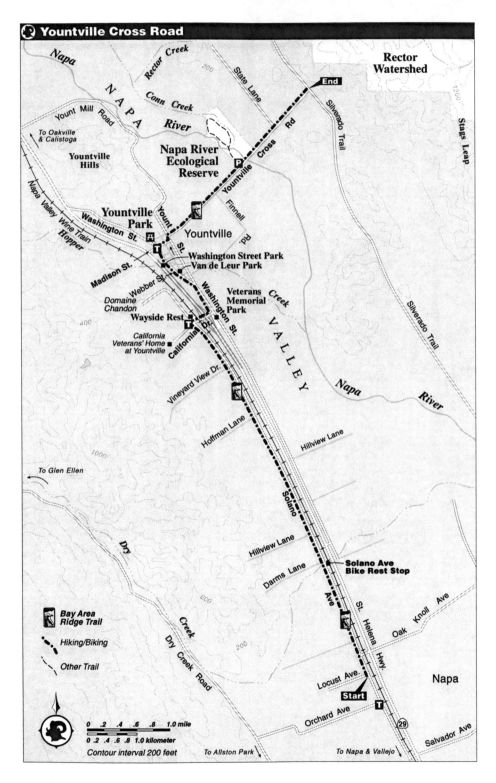

Yountville Cross Road

Napa

Rector Watershed

Rector Creek

State Lane

Conn Creek

Yount Mill Road

To Oakville & Calistoga

N A P A

River

Silverado Trail

Stags Leap

Yountville Hills

Napa River Ecological Reserve

End

Yountville Cross Rd

Finnell Rd.

Yountville Park

Yountville

Napa Valley Wine Train

Washington St.

Hopper

Yount St.

Washington Street Park
Van de Leur Park

Madison St.

Webber St.

Veterans Memorial Park

Creek

Domaine Chandon

Wayside Rest

Washington St.

California Veterans' Home at Yountville

California Dr.

V A L L E Y

Napa

River

Silverado Trail

Vineyard View Dr.

Hoffman Lane

Hillview Lane

To Glen Ellen

Dry

Solano

Hillview Lane

Darms Lane

Solano Ave Bike Rest Stop

Ave

St. Helena Hwy.

Oak Knoll Ave

Napa

Creek

Dry Creek Road

Locust Ave.

Start

Orchard Ave

29

Salvador Ave

Bay Area Ridge Trail

Hiking/Biking

Other Trail

0 .2 .4 .6 .8 1.0 mile
0 .2 .4 .6 .8 1.0 kilometer
Contour interval 200 feet

To Allston Park

To Napa & Vallejo

Yountville Cross Road

Length	2.5 miles one-way on Cross Road, plus 5.0 miles one-way south on Highway 29
Accessibility	Hikers and mountain bikers on entire route and equestrians on part of route
Agencies	Napa River Ecological Reserve and Napa County
Regulations	The reserve prohibits camping, cars, collecting, and alcohol use. Bike lanes are on the south side of the road in the landscaped corridor.
Facilities	None

Several east-west roads cross the Napa River in Napa County's wine country. The Yountville Cross Road, a dedicated Ridge Trail route, runs between the Silverado Trail and Highway 29, the St. Helena Highway.

Getting There

Traveling either north or south on the Silverado Trail, also known as Highway 121, turn east on the Yountville Cross Road. Or, from Highway 29, travel north on Solano Avenue (or St. Helena Highway) to the beginning of the trail at Campbell Avenue.

On the Trail

In its course around the San Francisco Bay region the Ridge Trail goes north through Marin and Sonoma counties, crosses the Napa Valley, and then swings south as it travels through Napa County. Here the trail follows the Napa River south through lush grape-growing country. Low signs displaying the Ridge Trail logo placed along the route reassures visitors that they are on the right trail.

Halfway across the valley on the Yountville Cross Road, look for signs marking the Napa River Ecological Reserve. A map of the reserve on a large sign at the north end of the parking area will orient you to this country. You can see that Conn Creek and Rector Creek join north of here and drain into the Napa River in a wide valley. Together they flow south to nourish this rich agricultural region. If you take the narrow trail northeast from the parking area, you will find a trail along the dike above the river bed, which is probably impassable in winter or after heavy spring rains. This area is a favorite birding site; reports of bald eagles, bluebirds, grebes, and many others lure bird lovers to this area.

When you get to Yountville on the west side of the valley, turn left (south) on Yount Street, go right on Madison Street, pass Yountville Park on your right, and in two blocks turn left on Washington Street. You will see two other parks in just a few blocks— Washington Street Park on your right and Van de Leur on the left, a few blocks beyond. Meanwhile, you are paralleling the Napa Valley Wine Train tracks. Then with Veterans Memorial Park on your left, turn right on California Drive, cross under Highway 29, and turn left on Solano Avenue in front of the Veterans Home, its golf course, and firehouse.

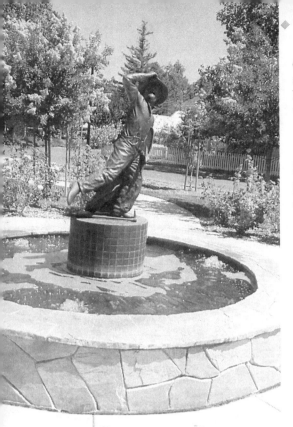

Statue of an early Napa County pioneer in Van de Leur Park

Graceful old trees shade the roadside and signs for well-known wineries affirm Napa Valley's reputation as a prominent wine-producing region.

◆ ◆ ◆

The next segment of the Bay Area Ridge Trail, the River-to-Ridge Trail, begins on the banks of the Napa River and John F. Kennedy parks.

River-to-Ridge Trail

Length 2.5 miles one-way to Skyline Wilderness Park, 0.75 additional miles to the main Skyline Park entrance

Accessibility Hikers and mountain bikers on sidewalks, equestrians in Skyline Wilderness Park

Agencies City of Napa and Skyline Park Citizens Association

Regulations Kennedy and Skyline parks are open daily from 9 AM to 1 hour before sunset (closed on Christmas Day). Skyline does not allow dogs and charges an entrance fee, which you can deposit in an "iron ranger" at the park entrance or at the southwest corner of the Napa State Hospital grounds if there's no guard in the park.

Facilities Kennedy Park has picnic tables, restrooms, parking, a marina and boat launch, and ball fields. Napa River Park has picnic tables, restrooms, parking, tent and RV camping, a marina and boat launch, fishing, archery, disc golf course, and ball fields. The Napa River Trail and the San Francisco Bay Trail go through the park as they follow the river from Highway 121 south to a 1.5-mile loop at south end of park. Skyline Park has picnic tables, camping, RV parking, a nature garden, an archery range, and a horse arena.

This neighborhood walk, bike, or horseback ride from the banks of the Napa River leads to the Ridge Trail route in the hills of Skyline Wilderness Park.

Getting There

JOHN F. KENNEDY PARK: From Highway 12 or 29 go east on Imola Avenue. After crossing the Napa River, turn right on Streblow Drive and continue to the Napa River Park. Parking is near playing fields and picnic areas.

SKYLINE WILDERNESS PARK: From Highway 29 or Highway 121 in Napa, go east on Imola Avenue. Look for the park entrance on the right (south) about 1 mile beyond entrance to Napa State Hospital.

On the Trail

The River-to-Ridge Trail provides a link between the San Francisco Bay Trail and the main route of the Ridge Trail in Napa County. It leaves the City of Napa's John F. Kennedy Park on the banks of the Napa River and heads east on a paved trail beside Streblow Drive. It then passes the Municipal Golf Course on the right and Napa Valley College on the left. Close to the trail on the grounds of the college is an early Napa home, the Streblow House, now refurbished as the Pelusi Recreation Building.

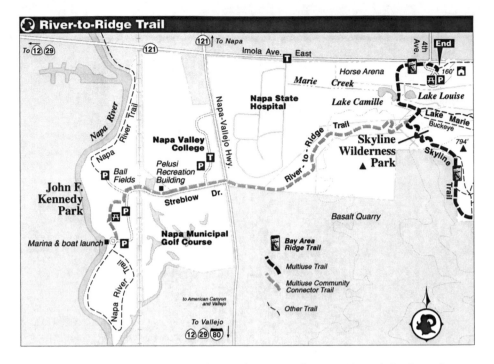

Continuing on the River-to-Ridge Trail you pass the city's Formal Gardens where the dedication of this trail was held on June 15, 2002. In spring look for beautiful roses, a special feature of this city park. Beyond the gardens the Ridge Trail route turns north on Highway 121, goes one block, crosses the highway at the traffic signal, and enters the southwest corner of the Napa State Hospital grounds. Here there is an "iron ranger" into which you can deposit your modest fees for this trip. Heading uphill the trail goes by a wide field that separates the trail from the nearby Youth Detention Center surrounded by a heavy, chain-link fence.

Farther along, Marie Creek flows through a forest of blue and valley oak trees on the east side of the trail and in sunny openings thickets of heatherlike chamise and baccharis (chaparral broom) fill the understory. Beyond, to the west, lies the gaping hole of a large quarry, seen through the trees. On clear days you can see the towers of the Golden Gate Bridge. As you rise higher on this trail, Sugarloaf Mountain appears in the east, and red tile roofs make orderly patterns in the City of Napa subdivisions below.

Continuing upward beside a deserted home site, its fireplace still standing, you enter a valley oak forest. Soon you reach the Skyline Trail in Skyline Wilderness Park. If you are going to the picnic tables, horse facilities, archery range, or parking areas in Skyline Wilderness Park, turn left (north) on the Skyline Trail. Shortly you pass the Buckeye Trail on your right and almost immediately turn left on Lake Marie Road. You go between Lake Camille and Lake Louise (chain-link fences on both sides of the trail) to reach Skyline Wilderness Park and the end of this leg of the Ridge Trail.

◆ ◆ ◆

If you are going to take the Bay Area Ridge Trail route through this park, turn right on this trail and follow it south through the park.

Skyline Wilderness Park and Napa Solano Ridge Trail

From the Park Entrance to the South Boundary

Length 10.1 miles round-trip, including the River-to-Ridge Trail segment

Accessibility Hikers, equestrians, and mountain bikers

Agencies Skyline Park Citizens Association and Bay Area Ridge Trail Council

Regulations Park is open from 9 AM to one hour before sunset Monday through Thursday and 8 AM to 1 hour before sunset Friday through Sunday (closed on Christmas Day). Current day-use fees apply, varying for different trail users. Swimming in the lake is prohibited, fishing is allowed. Dogs are prohibited from trails and the picnic area.

Facilities Parking, restrooms, and water at picnic area near park entrance; several picnic tables near Lake Marie, about 4 miles up the trail; horse arena, archery ranges, disc golf course, and Native Habitat Garden; tent camping and RV facilities

East of Napa State Hospital in the southern foothills of Napa Valley, this out-and-back trail is for hardy hikers and careful equestrians and mountain bikers. It is a narrow, often rocky trail with limited visibility. After a steep climb in the first mile, this trail ambles through oak forests and high grasslands to views of North Bay marshes and mountains and then continues beside a perennial stream to the far reaches of the park.

Getting There

From Highway 29 south of Napa, turn east on Imola Avenue. About 1 mile after passing Napa State Hospital, look for the park entrance on the right (south).

On The Trail

Skyline Wilderness Park was established in 1980 when 900 acres of Napa State Hospital grounds were declared surplus by the State of California. A dedicated local group, wishing to preserve the beautiful Marie Creek Canyon and its surrounding watershed, formed the nonprofit Skyline Park Citizens Association. It leases the land from the state and county and manages these foothill forests and grasslands for public enjoyment. Today, many trails thread through the park, including one to its highest point, 1685-foot Sugarloaf Mountain. The Skyline Trail, designated as a section of the Bay Area Ridge Trail, is the most westerly and longest route, reaching the southeastern park boundary

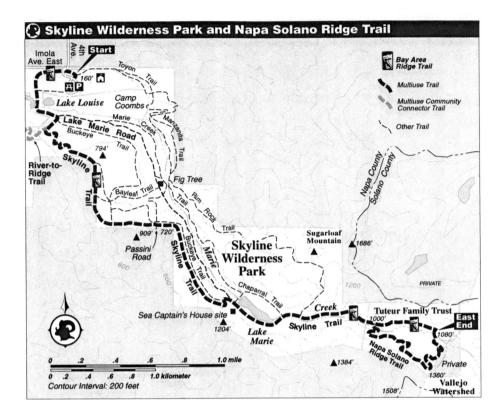

Skyline Wilderness Park and Napa Solano Ridge Trail

near the Solano County line. Plan for a round-trip of at least 10-plus miles, start early, especially on warm days; and take plenty of water.

To begin this trip, leave the picnic area near the park entrance, and bear right on gravel Lake Marie Road to cross a fenced causeway between two ponds, Lake Louise and Lake Camille, which are still part of the Napa State Hospital grounds. Lake Marie Road bends left (east), and in about 600 feet, after passing the Buckeye Trail, you turn right (southwest) off it onto the Skyline Trail.

The Skyline Trail zigzags up a steep hill studded with volcanic rock outcrops. At each bend west, the trail comes close to a low wall, built of these rocks gathered in early ranching days. In spring, native wildflowers, bright orange, yellow, and blue, accent the green grasslands; in summer, golden oats contrast with the dark lichen-covered rocks.

You now enter an oak-and-buckeye woods where the trail straightens and levels off a little, having gained almost 600 feet in elevation in less than a mile. As the trail heads south, lovely views open to the Napa marshlands edging San Francisco Bay. Beyond lies majestic Mt. Tamalpais. Not so attractive is the open jaw of an immense rock quarry, gnawing close to the park boundary.

At a trail junction the Bayleaf Trail arcs left (east), but the Skyline Trail keeps to the right here and at all trail junctions on the outward-bound trip, most of which are well-marked. Now you are on a high grassy meadow, where the light-pink blooms of bit-terroot are found in spring. Although bitterroot implies an unpleasant taste, California Indians considered it a delicacy when it was peeled and cooked.

The trail veers east through chaparral shrubs and ubiquitous poison oak, contours along the hillside, and heads down to a crossroads. Here a spur road from Lake Marie Road enters a private holding outside the park through the "Passini Gate."

Just across this road in an oak woodland, you start climbing to the high grasslands at the western edge of the park. When the weather is clear, you can see chaparral-covered Mt. George due north and Mt. Tamalpais southwest. Seen too, are hawks, scrub jays, woodpeckers, and towhees, just a few of the many birds the quiet hiker can observe in this wilderness park. In the soft dirt of the path, you will see the prints of many animals—deer, raccoons, bobcats, and even feral pigs.

Now 2.3 miles from the park entrance, you traverse a steep hillside where perennial Marie Creek cuts a deep cleft between this hillside and 1630-foot Sugarloaf Mountain. Here in a dense forest, the trailside is festooned with ferns.

Then in a small clearing, you come upon the skeleton of a house—a tall chimney and stonework foundations. Although known as the Sea Captain's House, local historians claim that it was originally built for the gatekeeper who tended the dam at Lake Marie, just a few hundred feet below. When the state decided it no longer needed the gatekeeper, it took down the house. A trail turnoff nearby goes down to the lake, but the Skyline Trail continues above it.

From here the trail follows an old, rocky roadbed through a mature oak-and-fir forest. It then descends to cross the creek upstream from the lake. Now on the north side of Marie Creek, look for some boulders to perch on while eating your knapsack lunch. This beautiful, remote wilderness truly befits the park's name.

Note a left turnoff (northwest) for the Chaparral Trail, an alternate route for your return trip. However, continuing on the Skyline Trail for the next 1.1 miles, you follow the meandering creek, leaving it only to skirt a sloping meadow. Then you cross to the south side of Marie Creek where a tributary joins it. On a gentle forest path, you soon reach a gate, where the trail once ended.

However, on September 24, 2005, the Tuteur Family Trust dedicated a 1.3-mile trail on their ranch as a segment of the Ridge Trail. This trail, known as the Napa Solano Ridge Trail, is the first section of the Ridge Trail to be built and managed by the Bay Area Ridge Trail Council, which raised the money to build the trail and oversees the volunteers who maintain and patrol it.

On this trail you cross Marie Creek on a fiberglass bridge and climb high on one side of the valley through chaparral and heritage oak trees. Trail users are asked to stay on the trail while admiring these majestic trees in order to reduce the spread of the sudden oak death pathogen that is found elsewhere in the park. The trail zigzags back down to the creek and crosses the second trail bridge before returning across the grasslands into the park. There may be cattle grazing, so please respect this property and the owner's animals.

It is planned that someday another segment of the Ridge Trail will continue south into Solano County to join other Bay Area Ridge Trail segments in Fairfield, Vallejo, and Benicia. In the meantime, retrace your steps along the route you just followed or return by any of several other trails that lead to the park entrance. The Chaparral and Marie Creek trails, for hikers only, and Lake Marie Road, multiuse, return to the entrance.

◆ ◆ ◆

For now, the next segment of the Bay Area Ridge Trail begins in the hills west of Fairfield.

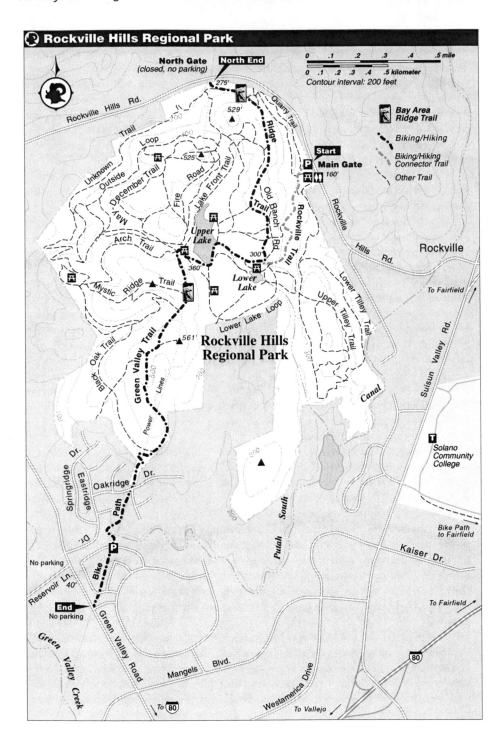

Rockville Hills Regional Park

North Gate
(closed, no parking)

North End

Start
Main Gate

Rockville Hills Rd.

Rockville

To Fairfield

Solano
Community
College

Bike Path
to Fairfield

Kaiser Dr.

To Fairfield

**Rockville Hills
Regional Park**

Upper
Lake

Lower
Lake

Green Valley Trail

Black Oak Trail

Mystic Ridge Trail

Arch Trail

Loop

Unknown Outside

May December Trail

Fire Road

Lake Front Trail

Old Ranch Trail

Rockville Trail

Lower Tilley Trail

Upper Tilley Trail

Lower Lake Loop

Quarry Trail

Ridge

Power Lines

Springridge Dr.

Eastridge Dr.

Oakridge Dr.

Bike Path

Reservoir Ln.

No parking

End
No parking

Green Valley Creek

Green Valley Road

Mangels Blvd.

Westamerica Drive

Putah South Canal

To Vallejo

To 80

80

0   .1   .2   .3   .4   .5 mile
0   .1   .2   .3   .4   .5 kilometer
Contour interval: 200 feet

Bay Area
Ridge Trail

Biking/Hiking

Biking/Hiking
Connector Trail

Other Trail

275'

529'

525'

160'

300'

360'

561'

40'

Rockville Hills Regional Park

From the East Entrance to Green Valley Road

Length 7.0 miles round-trip

Accessibility Hikers and mountain bikers

Agency City of Fairfield

Regulations Park is open from 8 AM to dusk. Bikers must wear helmets, stay on trails, and yield to hikers. Horses are prohibited.

Facilities Picnic tables near the Main Gate, at Upper Lake, and at end of the Upper Mystic Trail

Climb gently through these volcanic rock hills to a remote, grassy valley with a splendid stand of blue oaks. On your descent, you'll have views of Mt. Diablo, Elkhorn Peak, and the Twin Sisters. Most trees in the park are deciduous, so on a winter day these trails can be comfortably sunny, yet in summer, the predominant blue-oak forest offers welcome shade. This trip begins on a connector trail to the park's north entrance and then travels wide, unpaved service roads to a paved trail through a private subdivision.

Getting There

NORTH TRAILHEAD: From Interstate 80 take the Suisun Valley exit, and go north on Suisun Valley Road. Pass Solano Community College, and turn left on Rockville Hills Road. Rockville Hills parking area is on the left after 0.8 mile. Although the Bay Area Ridge Trail route begins from the north trailhead, 0.6 miles farther on Rockville Hills Road, use the parking at the main gate because there is no off-road parking on either side of the road.

SOUTH TRAILHEAD: There is no parking at the end of the trail on Green Valley Road.

On the Trail

From the Rockville Hills Regional Park's main gate on the park's eastern boundary, you take the 0.5-mile Quarry Trail that ascends north to join the main Bay Area Ridge Trail route on the park's north side. If you have a shuttle car, you could have a driver drop you off at the north trail entrance. Parking is prohibited at the north entrance.

The Bay Area Ridge Trail route follows the wide, paved road from the upper gate, which ascends through trailside cover of red-berried toyon, shiny-leafed manzanita, and shrubby coyote bush. Live oaks cling to steep hillsides above and below the trail, offering shade on warm days. In late spring, blue Douglas iris and light orange sticky monkey-flower fill the banks with color.

You climb around a northeast-facing hillside and pass a couple of left-branching trails to the main parking area. Stay on the paved trail and soon you will have views

The Crossroads Settlement of Rockville

The settlement of Rockville once lay on the old stage route between Benicia and Sacramento. In the early 1850s, it was nothing more than a group of summer encampments where settlers attended prayer meetings. Locals sought a more permanent prayer house and contributed money and volunteer labor to build a church on land given by an early pioneer family. The stone walls, quarried in the Rockville Hills, withstood the 1906 earthquake but fell into disrepair in the 1920s; in 1940 the church was restored as a pioneer monument. Today it stands just north of the Suisun Valley and Rockville Hills crossroads in the Rockville Public Cemetery, shaded by ancient oaks.

south across the farmlands to Suisun Bay and its fleet of unused, decommissioned Navy vessels moored there—the "mothball fleet." The low Potrero Hills lie northeast of the Suisun Bay marshes, partially surrounded by Rush Ranch, a 2000-acre estuarine nature preserve of the Solano County Farmlands and Open Space Foundation. In addition to protecting and restoring marshland and riparian habitats, this foundation strives to conserve agricultural lands and preserve key open space lands between Solano County's established communities.

Pass a right-branching trail, and continue on the paved road beneath sizable deciduous white oaks; their great branches arch over the trail to provide filtered shade. At the crest of the hill, look west to see a high, rocky ridge topped by tall towers supporting ribbons of electric transmission lines. The park's central valley lies between this ridge and your trail.

As you descend past some very large specimens of manzanita, you look down at the lakes nestled among stands of mature blue oaks. David Douglas, a botanist in the early days of western-states plant collecting, first identified these blue oaks, a species unique in that it can withstand the high summer temperatures and scant rainfall of these Inner Coast Range foothills. When blue oaks begin to leaf out in late spring, their thick, slightly lobed leaves take on the blue-gray color their name indicates.

About 1 mile from the trailhead, you meet the Rockville Trail, a connector trail to the main parking area that joins your trail from the left. A picnic site in a nearby knolltop grove of blue oaks offers vistas over the surrounding plain. The Bay

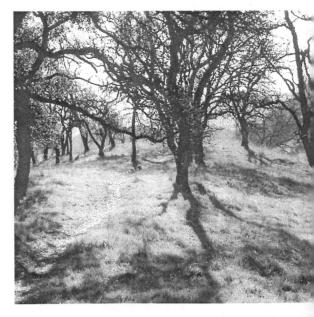

Rockville Hills Trail descends toward Green Valley.

Area Ridge Trail route swings right (west) from the junction and heads into grasslands on an unpaved trail. You pass close to Lower Lake and continue toward Upper Lake, your way brightened by masses of spring wildflowers, including low-growing, daisylike goldfields, bright yellow Johnny-jump-ups, and tall blue brodiaea.

At the top of Upper Lake's low dam, you may find tame, year-round resident ducks and geese that swim and waddle toward any hapless visitor who spreads out lunch at lakeside tables. Migratory water birds, winter visitors only, are less sociable. Birds of the surrounding blue-oak woodland—acorn woodpeckers, flickers, and western bluebirds—are even less interested in visitors, but their bright plumage will reward you with quick displays of color. Several picnic tables are placed around the lake offering places to enjoy your lunch and the sometimes aggressive waterfowl looking for a handout.

From the dam you can look across the lake to the rocky cliffs that form the backbone of the park. This rock formation, known as Sonoma Volcanics, is made up of undifferentiated volcanic and sedimentary rocks, ash, basalt, and andesite, dating from the late Miocene and Pliocene epochs, some 2 to 10 million years ago. Rockville Hills Regional Park marks the southern limit of a 40-mile-long band of Sonoma Volcanics.

Bear left at Upper Lake to follow the trail along the east side of the lake, pass one left-branching trail, and veer right around the south end of the lake. At a second trail intersection, you turn left to follow the Ridge Trail route toward the Green Valley Trailhead.

After a short, steep ascent, the trail reaches the ridgetop and levels off in a saddle. It then drops down to the Green Valley gate, which marks the entrance to a 100-acre donation from the adjoining subdivision developer. Go through the gate to a narrow trail on a thickly wooded, steep slope. Shiny-faced buttercups on tall stems herald spring here, and poppies last into summer.

You emerge on a high, treeless plateau, where you look due south to the 3849-foot summit of Mt. Diablo, rising prominently above the surrounding plain. Overhead, hawks circle lazily, searching the grasslands for their prey of mice, voles, and gophers. With luck, you may spot a pair of black-shouldered kites, frequent visitors to this area, identifiable by their long white tails and sharply pointed wings.

The trail veers right and then shortly bends left (south) across the plateau. If you continue straight (west) at this bend, you reach the edge of the plateau. From here, you have an uninterrupted view of Green Valley's lush fields; the mountains that serve as a natural boundary between Napa and Solano counties rise in the background. Twin-

The Creation of a Park

Rockville Hills Regional Park was once part of a large cattle ranch owned by the Masons, a local ranching family. In the 1970s, the City of Fairfield bought these rocky, wooded highlands to build a golf course. The city laid out golf-cart paths on the hills and in the interior valleys and improved existing stock ponds for irrigation, but Fairfield citizens defeated a bond issue to fund further development of the golf course, and the land became a city park instead. The Solano County Farmlands and Open Space Foundation took over the management of the 600-acre park in 1991 and installed picnic tables on shady knolls and beside level lakeside lookouts.

Side Trip to "Magic Valley"

For a short, delightful side trip into "Magic Valley," continue straight ahead at the Green Valley Trailhead sign on the Arch or Mystic Ridge Trail. Immense live oaks coexist with valley and blue oaks at the base of these north-facing slopes. You continue past a left-branching trail and veer south to reach a picnic table on a knoll overlooking Green Valley. The trail then turns east to rejoin the Ridge Trail, about 1 mile from the beginning of the "Magic Valley" side trip.

topped, 1330-foot Elkhorn Peak, fringed with a thatch of trees, stands due west. Visually follow this line of mountains north along undulating, tree-cloaked slopes, to the Twin Sisters in Solano County, each more than 2000 feet high.

Return to the main trail and continue across the plateau into a grove of ancient evergreen oaks, their branches sculpted by the prevailing northwest winds and their trunks 4 to 6 feet in diameter. Following the path through these widely spaced, venerable trees is like walking down a "grande allée" of some fabled estate of yesteryear. A pause here will give you time to bask in their shady grandeur and enjoy spring wildflowers or the bluish-white flowers of the soap plant on summer evenings.

Beyond the ridgetop, the wide trail descends a steep, east-facing hillside dotted with California buckeye trees. Their gnarled, white bark stands out against dry winter grasses, and their long, erect spikes of dense, pinkish-white blossoms scent the air in spring. From this hillside you see across a small valley to the park's eastern wooded ridge.

A short descent on a south-facing hillside takes you under power lines to a wide, fenced corridor that leads to a gate to a private housing development. Signs remind you to stay on the paved path and not to stray onto private streets or lawns in this private community. Continue a half mile on this urban trail to Green Valley Road.

Since there is no designated southern staging area and no parking on Green Valley Road, retrace your steps through Rockville Hills Park, or opt for an alternate route on the many other trails. In the late afternoon, red-winged blackbirds calling from the reeds in Lower Lake and swallows snatching insects in mid-air provide aerial entertainment.

◆ ◆ ◆

The next segment of the Bay Area Ridge Trail begins in Lynch Canyon in the vicinity of American Canyon.

Lynch Canyon Open Space

Length 3.0 miles

Accessibility Hikers, equestrians, and mountain bikers

Agency Solano County Parks and Recreation

Regulations Park is open from dawn to dusk Wednesday through Sunday.

Facilities Portable restroom at trail entrance

Climbs to a series of hilltops and subsequent descents into wide canyons make this a vigorous trip with around-the-compass views.

Getting There

From Interstate 80 in the vicinity of American Canyon use American Canyon Road exit, take McGary Road north paralleling I-80, and cross under the freeway on Lynch Road to parking at the entrance to the open space.

On the Trail

Lynch Canyon lies along the north side of Interstate 80 between Fairfield and Vallejo, its major ridge a scenic landmark for residents and travelers alike. Beginning in the early 1990s residents of this area, along with the Solano County Farmlands Open Space Foundation and local government agencies, worked to save this 1039-acre site for public open space. Through their efforts, it is now preserved as a historic site; a recreation resource for hikers, equestrians, and mountain bikers; and as an important link in the Bay Area Ridge Trail.

The Ridge Trail route starts from a valley just northwest of I-80 in the vicinity of American Canyon. Farm implements, an old barn, and the ranch's East Homestead remind one that this was a working ranch, long used for cattle grazing and farming. The Solano Land Trust's gate leads to a trip through an area where the Suisune Indians once hunted game—deer, antelope, and elk—for food, clothing, and shelter. Four grinding rocks found on the site were used by the Suisunes to make meal from acorns and other seeds.

Spring is an ideal time to visit this preserve when dazzling arrays of wildflowers cover the hillsides and the creeks are running full. A distinctive feature along the spine of the preserve is a loose aggregation of irregularly shaped rocks graced by wind-sculpted live oak and bay trees.

After going through the ranch gate at the staging area, your route borders Lynch Creek flowing under a canopy of oaks, bigleaf maples, and willows. You pass the Middle Valley Trail turnoff on your left and after going under the power lines, bear right over the grasslands to follow the creek to a reservoir. Here cows graze, frogs croak, and countless birds swoop over the lake to catch an insect or take a quick drink.

From the reservoir retrace your steps to the trail junction, and bear right (west) on the North Ridge Trail. Wend your way across the rolling grasslands toward a gap in the hills marked by an umbrella of live and valley oaks. After about a mile you reach a high

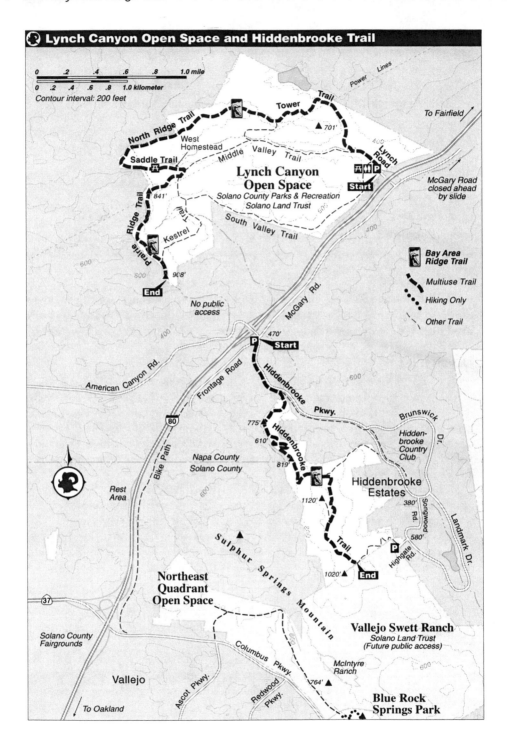

Lynch Canyon Open Space and Hiddenbrooke Trail

0 .2 .4 .6 .8 1.0 mile

0 .2 .4 .6 .8 1.0 kilometer

Contour interval: 200 feet

Power Lines

To Fairfield

North Ridge Trail

Tower Trail

▲ 701'

West Homestead

Middle Valley Trail

Lynch Road

Saddle Trail

Lynch Canyon Open Space
Solano County Parks & Recreation
Solano Land Trust

Start

McGary Road closed ahead by slide

841'

Ridge Trail

Prairie Trail

Kestrel

South Valley Trail

Bay Area Ridge Trail

Multiuse Trail

Hiking Only

Other Trail

908'

End

No public access

McGary Rd.

470'

P **Start**

American Canyon Rd.

Frontage Road

Hiddenbrooke Pkwy.

Brunswick Dr.

80

775'

Hiddenbrooke

610'

Hiddenbrooke

Hiddenbrooke Country Club

Napa County
Solano County

819'

Hiddenbrooke Estates

Bike Path

Rest Area

1120' ▲

380'

Songwood Rd.

Landmark Dr.

580'

P

Trail

Highgate Rd.

37

▲

Sulphur Springs Mountain

Northeast Quadrant Open Space

1020' ▲ **End**

Solano County Fairgrounds

Vallejo Swett Ranch
Solano Land Trust
(Future public access)

Columbus Pkwy.

McIntyre Ranch

Vallejo

Ascot Pkwy.

Redwood Pkwy.

764' ▲

Blue Rock Springs Park

To Oakland

Chief Solano and General Mariano Vallejo

Chief Solano and his Wintun people may have been hiding near the base of the steep, rocky ridge along the present-day Middle Valley Trail when General Mariano Vallejo first encountered them in the 1830s. Eventually Vallejo and Solano became friends and cooperated to quell other tribes but then Solano disappeared. Twelve years later he paid a surprise visit to General Vallejo in his Sonoma home, and the two were joyfully reunited. Unfortunately, their friendship ended when Solano caught pneumonia and died shortly thereafter.

point at the Solano and Napa County boundary from which you can see in the distant north the Two Sisters surmounting another leg of the Ridge Trail. To the west stretch the vast Napa Marshlands, now preserved as open space, and Mt. Tamalpais soars in the distance.

Your trail zigzags downhill past oak trees clinging to huge rocks. (Perhaps the rocks maintain moisture that the trees' roots seek out.) The trail, now called the Saddle Loop Trail, swings west, then east, crosses the creek you met at the beginning of the trip, and west again. It rises to 841 feet as it turns south—and becomes the Prairie Ridge Trail. This trail rises to a 908-foot high point from which you can look ahead to a ridge dotted with large boulders that seem like sentinels guarding the valley below. South of this rugged ridge you can see the highest point of the Hiddenbrooke Trail and on beyond, Mt. Diablo.

Since the Prairie Ridge Trail ends at the southern boundary of the Lynch Canyon Open Space, watch for the junction with the Kestrel Trail and turn left (north) on it. Shortly, the Kestrel Trail bends west and in another mile becomes the South Valley Trail. But you take the Middle Valley Trail, bear right (northeast) on it, and continue to the next junction where the Middle Valley Trail goes off to the right. On this leg of the Middle Valley Trail you follow the creek for more than a mile, in and around rocks and under the shade of hardy oaks, until you meet Lynch Road. Here you bear right to return to the staging area where you began this trip.

◆ ◆ ◆

The next segment of the Bay Area Ridge Trail begins about 1.5 miles southeast of Lynch Road on the Hiddenbrooke Trail.

Hiddenbrooke Trail

From McGary Road to Trail's Southern Terminus

Length 5.0 miles round-trip

Accessibility Hikers, equestrians, and mountain bikers

Agency Hiddenbrooke Estates

Regulations Hiddenbrooke community is open from 6 AM to dusk and prohibits dogs.

Facilities None

see map on p.104

These rolling grasslands offer expansive views of San Francisco and San Pablo bays and the mountains that encircle them, from Mt. Tamalpais to Mt. Diablo. You'll gain 550 feet on short, steep climbs along this broad, exposed trail. Take this trip on cool summer mornings or late afternoons; some spots are muddy after heavy rains.

Getting There

From Interstate 80 northeast of Vallejo and west of Fairfield, take the American Canyon Road exit east onto Hiddenbrooke Parkway. Immediately turn right and park in the area at the entrance to the community. There are also two parking spaces on Hiddenbrooke Parkway just inside the gates to the community. Follow the paved sidewalk with a landscaped border along Hiddenbrooke Parkway for 0.5 mile to the trailhead on the right. A signpost bears Bay Area Ridge Trail insignia.

On the Trail

Your trip begins on an unpaved trail that runs between the tree-lined, landscaped border of the Hiddenbrooke Parkway and the fenced property line. As you climb upward beside graceful, gray-green olive trees, look right over the adjoining grasslands and ahead to the first hill. At the top of the first rise, veer to the right, away from the parkway, and round the south side of this hill. The trail then climbs a steep hill along the property-line fence to reach your first viewpoint. Across a wide canyon ahead, you glimpse a distinctive clump of wind-sculpted trees that top an otherwise bald hill. On a clear day, you can see west across the community of American Canyon to the Napa River, as it flows south past the former Mare Island Naval Shipyard. Slightly northwest of the island, the Napa-Sonoma Marshes Wildlife Area, fed by several arms of the Napa River, extends to the shores of San Pablo Bay. Across the water are the low hills of Napa County and the taller peaks of the North Bay.

The trail turns left, descends along the fence line, and then climbs again to a zigzag cattle gate, just wide enough for hikers and for bikes held vertically. (Equestrians use the patrol gate, and please close it behind you.) Look due north to locate the distinctive double points of Twin Sisters rising above the surrounding plain. You drop into a small valley where clumps of oak and bay trees hug a rocky ridge 10 feet above the trail. Veined with red-brown ore, the rocks recall the mining days of this region, when mercury was extracted for processing the gold found in the Sierra foothills. The mines are now closed and sealed, but one gave its name—St. Johns Mine Hill—to a nearby knoll on private property.

You round a shoulder of the trip's central hill and ascend its south side, past a cow path on the left. Then turn left sharply onto the wide trail beneath the brow of the central hill. Continue to a gap in the hills, where you can see south to Suisun Bay and Mt. Diablo beyond it. To the north lie the expansive green fairways and greens of the Hiddenbrooke Golf Course and the homes along the meandering roads of Hiddenbrooke Estates. In early spring, you may see bright yellow tufts of a ground-hugging plant commonly known as hog fennel.

Soon you reach a junction marked END RIDGE TRAIL SEGMENT. A short path leads to 360-degree views of the Bay Area from the trip's highest point at 1020 feet. Follow this path to the preserve boundary; after a winter storm has cleared the air, you will see east to the snowy Sierra peaks and west to the Golden Gate, spanned by the famous bridge. You can identify the prominent mountaintops around the bay and trace the circular Bay Area Ridge Trail on or near them, beginning just north of the bridge with Mt. Tamalpais, then to Mt. Burdell, Sonoma Mountain, Mt. Diablo, Mission and Monument peaks, Mt. Madonna, Loma Prieta, Mt. Umunhum, Black Mountain, Kings Mountain, and back to the bridge. You can also look south to a broad valley where a proposed route of the Ridge Trail would head toward the McIntyre Ranch and the existing Blue Rock Springs and Vallejo-Benicia Buffer Trail. Descend from the rocky high point of this trip, and retrace your steps to the parking area, noting unique aspects of the immediate terrain and of the Bay Area beyond.

◆ ◆ ◆

The next segment of the Ridge Trail begins in Blue Rock Springs Park in the vicinity of American Canyon.

Deer near Hiddenbrooke Trail

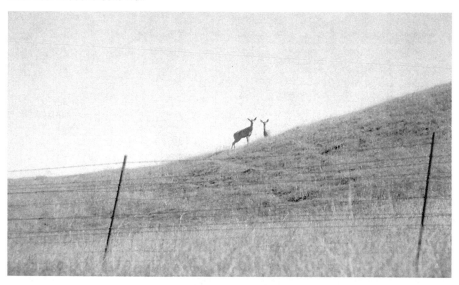

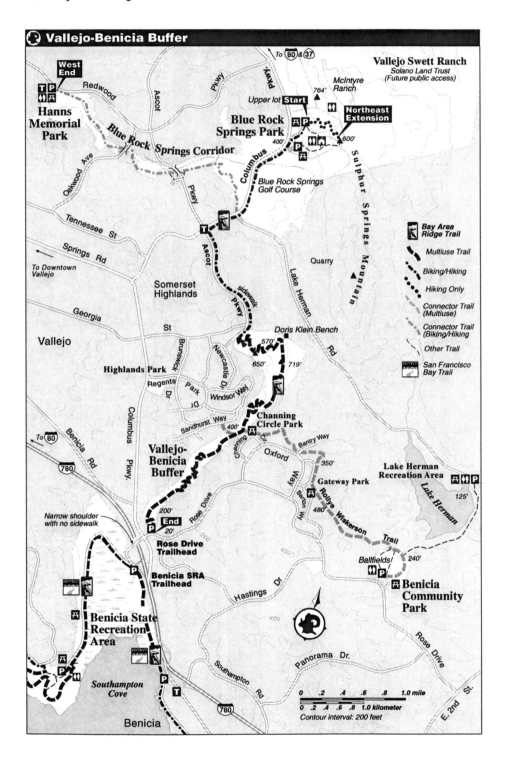

Vallejo-Benicia Buffer

Vallejo Swett Ranch
Solano Land Trust
(Future public access)

To 80 & 37

West End

Redwood

Ascot Pkwy

Pkwy

McIntyre Ranch
764'

Upper lot **Start**

Blue Rock Springs Park

Hanns Memorial Park

Blue Rock Springs Corridor

Columbus

Northeast Extension

600'

400'

Oakwood Ave

Blue Rock Springs Golf Course

Sulphur Springs Mountain

Tennessee St

Springs Rd

Ascot Pkwy

Quarry

To Downtown Vallejo

Bay Area Ridge Trail

Somerset Highlands

sidewalk Pkwy

Lake Herman Rd

Multiuse Trail

Biking/Hiking

Hiking Only

Georgia

St

Doris Klein Bench

Connector Trail (Multiuse)

Vallejo

Brunswick

Newcastle Dr

570'

650' 719'

Connector Trail (Biking/Hiking)

Other Trail

Highlands Park

Regents

Park Dr

Windsor Way

San Francisco Bay Trail

Dr

Sandhurst Way

Channing Circle Park

Columbus Pkwy

400'

Channing Cir

Oxford

Bantry Way

350'

Lake Herman Recreation Area

To 80

Benicia Rd

Vallejo-Benicia Buffer

780

Rose Drive

Way

Gateway Park

Rollye Wiskerson

Baxton Wy

480'

Lake Herman

125'

Narrow shoulder with no sidewalk

200'

End

20'

Trail

Rose Drive Trailhead

200

Ballfields

240'

Benicia SRA Trailhead

Hastings Dr

Benicia Community Park

Benicia State Recreation Area

400

Southampton Cove

Southampton Rd

Panorama Dr

Rose Drive

E. 2nd St

Benicia

780

0   .2   .4   .6   .8   1.0 mile
0 .2 .4 .6 .8 1.0 kilometer
Contour interval: 200 feet

Vallejo-Benicia Buffer

From Blue Rock Springs Park to Rose Drive

Length   5.9 miles, including 1.0-mile round-trip on northeast extension, 1.9 miles on sidewalks and bike lanes, and 3.0 miles one-way on Buffer Trail

Accessibility   Hikers, equestrians, and mountain bikers

Agencies   Greater Vallejo Recreation District and California Department of Parks and Recreation

Regulations   Because of a fire in 2007, Blue Rock Springs Park is open only for docent-led tours led by the Solano Land Trust (707-432-0150). The Buffer and Rollye Wiskerson connector trails are open from dawn to dusk.

Facilities   Water, restrooms, and telephone at Blue Rock Springs Park

Take this varied trip along the ridgeline greenbelt between Vallejo and Benicia. Begin on a short round-trip to a rocky ridge, and return to the rolling green lawns and shady picnic areas of Blue Rock Springs Park to follow a paved path or bike lane to the Buffer Trail. Meander through the open space easement, up and down hilly grasslands, toward Benicia State Recreation Area. Little shade protects you from the hot summer sun on this unpaved trail, which gains 300 feet and loses 540 feet; the ridge may be windy or foggy.

Getting There

NORTH TRAILHEAD, BLUE ROCK SPRINGS PARK: From Interstate 80, take Columbus Parkway east for 2.5 miles, and turn left (east) into the parking lot with ample space. Use the upper lot for the northeast hillside leg.

SOUTH TRAILHEAD, ROSE DRIVE: From Interstate 780 east (Vallejo-Benicia Freeway), take the Benicia State Park Road exit, bear right, and circle around to cross over the freeway. Continue to Columbus Parkway, and cross it onto Rose Drive. Park on the first block on the west side of the street only. Trail entrance on north side of day-care center. From I-780 west (Vallejo-Benicia Freeway), take the Columbus Parkway exit, and turn right (northeast) on Rose Drive. Find the parking lot and trail entrance as above.

On the Trail

This trip over General Mariano Vallejo's former lands begins in Blue Rock Springs Park, once the site of an elegant home and lavish gardens built by his son-in-law General Frisbie. It later became a popular picnic place and is now managed by the Greater Vallejo Recreation District; its green lawns, spring-fed pond, picnic tables, and big trees attract visitors year-round.

Northeast Extension

A short Bay Area Ridge Trail segment extends the Vallejo-Benicia Buffer a half mile north toward the Hiddenbrooke Trail. On the planned Ridge Trail route, the Hiddenbrooke Trail will eventually connect to Blue Rock Springs Park via McIntyre Ranch. In the meantime, this short but interesting round-trip offers an opportunity to climb to the rocky ramparts in the northeast corner of the park. Although this park was temporarily closed in 2007 by a fire, it's now open for docent-led tours through Solano Land Trust.

The trail begins on the park's north side; to reach it, park in the upper parking area, or follow the sidewalk north from the lower lot. **Hikers** continue on the sidewalk or a paved park path past the green lawns to a grassy hillside. Just beyond three young pine trees on your right, climb the wooden steps outlined by native rocks. The trail soon bears right around the developed park's perimeter.

Hikers pass through a zigzag cattle gate on your left after 0.1 mile to begin your uphill route. Seven switchbacks (dangerously ignored by bikers speeding downhill) climb to the summit of a rocky ridge. Along the way, two sturdy benches built and installed by Gregory Basham, an Eagle Scout of Vallejo Troop 12, offer the opportunity to pause and enjoy the North Bay ambience; you have fine views of the bay and surrounding hills, the golf course, and the Vallejo-Benicia Buffer route. Uphill from these benches, a wall of huge rocks with crenellations is reminiscent of ancient fortresses; on your left, these ragged outcrops top another hill. These hills and those you passed on the Columbus Parkway are part of the Sulphur Springs Mountain chain.

You reach the summit after about a third of a mile; turn around to survey your climb, and then continue on the trail through an opening in the high rock wall ahead of you. Despite the harsh terrain, a few rangy live oaks, some hardy toyon bushes, and a buckeye tree grow in clefts between the rocks. Wend your way carefully to the other side, where small boulders scattered among trees offer perches from which you can survey the wide views southeast. You can see and hear the trucks and bulldozers in a rock quarry nearby. To the left is a canyon between the hills, a possible future Ridge Trail route northward. After you have enjoyed the views, retrace your steps to the parking area.

South to the Buffer Trail

To continue on the Ridge Trail route toward the Vallejo-Benicia Buffer, find the path just south of the park entrance road. **Hikers** follow it to a paved sidewalk, and **mountain bikers** use the bike lane along the east side of Columbus Parkway, bordered by the municipal golf course. You pass Lake Herman Road and reach Ascot Parkway, where you turn left at the signaled crossing. Young trees and clipped green lawns dot the well-landscaped banks along Ascot Parkway. This segment of the Ridge Trail was not damaged by the 2007 fire that affected Blue Rock Springs Park.

Buffer Trail

After less than a mile on the parkway, you pass Georgia Street and look for a landscaped entry in front of a weathered-gray fence on the east side of the street. **Hikers** and **mountain bikers** turn left to begin the Buffer Trail, signed as the BAY AREA RIDGE TRAIL route. Manzanita, toyon, coffeeberry, and springtime blue lupine, all native California plants installed by volunteers, fill the space beside the trail for the first 50 feet.

General Mariano Vallejo

As you begin your trip over the lands north of Carquinez Strait, consider that they were once part of a vast, 11-square-league (approximately 99 square miles) land grant encompassing most of present-day Vallejo, Benicia, and Cordelia. Known as Rancho Soscol, the grant was awarded in 1844 by Governor Micheltorena to General Mariano Vallejo for his military service and generous loans to the Mexican government. In 1847 the present-day Carquinez Strait town of Benicia was named Francesca, after General Vallejo's wife. When the older settlement of Yerba Buena was renamed San Francisco, Francesca changed its name to Benicia, another of Señora Vallejo's names.

Although today's thriving City of Vallejo was named for the general, he never resided there. Instead, he lived comfortably and well in Sonoma, protected by his army of Mexican soldiers. Nevertheless, General Vallejo worked hard to make Vallejo the second California state capital and contributed land and a building to house the state legislature. On January 5, 1852, the legislature met in the new Vallejo capitol building, but their stay was short. By January 12 of that year, the dissatisfied legislature moved to Sacramento, returning to Vallejo only for a brief stay in 1853 due to floods in Sacramento. However, the legislature did compliment Vallejo for his generosity by naming today's city after him, even though Vallejo himself had suggested the name "Eureka."

Vallejo and subsequent landowners ran cattle over these hills and shipped hides through the Carquinez Strait to San Francisco and on to world ports. Today, the cattle are gone and houses cover the hillsides, except for a 500-foot-wide easement between the cities of Vallejo and Benicia. This ridgeline greenbelt is called a buffer and serves as open space joining the two cities bearing the Vallejo family names.

The single-track trail zigzags to the 640-foot summit of the first of this trip's many hilltops. Before you lies the long sweep of the greenway's undulating terrain that stretches almost to the shores of Southampton Bay on Carquinez Strait. The homes that edge both sides of the Buffer highlight the importance of activists' persistent efforts to convince the Vallejo and Benicia councils to create this linear open space, which now serves as a trail and a wildlife corridor.

Beyond the first hilltop, the trail heads north into a swale. Then after a long traverse and switchback, it reaches the highest point on the trip. You have views of impressive bodies of water from this vantage place: due east is Lake Herman, the local water supply; beyond, the Navy's mothball fleet floats on the quiet waters of Suisun Bay; below you to the south, a third of California's water surges through Carquinez Strait, drained from the Sierra Nevada into the San Joaquin and Sacramento rivers. Beyond the strait, San Francisco Bay spreads out over a vast expanse of tidelands, marshes, sloughs, and open waters. On a clear day you can see the towers of the Golden Gate Bridge under which these waters flow to the Pacific.

Blue Rock Springs Corridor

Connecting Hanns Memorial Park and Blue Rock Springs Park, this 2.1-mile segment of the Bay Area Ridge Trail passes a school, two other parks, and a golf course adjacent to the corridor. At trail's end there are picnic sites, play areas, and a golf course managed by the Greater Vallejo Recreation District. From Hanns Memorial Park **hikers** and **mountain bikers** travel east through more than a mile of dedicated parkland beside Blue Rock Springs Creek. You will be serenaded with birdsong in quiet morning hours and shaded by creekside trees on hot afternoons. Passing through a residential neighborhood and beside a school, you then turn south beside the Blue Rock Springs Golf Course fence. Here you join the Vallejo-Benicia Buffer Trail, also part of the Ridge Trail, and go northeast along Columbus Parkway to reach Blue Rock Springs Park.

For the next half mile, you follow a wide track south over the hilltops. A Ridge Trail sign directs you right (west) on a narrower trail, built by a team of volunteers. Continue downhill on a gentle grade along the west-facing hillside. When you reach a concrete-sided drainage ditch with a V-shaped cross section, again head south, paralleling the ditch.

In spring, these rolling grasslands are ablaze with orange poppies and blue lupines. As the season progresses, yellow-flowered mule ears on strong, erect stems add their color to the hillsides. Heavenly blue brodiaea and lemon-yellow mariposa lilies are special floral treats that peek through the grasses in early June. The roasted bulbs of these plants were favorite foods of the local Native American tribes.

The Rollye Wiskerson Trail joins your route from the east; built and named for the Solano County master trail-builder, this trail runs along the north edge of a residential neighborhood and connects three community parks to the Buffer Trail.

Past the junction, your trail is again a wide track that undulates up and down along the fence line. Veer right (south) on a single-track trail to avoid a very steep hill. Follow the contour of the hillside and round a couple of switchbacks. You then dip into a little valley and trend left, into the Benicia side of the easement, where pretty gardens and colorful children's play equipment hug the fence line.

On three more switchbacks, you climb to the crest of another hilltop; from there you have good views of Southampton Bay and the Benicia State Recreation Area, where other legs of the Ridge Trail hug the waterfront. If the day is clear, you'll see, and sometimes hear, ships on the fast-flowing waters of Carquinez Strait. The trail zigzags along the fence line, with moderate undulations over the last hilltops, and finally descends steeply to the trail's end at Rose Drive in Benicia. If you are returning to Blue Rock Springs Park, allow plenty of time for the uphill trip, especially on hot summer days.

◆ ◆ ◆

There is a short gap between Rose Drive and the beginning of the next segment of the Bay Area Ridge Trail along the Benicia Waterfront.

Vallejo-Benicia Waterfront

From Benicia State Recreation Area East to Benicia Point at F Street and West to Carquinez Bridge Overlook

Length 3.5 miles east on Benicia Waterfront Trail to Benicia Point, 3.5 miles west on Vallejo Waterfront Trail to Al Zampa Bridge Overlook

Accessibility Hikers, equestrians, mountain bikers, and wheelchair users (hikers only on Carquinez Overlook Trail)

Agencies Cities of Vallejo and Benicia and California State Parks Department

Regulations Benicia State Recreation Area is open from 6 AM to 30 minutes after sunset, charges an entrance fee, and prohibits dogs. Bikes are prohibited on Carquinez Overlook Trail. A state fishing license is required for those 16 years and older. City of Benicia Waterfront and City of Vallejo trails are open during daylight hours. Bikes are prohibited on unpaved trails.

Facilities Water and restrooms at Benicia State Recreation Area; water, restrooms, and telephone at 9th Street Park

Take a trip through Mexican and early California history on two routes that follow the Carquinez Strait waterfront through the thriving towns of Benicia and Vallejo. Enjoy brisk breezes and occasional fog as you watch the San Joaquin and Sacramento rivers funnel into San Francisco Bay. This route travels mostly level trails, including sidewalks, paved and unpaved trails, and foot paths.

Getting There

BENICIA STATE RECREATION AREA: From Interstate 80 take Interstate 780 (Vallejo-Benicia Freeway) to the exit marked Benicia State Recreation Area. Follow the road as it curves right, jog to the left (south), and turn right into recreation area.

On the Trail

East to Historic Benicia and Around Benicia Marina

All trail users head southeast on the paved trail from the recreation area that skirts the marshlands around Southampton Bay. Among the shorebirds and waterfowl that feed in the marshes, you may see the 30-inch-tall, stately white egret. You will certainly see many runners, strollers, and mountain bikers on this trail.

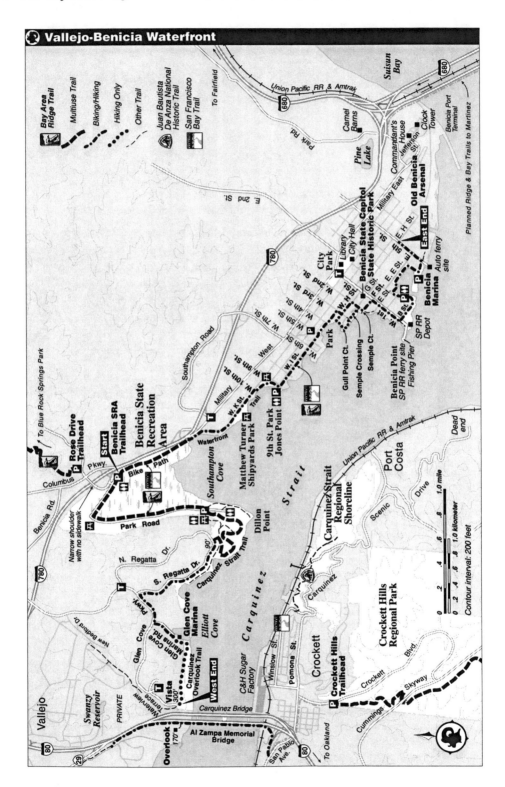

Vallejo-Benicia Waterfront

Legend:
- Bay Area Ridge Trail
- Multiuse Trail
- Biking/Hiking
- Hiking Only
- Other Trail
- Juan Bautista De Anza National Historic Trail
- San Francisco Bay Trail

Suisun Bay

680

Union Pacific RR & Amtrak

To Fairfield

Park Rd.

Camel Barns

Pine Lake

Commandant's House

Jefferson St.

Clock Tower

Benicia Port Terminal

Old Benicia Arsenal

East End

Auto ferry site

Planned Ridge & Bay Trails to Martinez

E. 2nd St.

Military East

E. H. St.

780

Benicia State Capitol State Historic Park

City Park

Library

City Hall

G St.

Benicia Marina

W. 2nd St.

W. 3rd St.

W. 4th St.

W. 5th St.

Gull Point Ct.

Semple Crossing

Semple Ct.

Benicia Point
SP RR ferry site
Fishing Pier

SP RR Depot

Southampton Road

West

Park

W. 6th St.

W. 7th St.

W. 9th St.

W. 10th St.

W. K St.

W. J St.

To Blue Rock Springs Park

Rose Drive Trailhead

To Blue Rock Springs Park

Start
Benicia SRA Trailhead

Benicia State Recreation Area

Columbus Pkwy.

Bike Path

Park Road

Military

Watertown

Matthew Turner Shipyards Park

9th St. Park
Jones Point

Southampton Cove

Dillon Point

Carquinez Strait

Union Pacific RR & Amtrak

Port Costa

Dead end

Scenic Drive

1.0 mile

Benicia Rd.

Narrow shoulder with no sidewalk

780

N. Regatta Dr.

S. Regatta Dr.

Carquinez Strait Trail

Carquinez Strait Regional Shoreline

Carquinez

Crockett Hills Regional Park

Contour interval: 200 feet

Vallejo

Swanzy Reservoir

New Bedford Dr.

PRIVATE

Glen Cove Pkwy.

Glen Cove Marina Rd.

Glen Cove Marina
Elliott Cove

Carquinez Overlook Trail

West End

Vista 300'

Maryview Terrace

C&H Sugar Factory

Winslow St.

Pomona St.

Crockett

Crockett Hills Trailhead

Blvd.

Crockett

Skyway

Cummings

80

29

Overlook 170'

Al Zampa Memorial Bridge

Carquinez Bridge

San Pablo Ave.

80

To Oakland

Touring Historic Benicia

The centerpiece of Benicia's attractions stands at West 1st and G streets—an imposing, red brick building with white, two-story columns: California's third capitol. Although the legislature convened here only in 1853, the building is now faithfully restored and open as a state historic park. The Fischer-Hanlon house, a fine example of Victorian architecture, is next door. Until recently, it was occupied by the original owner's descendants; it is now open for tours.

You are in the heart of Benicia's old town, where saloons, hotels, and the 1847 Von Pfister adobe bring to life the years before and after the Gold Rush. If you continue down West 1st Street to Benicia Point, you'll see where 400-foot-long barges once ferried trains across to Port Costa. Cars were also ferried across the strait until the Benicia-Martinez Bridge was built. In just a few minutes' walk, you'll reach the 1850s military buildings—the Benicia Arsenal with its landmark clock tower, the Camel Barn Museum, and the Commandant's House.

Today, Benicia bustles with activity that matches its lively past—huge ships unload Japanese cars at the port, and slick condominiums, shopping malls, and subdivisions line the hillsides and crowd its shores. However, open space trails along the waterfront and through the Vallejo-Benicia Buffer join these cities and former capitals of California that bear General Mariano Vallejo's family names.

Across Southampton Bay to the south, Dillon Point juts into the strait, named for a rancher who, in 1855, bought the 400 acres that now lie within the state recreation area. Patrick Dillon's homesite is marked by towering eucalyptus, and a few of the fruit trees from the orchards he planted remain, but his vineyard, quarry, and brickyard are gone.

Equestrians and **wheelchair users** end this segment at the east boundary of the State Recreation Area at K Street, while **hikers** and **mountain bikers** continue on the sidewalk, the Waterfront Trail. Near West 14th Street, you reach the first of many historical sites. A sign tells of the famous 1889 boxing match between James J. Corbett and "Battling Joe" Choynski. The first rounds were fought in Fairfax, and the fight was continued a week later on a barge in Southampton Bay.

Turn right (south) on West 12th Street to the Matthew Turner Shipyards Park, where you'll have your first close-up view of the Carquinez Strait. In 1900, 169 ships were launched here; today you'll find benches, picnic tables, pretty gardens, and another historical marker. Across the strait lies Port Costa, once an important depot for transporting grain by barge, ship, and rail. The Southern Pacific Railroad still runs transcontinental freight, and Amtrak operates a fleet of passenger trains on waterfront tracks.

Now return to K Street, where a bluff-top path runs diagonally across the 9th Street Park to Jones Point. Commodore Thomas Jones was founder of the U.S. Naval Academy and Commander of the Pacific Fleet in the 1840s. Southampton Bay is named for one of his supply ships. Jones feared war with Mexico and advocated a port here in Benicia's deep offshore waters. Modern-day sailors launch their craft beside Jones Point to ply these same waters.

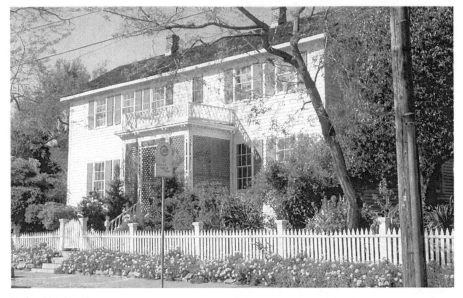

Fischer-Hanlon House

Follow I Street beyond the park, past houses with charming gardens. In the 1860s, two tanneries near here processed hides from vast inland cattle ranches. Each hide was marked with the ranch's unique registered brand. Farther on, barriers exclude motor vehicles from I Street, but Ridge Trail signs assure bikers and pedestrians that they can pass. At 4th Street, you'll find picnic tables and children's play equipment that overlooks a small crescent-shaped bay.

Turn right (south) on West 3rd Street, and continue two blocks to Gull Point Court. **Hikers** can descend to Semple Crossing, one street below, on a stairway near a handsome, restored Victorian house. **Mountain bikers** follow Gull Point Court to Semple Crossing.

From Semple Crossing, **hikers** use the sidewalks to West F Street and then follow 1st Street to Benicia Point where there is a fishing pier, parking, and the old Southern Pacific Depot. The sidewalk continues into and around the Benicia Marina and east to another pier at the end of East 5th Street.

For those who have walked or biked from the Carquinez Overlook Trail east along the Carquinez Strait waterfront, it's time to turn around or perhaps have a picnic by the marina. There is parking near the pier, and from the pier you can see across to the Martinez Regional Shoreline, its marina, and the new bridge to Martinez. Or take a different route back via the nearby historic Benicia State Capitol building.

West to the Carquinez Bridge Overlook

To take the waterfront trail west, **all trail users** again begin at the entrance to Benicia State Recreation Area. Follow the paved park road (**hikers** and **equestrians** on the shoulder) as it skirts the marshes and western shore of Southampton Bay on its way to Dillon Point, about 1.5 miles from the entrance gate. Here is a picnic area and parking lot where trails go off right and left, but the Ridge Trail route (multiuse) goes almost due south out to Dillon Point where there is yet another parking area. Here the multiuse trail, the Benicia Bay Trail, and also Bay Area Ridge Trail route, meanders westward up and around two high points. Look due west from the crest of the second hill for a view of the Carquinez Bridge and your route along the town of Vallejo's bluffs, high above the strait. **Equestrians** and **wheelchair users** end their trip at the South Regatta Drive Gate.

To continue, **hikers** and **mountain bikers** take the short trail that descends to a gate to South Regatta Drive. (Don't veer off into the long swale on your left.) Turn left and follow sidewalks through several subdivisions to Glen Cove Parkway. For the first half mile, you have an unobstructed view out to the strait and its maritime traffic; then you see west through the trees to Glen Cove and the City of Vallejo's Waterfront Park.

Continue on South Regatta Drive to Glen Cove Parkway—0.9 mile from the Benicia State Recreation Area gate—and turn left. Pass Vallejo's Glen Cove Park, with attractive plantings and brightly painted children's play apparatus. After just 0.2 mile on Glen Cove Parkway, turn left again on Glen Cove Marina Road, and go 0.1 mile downhill to a cul-de-sac and the entrance to the Glen Cove Marina.

The Victorian yacht club at this marina once served as the residence for personnel at the Carquinez Lighthouse and Life Saving Station, and was formerly situated just west of an early version of the Carquinez Bridge at the mouth of the Napa River. After the lighthouse was automated in 1955, the building was sold and barged to its present site at Elliot Bay in 1957. The three-story building, painted white with gray trim, now presides over the yacht basin.

Bikers end their trip here at the marina, and **hikers** continue from the west shore of the yacht basin, where a crushed granite path heads up a broad easement. From this bluff-top path above the strait, you look down on tankers and freighters from ports around the world, barges, naval vessels, and pleasure craft. On a foggy day, the horns of ships and the bells of buoys reverberate eerily from the strait's watery canyon. High above the strait, the Carquinez Bridge carries its noisy load of land-based, eastbound traffic.

Connecting trails from pocket parks in the adjoining subdivision intersect with this segment of the Bay Trail and the Bay Area Ridge Trail. The trail ends at a dramatic vista point below the bridge, near Waterview Terrace. The swiftly moving waters of the strait join San Pablo Bay, with Mt. Tamalpais and the Coast Ranges as a backdrop. West of the newest span across the strait, the Al Zampa Memorial Bridge, there are two historic maritime facilities—the Mare Island Naval Shipyard and the California Maritime Academy. On the return trip, you'll see the port communities of Vallejo, Benicia, and Martinez with Mt. Diablo in the distance. This waterfront trail, also the route of the Bay Trail, crosses the river to Martinez on a bridge that is being retrofitted for two-way bike and pedestrian traffic.

◆ ◆ ◆

To learn more about the Al Zampa Bridge, check out the description of the next segment of the Ridge Trail, which crosses it.

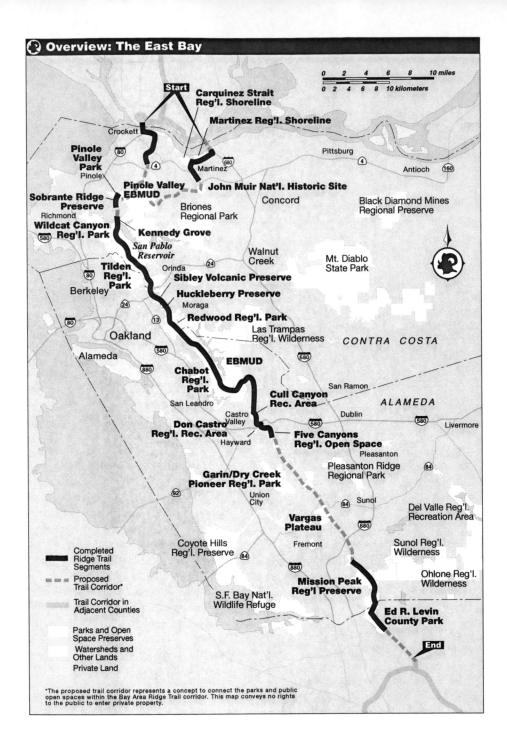

Start

Carquinez Strait Reg'l. Shoreline

Martinez Reg'l. Shoreline

Crockett

Pittsburg

Pinole Valley Park
Pinole
80

4
Martinez
680

Antioch
160

Pinole Valley EBMUD

John Muir Nat'l. Historic Site

Concord

Black Diamond Mines Regional Preserve

Sobrante Ridge Preserve
Richmond

Briones Regional Park

Wildcat Canyon Reg'l. Park
580

Kennedy Grove

San Pablo Reservoir

Walnut Creek

Mt. Diablo State Park

Orinda
24

Tilden Reg'l. Park
Berkeley
80

Sibley Volcanic Preserve

Huckleberry Preserve
Moraga

24

Redwood Reg'l. Park

Las Trampas Reg'l. Wilderness

CONTRA COSTA

Oakland
13
580

EBMUD

Alameda

880

Chabot Reg'l. Park

San Ramon

680

ALAMEDA

San Leandro

Cull Canyon Rec. Area

Castro Valley

Dublin

580

580

Livermore

Don Castro Reg'l. Rec. Area
Hayward

Five Canyons Reg'l. Open Space

Pleasanton

Garin/Dry Creek Pioneer Reg'l. Park
92

Union City

Pleasanton Ridge Regional Park
84

84
Sunol

Del Valle Reg'l. Recreation Area

Vargas Plateau
680

Coyote Hills Reg'l. Preserve
84

Fremont

Sunol Reg'l. Wilderness

880

Ohlone Reg'l. Wilderness

Completed Ridge Trail Segments

Proposed Trail Corridor*

Trail Corridor in Adjacent Counties

Parks and Open Space Preserves

Watersheds and Other Lands

Private Land

Mission Peak Reg'l Preserve

S.F. Bay Nat'l. Wildlife Refuge

Ed R. Levin County Park

End

0 2 4 6 8   10 miles
0 2 4 6 8   10 kilometers

*The proposed trail corridor represents a concept to connect the parks and public open spaces within the Bay Area Ridge Trail corridor. This map conveys no rights to the public to enter private property.

118

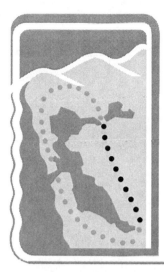

THE EAST BAY

Al Zampa Memorial Bridge. 121

Martinez City Streets to Carquinez Strait Regional Shoreline 123

Carquinez Strait Regional Shoreline to John Muir National Historic
Site on the Hulet Hornbeck Trail 127

Mount Wanda Trail 130

Crockett Hills Regional Park. 133

Sobrante Ridge Regional Preserve. 135

Kennedy Grove to Tilden Regional Park 139

Tilden Regional Park to Redwood Regional Park 145

Redwood and Anthony Chabot Regional Parks 151

Anthony Chabot Regional Park 155

East Bay Municipal Utility District Lands to Independent School . .161

Independent School to Five Canyons. 165

Mission Peak Regional Preserve and Ed R. Levin County Park. . . . 169

Al Zampa Memorial Bridge

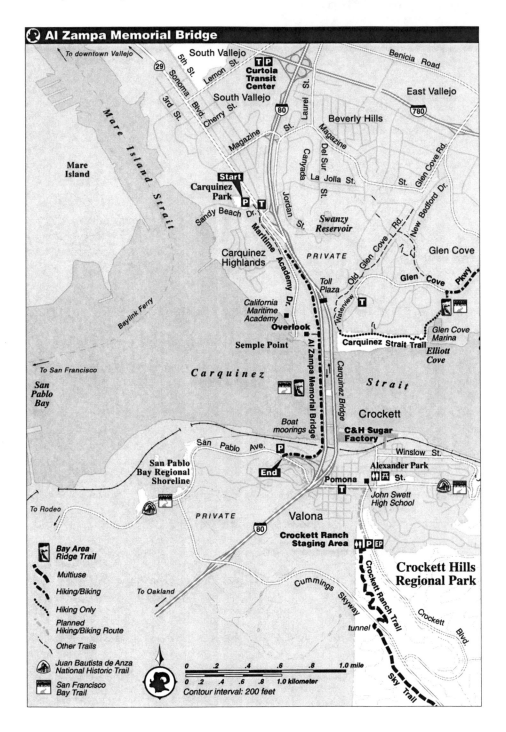

To downtown Vallejo

29

Mare Island Strait

Mare Island

South Vallejo

5th St.
Lemon St.
Sonoma Blvd.
3rd St.
Cherry St.
Magazine

South Vallejo

Curtola Transit Center

80

Laurel St.

Benicia Road

East Vallejo

780

Beverly Hills

Magazine St.

Canada

Del Sur St.
La Jolla St.

Glen Cove Rd.

New Bedford Dr.

Start
Carquinez Park

Sandy Beach Dr.

Jordan St.

Maritime Academy Dr.

Swanzy Reservoir

PRIVATE

Old Glen Cove L Rd.

Glen Cove

Carquinez Highlands

Toll Plaza

Glen Cove Pkwy

Waterview

Glen Cove Marina

California Maritime Academy

Overlook

Baylink Ferry

To San Francisco

San Pablo Bay

Semple Point

Al Zampa Memorial Bridge

Carquinez Strait Trail

Elliott Cove

Carquinez

Carquinez Bridge

Strait

Crockett

Boat moorings

C&H Sugar Factory

San Pablo Ave.

San Pablo Bay Regional Shoreline

End

Pomona

Alexander Park
St.

Winslow St.

John Swett High School

To Rodeo

PRIVATE

Valona

80

Crockett Ranch Staging Area

Cummings Skyway

Crockett Ranch Trail

Crockett Hills Regional Park

Crockett Blvd.

tunnel

Sky Trail

To Oakland

Legend

Bay Area Ridge Trail

Multiuse

Hiking/Biking

Hiking Only

Planned Hiking/Biking Route

Other Trails

Juan Bautista de Anza National Historic Trail

San Francisco Bay Trail

0   .2   .4   .6   .8   1.0 mile
0 .2 .4 .6 .8 1.0 kilometer
Contour interval: 200 feet

Al Zampa Memorial Bridge

On Carquinez Strait Bicycle and Pedestrian Pathway

Length   1.6 miles one-way

Accessibility   Hikers, bicyclists, dog-walkers (with dogs on leash), strollers, and exercise buffs

Agency   California Department of Transportation

Regulations   Motorized vehicles are prohibited. All dogs must be on leash. Cyclists must call out to those they wish to pass.

Facilities   Carquinez Park, a half mile beyond the bridge's north end, has rolling lawns, picnic tables, restrooms, and parking. The bridge's south end has a parking lot adjacent to Dead Fish Restaurant, which has many spaces when the restaurant is closed.

Join strollers, exercise buffs, dog walkers, and commuters on a high suspension bridge over the wide waters of Carquinez Strait where the Sacramento and San Joaquin rivers flow to San Francisco Bay.

Getting There

FROM THE NORTH: Take Interstate 80 in the vicinity of Vallejo, take Highway 29 South (Sonoma Boulevard), and turn left at Sandy Beach Road to Carquinez Park on the west side of the road. Park in one of the several parking areas. Walk or ride three blocks to the pedestrian/bicycle entrance to the bridge on the left.

FROM THE SOUTH: Take Interstate 80 toward the Al Zampa Bridge, take the Pomona Street off-ramp, and then go left under the highway to parking at the large Caltrans lot near the restaurant currently known as the Dead Fish. The sidewalk to the bridge is well marked. Follow it going north onto the bridge. The pedestrian/biker route is on the west side of the bridge with fine views of the river and surrounding countryside.

On the Trail

From Carquinez Park go downhill for a few blocks to the bridge trail entrance graced with native plants and marked by a large Ridge Trail and Bay Trail sign, a map of the trail, and a low, blue metal bench.

At the beginning your trail is wide and separated from the vehicular traffic by a 5-foot concrete wall topped by a black chain-link fence on each side of the trail. Shortly, off to the west of the trail, you pass a large open field flanked by tall eucalyptus trees that provide late afternoon shade. This bridge, the second to cross the strait, was opened in November 2003, replacing an earlier bridge that is being removed. Look for the Alfred Zampa Memorial Bridge plaque, which tells the story of the Crockett native, an ironworker who worked on all the bridges that cross San Francisco Bay. A survivor of a fall into the safety net during the building of the Golden Gate Bridge, he helped form the "Halfway to Hell Club" for bridge-building survivors.

On your right is a high, concrete wall incised with nautical themes. This wall then becomes the backdrop for a semicircular platform from which you can see the many forms of river traffic—two-man racing sculls, kayaks with outriggers, sleek sailboats, small fishing boats, ocean-going vessels and merchant ships. Almost at water's edge transcontinental trains speed along tracks on the west side of the strait.

Below are the buildings and small boat anchorage of the Maritime Academy, a training school for the U.S. Merchant Marine fleet. About halfway across you pass the sign that marks the watery boundary of Contra Costa and Solano counties. The vehicle traffic roars by faster and noisier than the Carquinez water—one-half going west, the other east. You, however, continue on your pedestrian or bicycle route to the south side of the bridge with plenty of opportunity to watch the maritime traffic float almost noiselessly on their watery route.

The vehicle and pedestrian off-ramps turn west, while those continuing toward San Francisco go straight ahead, and shortly end at the Dead Fish Restaurant parking lot, which is also the car park for carpoolers. Here you turn around for the 1.6-mile trip back to the north side of the Carquinez Strait. There is always some activity on the water plus plenty of auto-generated noise from the lanes beside you. Now you have a better look at the Maritime Academy and the houses, wharves, and docks on the north side of the strait.

◆ ◆ ◆

If you are continuing on the Ridge Trail to the north, find the crosswalk, and go to the ramp that takes you to the lower level and the Ridge Trail segment on the east side of the strait.

Martinez City Streets to Carquinez Strait Regional Shoreline

From George M. Miller, Jr., Bridge to Martinez Regional Shoreline and East Staging Area

Length	2.0 miles one-way
Accessibility	Hikers and mountain bikers
Agencies	City of Martinez and East Bay Regional Park District
Regulations	The City of Martinez requires bikers under age 18 to wear helmets. Martinez Regional Shoreline is open from 5 AM to 10 PM, unless otherwise posted.
Facilities	Fishing pier, picnic tables, water, and restrooms at Martinez Regional Shoreline

Take a walk or bike ride along the Carquinez Strait shoreline, and discover the area's rich history, from early Spanish explorers and rancheros to Gold Rush miners; and from sea captains of grain ships and oil tankers to the founders and public leaders of Contra Costa County's capital city. This route follows sidewalks and bike lanes with only 100 feet in elevation gain.

Getting There

EAST TRAILHEAD: From Interstate 680 south of Benicia Bridge, take the Marina Vista exit. Follow it to on-street metered parking; or to park in Hulet Hornbeck Regional Shoreline, continue to Ferry St., turn right, and cross railroad tracks. Turn right on Joe DiMaggio Street and then left on North Court Street to several parking areas.

WEST TRAILHEAD: From Interstate 80 or Interstate 680 in Contra Costa County, take Highway 4 (John Muir Parkway) to Martinez. Take the Alhambra Avenue exit, and go 1.75 miles north through Martinez. Turn left on Escobar, right on Talbart, and then veer left on Carquinez Scenic Drive. Just after you pass the cemeteries, turn left into East Staging Area. From I-680 south of Benicia Bridge, take Marina Vista west, turn left on Berrellesa and right immediately on Escobar. Turn right on Talbart, veer left on Carquinez Scenic Drive, and then turn left into East Staging Area.

On the Trail

The Ridge Trail route starts at Mococo Road, about a quarter mile west of the Benicia Bridge, but since there is no parking at Mococo Road, you must start your trip by going east from Marina Vista Avenue or from Martinez Regional Shoreline. **Mountain bikers** should use Escobar Street going east to Mococo.

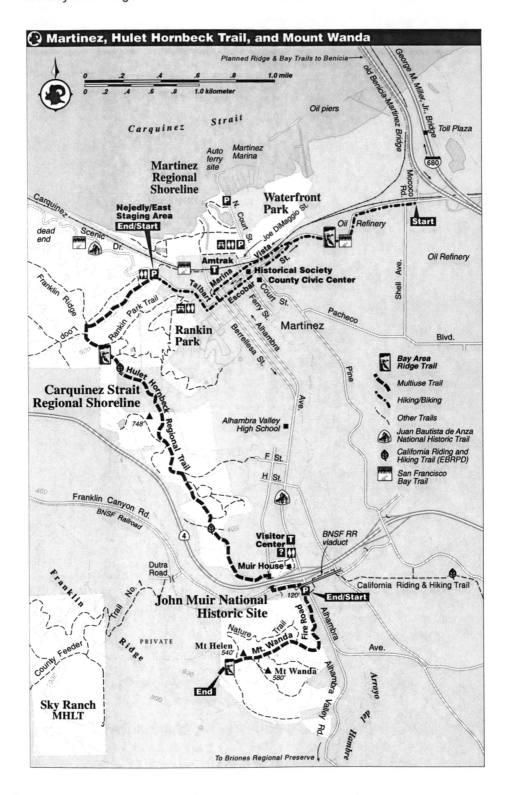

Martinez, Hulet Hornbeck Trail, and Mount Wanda

Planned Ridge & Bay Trails to Benicia →

George M. Miller, Jr. Bridge

Old Benicia-Martinez Bridge

Toll Plaza

680

Oil piers

Carquinez Strait

Auto ferry site

Martinez Marina

Martinez Regional Shoreline

Nejedly/East Staging Area
End/Start

dead end

Scenic Dr.

Court St.

Joe DiMaggio St.

Waterfront Park

Oil Refinery

Start

Oil Refinery

Franklin Ridge Loop

800

Rankin Park Trail

Amtrak

Marina Vista St.

Talbart

Escobar St.

Ferry St.

Court St.

Alhambra

Shell Ave.

Historical Society
County Civic Center

Pacheco

Blvd.

Rankin Park

Berrellesa St.

Martinez

Pine Ave.

Carquinez Strait Regional Shoreline

Hulet Hornbeck Regional Trail

748^

600

Alhambra Valley High School

| | **Bay Area Ridge Trail** |
| Multiuse Trail |
| Hiking/Biking |
| Other Trails |
| **Juan Bautista de Anza National Historic Trail** |
| **California Riding and Hiking Trail (EBRPD)** |
| **San Francisco Bay Trail** |

400

Franklin Canyon Rd.
BNSF Railroad

4

400

F St.

H St.

600

Visitor Center

Muir House

BNSF RR viaduct

Dutra Road

John Muir National Historic Site

Trail No. 1

Franklin Ridge

County Feeder

PRIVATE

600

120'

End/Start

California Riding & Hiking Trail

Alhambra Ave.

Nature Trail

Mt Helen
540'

Mt. Wanda

Fire Road

Arroyo del Hambre

End

Mt Wanda
580'

Alhambra Valley Rd.

300

Sky Ranch MHLT

To Briones Regional Preserve →

0   .2   .4   .6   .8   1.0 mile
0   .2   .4   .6   .8   1.0 kilometer

Historic Martinez

The Martinez Museum is housed in the Moore house, a historic building on the corner of Escobar and Ferry streets. You can view artifacts from the town's long history and pick up a brochure for a walking tour of the historic buildings in Martinez. Learn about Don Ignazio Martinez, who received 17,000 acres in this valley for his military services to the Mexican government. His daughter, Susana, who inherited some of this acreage, married San Francisco businessman William Smith. Smith first surveyed and laid out 20 of the land-grant acres for the original city of Martinez.

Martinez was the first city in present-day Contra Costa County. With the onset of the Gold Rush, it grew into a busy port and became the county seat in 1851. Ocean-going vessels carried grain grown in the Central Valley from Martinez docks to international ports. The completion of the transcontinental railroad through Martinez in 1876 brought the "iron horse" into Martinez. Shell oil established its refineries and pipelines here in 1915. The city continues to be an important shipping center and governmental center.

Today, this Bay Area Ridge Trail segment follows the shoreline route used by explorers and early settlers. The route was dedicated as a joint Ridge Trail and Bay Trail segment on November 7, 1998.

Mountain bikers start your westward trip at Mococo Road on the Marina Vista bike lanes. **Hikers** begin at Shell Avenue, 0.1 mile west, on the paved sidewalk along Marina Vista's south side. **Hikers** and **bikers** travel near railroad tank cars on sidings and loaded freight trains passing refineries and oil storage tanks. Huge pipes snake along the hillside and then form shiny, high bridges over the thoroughfare to reach storage tanks and railroad tank cars. Sounds of switching engines and sights of parked tanker cars on sidings plus oil refinery odors offer a different ambience from rural parkland trips.

Tall Italian cypresses soon camouflage the refinery, and dense plantings partially shield the view of the railroad tracks. About a half mile beyond Shell Avenue your route swings south, away from the tracks, and hugs the hillside below the refineries. It curves northwest and passes below hillside homes with porches that overlook the strait.

At Miller Street, tall eucalyptus mask the railroad view; after Huntington Drive, Marina Vista splits at a **Y** and becomes a one-way street going west. **Hikers** can safely cross to the north side of Marina Vista at Miller Street or continue west on Escobar Street. After the split, a landscaped island lies between Marina Vista and Escobar streets. On a hillside to your left, a large Victorian house and summer cottages of several vintages have broad views of the strait and the Benicia hills beyond.

Soon you reach the busiest section of town, where county and city government buildings—courthouses, office buildings, and finance and postal departments—fill several square blocks. When I walked this trail, local shoppers and government employees on their lunch breaks strolled the streets between Ward and Marina Vista, giving a lively feel to the heart of the city. The historic Moore house, on the corner of Escobar and Ferry streets, is now the Martinez Museum, a charming, white, two-story structure with a covered veranda and double-gabled roof.

From Marina Vista and Escobar streets, turn north on either Ferry or Berrellessa streets to reach the East Bay Regional Park District's Martinez Regional Shoreline. Its picnic tables and shorefront benches offer attractive places to rest along your Ridge Trail route. Friends and family could join you here for a picnic or snack and a chance to watch the waterfowl on ponds or the ships and pleasure boats that ply the swift waters of Carquinez Strait. A former ferry dock that is now used as a fishing pier might intrigue anglers.

When you leave this excellent shoreline park, follow Marina Vista westward past the old, wood-sided Southern Pacific Railroad station to the newly built Amtrak station. Then turn left (southeast) on Berrellesa; after two blocks, go right (west) on Escobar. Turn right again at Talbart Street after two more blocks, and ascend past small homes of Victorian and early 20th-century vintage. Three blocks farther, at Foster Street, veer left onto Carquinez Scenic Drive, and pass cemeteries on the right and left. William Smith, son-in-law of Don Ignazio Martinez, is buried in Alhambra Cemetery, on the right. After you pass Rankin Park on the left, watch for the entrance to the East Staging Area of Carquinez Strait Regional Shoreline, where this segment of the Bay Area Ridge Trail ends.

Now that the new Benicia-Martinez bridge bicycle and pedestrian lanes are completed, Ridge Trail and Bay Trail users are able to travel along several continuous segments of trail in Solano County and cross the bridge to join this trail in Martinez and others in Contra Costa County.

◆ ◆ ◆

The next Bay Area Ridge Trail segment continues southeast from this staging area to the John Muir National Historic Site.

Ships of varied hues and sizes at the Martinez Marina

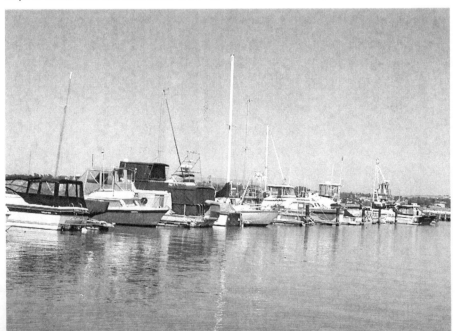

Carquinez Strait Regional Shoreline to John Muir National Historic Site on the Hulet Hornbeck Trail

From East Staging Area to John Muir National Historic Site

see map on p.124

Length 3.0 miles

Accessibility Hikers, equestrians, and mountain bikers

Agencies East Bay Park Regional Park District and National Park Service

Regulations The Hulet Hornbeck Trail is open from 8 AM to a half hour after sunset. Dogs permitted in staging area on leash and must be under voice control in open space. John Muir National Historic Site is open from 10:30 AM to 4:30 PM Wednesday through Sunday and charges an entrance fee.

Facilities Restrooms at East Staging Area, water and restrooms at historic site

Roam rolling ridgelands in northern Contra Costa County on a trail named for longtime East Bay Regional Open Space District planner and trail enthusiast Hulet Hornbeck. It follows the old California Riding and Hiking Trail, a round-the-state trail system planned in the mid-1900s. One of the few remaining segments of this trail it follows wide, unpaved service trails along the exposed ridge south of the Carquinez Strait and ends in the Alhambra Valley of Martinez, where you can visit John Muir's home. The first and last legs of the trail are short and steep.

Getting There

By Car

NORTH TRAILHEAD, CARQUINEZ SHORELINE: From Interstate 80 or Interstate 680 in Contra Costa County take Highway 4 (John Muir Parkway) to Martinez. Take the Alhambra Avenue exit, and go 1.75 miles north through Martinez. Turn left on Escobar Street and right on Talbart, and then veer left on Carquinez Scenic Drive. Just after you pass the cemeteries, turn left into the East Staging Area.

SOUTH TRAILHEAD, JOHN MUIR NATIONAL HISTORIC SITE: From Interstate 80 or Interstate 680 in Contra Costa County take Highway 4 (John Muir Parkway) to Martinez. Take the Alhambra Avenue exit, turn north on Alhambra Avenue, and immediately look for the historic site on your left at 4202 Alhambra Avenue. Parking is limited here, but additional parking is available at the southwest corner of Alhambra Avenue and Franklin Canyon Road with access to the trail from Franklin Canyon Road through a tunnel under Highway 4.

By Bus

A Contra Costa County Connection bus runs to Alhambra Avenue and Marina Vista and to Alhambra Avenue and Franklin Canyon Road from BART stations daily, except Sundays.

On the Trail

The original name for this valley, derived from an 1842 land grant, was Cañada del Hambre y las Bolsas del Hambre, or the Valley of Hunger. It was renamed Alhambra Valley when Mr. and Mrs. Strentzel, parents of John Muir's wife, settled here in the 1880s. **Hikers, equestrians,** and **mountain bikers** begin this trip from the East Staging Area (also known as the Nejedly Staging Area); head uphill toward the East Bay Regional Park District's green gate, emblazoned with a prominent Bay Area Ridge Trail sign. (An alternate route through adjoining Rankin Park takes off to the left behind the uppermost picnic table.) Close the gate to the EBRPD Trail, and take the path that cuts across a wide flat. You soon enter a glade of bay and buckeye trees, where toyon and poison oak grow in the understory.

You begin a steady ascent through oak woodlands, beside a seasonal creek, and gain more than 500 feet in elevation in less than a half mile. You emerge into grasslands on a couple of switchbacks but soon return to shaded woodland. In winter, you may find burnished, brown buckeye balls (seedpods) and deer or bobcat prints on the trail. In spring, you may see the long, wavy leaves of soap plant promising evening blooms of delicate, bluish-white flowers on tall stalks. After a series of three steep pitches followed by short, level stretches, you reach a gate at the Franklin Ridge Loop Trail. If you detour to the right and circle the knoll, you'll find picnic sites overlooking the strait and a view west of Mt. Tamalpais.

John Muir National Historic Site

Stop at the John Muir National Historic Site to learn more about the life of the father of the U.S. National Park System. At the visitor center, you can watch a video about his life from his childhood in Wisconsin to his trip in Yosemite with President Theodore Roosevelt. You can visit the Muir family Victorian house and grounds, with orchards, barns, and the old Vicente Martinez adobe.

Although John Muir's real love was the Sierra Nevada, he often wandered these hills with his daughters, Wanda and Helen, and set aside special hilltops for evening strolls with them. Muir surely would have appreciated the Bay Area Ridge Trail Council's efforts to join Bay Area open spaces with a regional ridgeline trail. As he wrote, "Everybody needs beauty as well as bread, places to play in and pray in where Nature may heal and cheer and give strength to body and soul alike."

From the desk in his study, Muir wrote many of the books and articles that inspired political action to save wildlands and wildlife. He helped establish a national conservation policy, reflected today in environmental legislation and in the excellent U.S. National Park System.

To proceed southeast on the Hulet Hornbeck segment of the Ridge Trail, bear left at the gate; at the next fork, take the graveled road on the right, and descend into a saddle between grassy, rounded hilltops. A pastoral scene of orchard, windmill, and water tank lies in the valley to your left, reminiscent of the farming that flourished in this area when John Muir and his family lived here.

Your route ahead rises to grass-covered hilltops followed by dips into hollows of evergreen oaks. Enjoy views from the hilltops: on your left, the Carquinez Strait, Benicia-Martinez Bridge, and the Navy's mothball fleet in Suisun Bay; the Benicia foothills rise across the strait, crossed by the Vallejo-Benicia Buffer leg of the Ridge Trail. Kestrels may flutter overhead, while red-tailed and northern harrier hawks ride the updrafts, each bird searching for prey. Orange poppies and blue-eyed grass brighten the trail in spring.

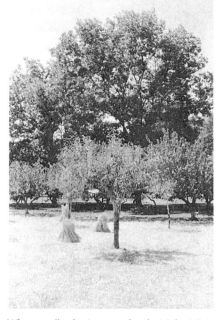

Wheat stalks dry in an orchard at John Muir National Historic Site.

You go through another gate, beyond which you are on an EBRPD trail easement through private property. Signs remind you to stay on the trail. A Ridge Trail sign directs you right, past a brown barn; a yellow house is on your left. You soon reach the trip's highest point. Mt. Diablo's twin summits loom ahead and are in sight for the rest of the trip; the view is fine at sunset, when a soft, pink glow cloaks the mountain. From the next hilltop you can see south to a succession of gently rounded hills that rise above tree-filled canyons. Franklin Ridge tops the canyon of the same name; Edward Franklin lived in the canyon from 1853, when he bought a portion of the Ignacio Martinez estate, until 1875.

After crossing under tall transmission towers and power lines, follow a Bay Area Ridge Trail sign that directs you onto a narrow, paved road into a tight canyon. Where the paving veers right, you continue straight ahead on a dirt trail; the town of Martinez lies below. From the top of a steep hill, you make a quick descent on a Caltrans easement above Highway 4, the John Muir Parkway. (Bicyclists should dismount.) The trail ends at a fenced cross trail, where you can go left to the John Muir National Historic Site.

To reach the southern trailhead of this Ridge Trail route, turn right and continue on the Hulet Hornbeck Trail and the California Riding and Hiking Trail through a tunnel under the John Muir Parkway to Franklin Canyon Road. Turn left (east) to reach the parking area at its junction with Alhambra Avenue, where you could have a shuttle waiting. Otherwise, your route back to the East Staging Area on the Hulet Hornbeck Trail will afford fine views west, north, and east.

◆ ◆ ◆

The next Bay Area Ridge Trail segment, to the summit of Mt. Wanda, begins at the Alhambra Avenue parking area across Highway 4 in John Muir National Historic Site.

Mount Wanda Trail

From Franklin Canyon Road and Alhambra Avenue in Martinez to Summit of Mount Wanda in John Muir National Historic Site

see map on p.124

Length   1.0 mile

Accessibility   Hikers, equestrians, and mountain bikers

Agency   National Park Service

Regulations   Site is open from 8 AM to a half hour after sunset. Dogs are permitted in staging area on leash and must be under voice control in open space.

Facilities   Water and restrooms

A short, but unrelentingly upward trip, with an elevation gain of 460 feet, to vast views of Carquinez Strait and surrounding hills from a hilltop often visited by John Muir and his daughters.

Getting There

By Car

From Interstate 80 or Interstate 680 in Contra Costa County take Highway 4 (John Muir Parkway) to Martinez. Take the Alhambra Avenue exit and park on the southeast corner of its intersection with Franklin Canyon Road and the foot of trail to Mt. Wanda. Parking at the site is limited, but additional parking is available at 4202 Alhambra Avenue.

By Bus

A few Contra Costa County Connection buses service downtown Martinez.

On the Trail

Leave the parking area on a service road that follows the east edge of the park property. Dense growth of bay, buckeye, and oak trees overarch the trail and offer sites for the birds you may hear singing in the trees or the squirrels that scatter as you approach. Blue brodiaea on long stems bloom above patches of dainty white woodland stars. In sunny openings look for bright, shiny-faced, yellow buttercups amid patches of low-growing, yellow-flowering pineapple plant, the latter often considered a weed.

When you emerge from the woods at the top of the hill, the view of Carquinez Strait and its surrounding cities, Benicia and Martinez, is well worth the climb. You will be repeatedly impressed by the magnificence and magnitude of this confluence of rivers that drain the Sierra Nevada and foothills of Central California.

On April 21, 2007, the Bay Area Ridge Trail Council dedicated this trip as a segment of the Ridge Trail. West of this site is Mt. Helen, which Muir named for Helen,

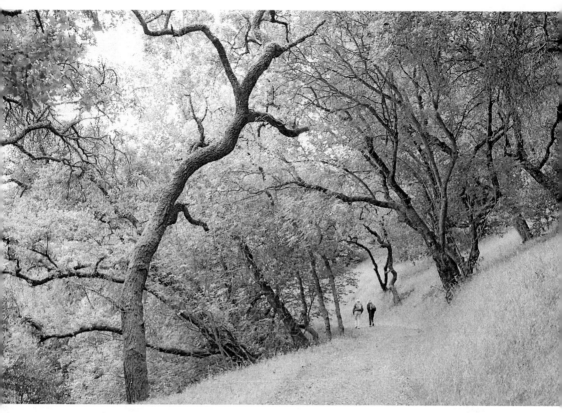

Mt. Wanda Trail   *Elizabeth Byers*

one of his daughters. It is said that Muir enjoyed strolling these hills with his daughters. You too, can enjoy this hilltop on a trail that circles the site. Take the trail on which you reached this site and walk through a grove of liveoaks, madrones, and deciduous blue oaks. The latter are of unusual height and girth with strikingly blue leaves in early spring. Then return downhill on the trail to the parking area.

◆ ◆ ◆

The next leg of the Ridge Trail begins in Crockett Hills Regional Park.

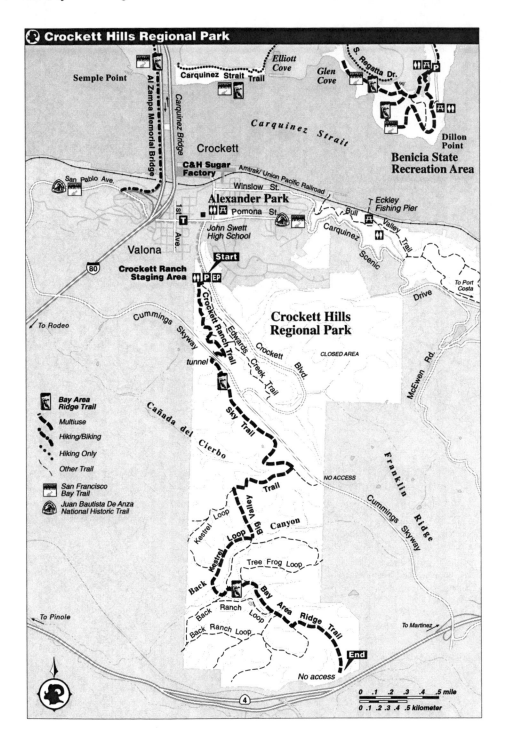

Crockett Hills Regional Park

Semple Point

Elliott Cove

Carquinez Strait Trail

S. Regatta Dr.

Glen Cove

Al Zampa Memorial Bridge

Carquinez Bridge

Carquinez Strait

Dillon Point

Benicia State Recreation Area

Crockett

C&H Sugar Factory

Amtrak/ Union Pacific Railroad

Winslow St.

San Pablo Ave.

Alexander Park

Pomona St.

Eckley Fishing Pier

Bull

John Swett High School

Carquinez Scenic

Valley Trail

1st Ave.

Valona

Start

80

Crockett Ranch Staging Area

EP

Drive

To Port Costa

To Rodeo

Cummings Skyway

Crockett Ranch Trail

Crockett Blvd

Crockett Hills Regional Park

CLOSED AREA

McEwen Rd.

tunnel

Edwards Creek Trail

Cañada del Cierbo

Sky Trail

Trail

NO ACCESS

Franklin Ridge

Cummings Skyway

Legend
- **Bay Area Ridge Trail**
- Multiuse
- Hiking/Biking
- Hiking Only
- Other Trail
- San Francisco Bay Trail
- Juan Bautista De Anza National Historic Trail

Kestrel Loop

Big Valley

Canyon

Loop

Kestrel

Tree Frog Loop

Back

Bay Area Ridge Trail

Back Ranch Loop

To Pinole

Back Ranch Loop

To Martinez

End

No access

4

0 .1 .2 .3 .4 .5 mile

0 .1 .2 .3 .4 .5 kilometer

Crockett Hills Regional Park

From Crockett Ranch Staging Area to Trail's End at Highway 4

Length 4.5 miles one-way (no outlet on Highway 4)

Accessibility Hikers, equestrians, and mountain bikers

Agency East Bay Regional Park District

Regulations East Bay Regional Park District rules apply, meaning that dogs must be on a leash 6 feet or shorter.

Facilities Water, restroom, and picnic table at staging area

Climb to high grasslands for East Bay views from Carquinez Strait west to Mt. Tamalpais and north to Hood Mountain and Bald Mountain on the Ridge Trail route.

Getting There

From Interstate 80 in Crockett take Pomona Street east, almost immediately turn right (south) on Crockett Boulevard, and drive about a half mile to a staging area on the right.

On the Trail

From the staging area **all users** go uphill to a gate that leads to the trail. After going through the gate (please close it to keep the cattle in), bear left on the wide Crockett Ranch Trail. Shaded by coast live oaks and edged by wild cucumber vines and tangles of poison oak, this half-mile trail rises steeply to its summit. Here you go through a low tunnel under the Cummings Skyway—equestrians should dismount. The tunnel leads to the Sky Trail, a wide service road and the Bay Area Ridge Trail route. Turn left (east) ambling along rolling, grassy hillsides high above the Carquinez Strait. The trail rounds low ridges clothed with wild grasses, green and dotted with wildflowers in spring and golden brown in summer. Occasional clumps of live oaks beside the route offer welcome patches of shade on hot days.

Far to the southwest rises Mt. Tamalpais, in sight for most of the outbound trip. To the north lies the Al Zampa Memorial Bridge crossing the Strait to Vallejo, once the capital of the young State of California, and to points north and east. Tugboats and seagoing ships ply the strait's waters, which come from the San Joaquin and Sacramento, California's two great rivers that drain its central valleys. The East Bay Regional Park District's Carquinez Regional Shoreline stretches for 2 miles along this side of the strait, a recreational boon for area residents and visitors.

After about 1 mile, watch for the Big Valley Trail, and turn right (southwest) on it. The land drops away steeply on your right, and a long knoll rises about 200 feet above you on the left. Then the Big Valley Trail, your Ridge Trail route, goes left in a little draw above an intermittent creek. Here you join the Kestrel Loop Trail going south. You make a sharp left turn, descend to cross the intermittent creek, and then climb to regain lost elevation. Contouring along a southeast-facing hillside at about the 600-foot level you

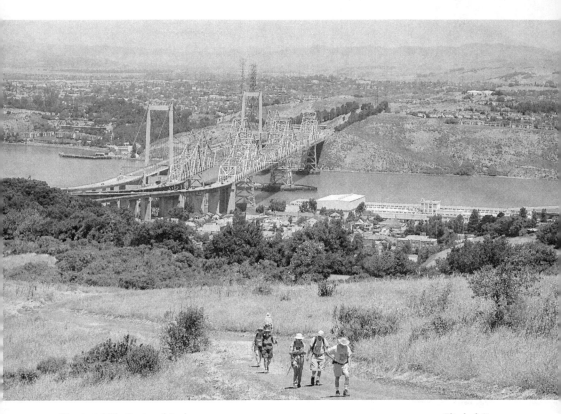

Crockett Hills Regional Park   *Elizabeth Byers*

head eastward for almost a mile. Here the trail ends at the park boundary on Highway
4. Until the trail is extended beyond this point, you must turn around and retrace your
steps, making this a 9-mile round-trip.

Retracing your outbound route you see north to the big stacks of the California and
Hawaiian Sugar Refinery Company, longtime landmarks in the town of Crockett. (The
Starr Flour Mill, too, was an early Crockett enterprise. You can you see its remnants off
to the north.) Today, due north on this side of the strait is the EBRPD Eckley Park and
Fishing Pier, where once the thriving Eckley Ferry operated to cross the strait. These
rolling grasslands were probably Native American hunting and gathering grounds and
later became 19th-century ranchlands. At the Crockett Ranch staging and picnic area
you can see the original barn, milk house, and corrals, reminders of an earlier, different
way of life.

The next segment of the Ridge Trail begins southwest across the Contra Costa hills
in Sobrante Ridge Regional Preserve.

Sobrante Ridge Regional Preserve

From Pinole Valley Park to Conestoga Way

Length	2.2 miles, plus 1.2 miles on connector trail from Pinole Valley Park; 0.7 mile on connector trail from Coach Drive
Accessibility	Hikers, equestrians, and mountain bikers
Agency	East Bay Regional Park District
Regulations	Motor vehicles are prohibited. Bikes are prohibited on the Manzanita Trail and Sobrante Ridge Trail.
Facilities	Water, restrooms, and telephone at Pinole Valley Park and water at Coach Drive

Climb to high grasslands and shaded woodlands on a narrow, shady trail from Pinole Valley Park that gains 640 feet in the first mile; on cool days, take the exposed alternate trail from Coach Drive for an easier climb of 200 feet in 0.7 mile. On the wide, partially shaded ridgetop trail, you'll take in remarkable views of the mountains that ring the bay; the narrow southern leg descends 320 feet in less than a mile.

Getting There

NORTHERN TRAILHEAD, PINOLE VALLEY PARK: From Interstate 80, turn east onto Pinole Valley Road, go about 1.5 miles to the park entrance on the right and park near the playing field. Follow signs across the creek and pass through a picnic area to the trail entrance at the base of a hill.

EASTERN TRAILHEAD, COACH DRIVE: From Interstate 80 in San Pablo take San Pablo Dam Road, go 4 miles to Castro Ranch Road, and turn left (northeast), continue past trail entrance on Conestoga Way, and turn left (southwest) on Carriage Drive. Turn right (north) on Coach Drive, and continue to its terminus and off-street parking.

SOUTHERN TRAILHEAD, CONESTOGA WAY: From Interstate 80 in San Pablo take San Pablo Dam Road, go 4 miles to Castro Ranch Road, and turn left (northeast). Go about 1 mile, turn left on Conestoga Way, and in 0.1 mile look for the trail entrance on the left. Park on the street.

On the Trail

As of this writing, this trip's official route begins in Pinole Valley Park on the Pinole Valley Connector Trail and joins the main Bay Area Ridge Trail route on the Sobrante Ridge Trail, which ends at Conestoga Way. (You can also reach the northeast leg of the main Ridge Trail route from Coach Drive on a shorter, sunnier climb to the ridge.) A future Ridge Trail extension northeast will cross East Bay Municipal Utility

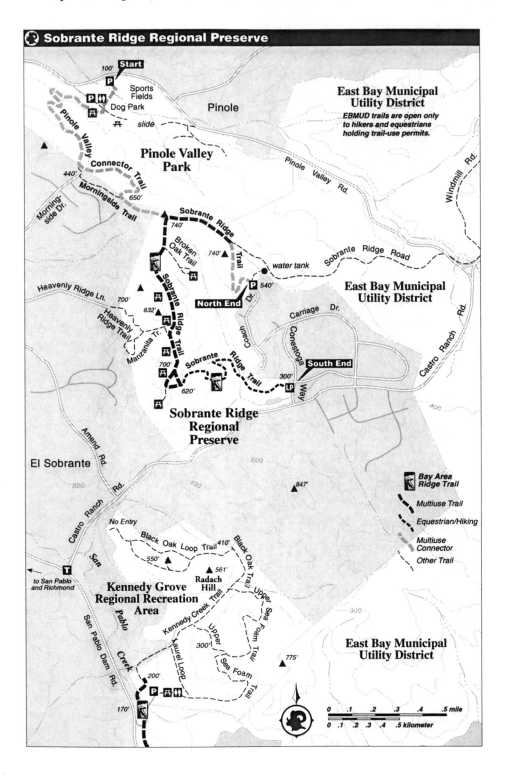

Sobrante Ridge Regional Preserve

100' Start

P

Sports
Fields

P M

Dog Park

Pinole

slide

Pinole Valley

Pinole Valley
Park

Pinole Valley Rd.

East Bay Municipal
Utility District

EBMUD trails are open only
to hikers and equestrians
holding trail-use permits.

Windmill Rd.

Connector Trail

440'

Morningside Trail

650'

Morning-
side Dr.

Sobrante Ridge

740'

Broken
Oak Trail

740'

Trail

water tank

Sobrante Ridge Road

P 540'

East Bay Municipal
Utility District

Heavenly Ridge Ln.

700'

Heavenly
Ridge Trail

832'

Sobrante Ridge Trail

North End

Dr.

Carriage Dr.

Manzanita Tr.

700'

Sobrante

Ridge Trail

Coach

Conestoga

Way

South End

300'

LP

Castro Ranch Rd.

620'

Sobrante Ridge
Regional
Preserve

Amend Rd.

El Sobrante

200

Castro Ranch Rd.

San

400

600

400

847'

Bay Area
Ridge Trail

Multiuse Trail

Equestrian/Hiking

Multiuse
Connector

Other Trail

No Entry

Black Oak Loop Trail 410'

550'

Black Oak Trail

561'

Radach
Hill

Upper Sea Foam Trail

to San Pablo
and Richmond

T

Kennedy Grove
Regional Recreation
Area

Kennedy Creek Trail

Upper

300'

Sea Foam

Upper Sea Foam Trail

300

775'

East Bay Municipal
Utility District

San Pablo

Pablo

Laurel Loop

Creek

San Pablo Dam Rd.

200'

P

170'

0   .1   .2   .3   .4   .5 mile

0   .1   .2   .3   .4   .5 kilometer

Leftover Land

Sobrante Ridge Preserve's 277 acres cover part of the land grant that was deeded to Juan José Castro by the Mexican government in 1841. It was probably named Sobrante, meaning "leftover or surplus," because of its position between two other land grants. After the break up of Castro's rancho, several owners used the property. One owner, Cutter Labs, maintained it as pasture land for horses and cows used in the manufacture of vaccines. A later owner deeded the present ridgetop and lands on its east side to the East Bay Regional Park District in return for permission to develop on the lower western slopes.

District lands to connect this trail with the Mount Wanda Trail in John Muir National Historic Site.

Hikers, equestrians, and **mountain bikers** begin at the parking area at Pinole Valley Park and pass the playing fields and restrooms to a picnic area in a dense grove of bay trees. The park office is in a white Victorian-style building on your left by the picnic area. Beyond the picnic tables, a narrow, multiuse trail zigzags uphill through oak and bay woodlands; ferns drape the banks and dainty white woodland stars and yellow buttercups bloom in the low underbrush. Farther uphill, the trail emerges from the woods to sunny clearings with swaths of wildflowers.

At the top of the ridge, you turn left (east) to merge with the Morningside Trail and continue into the preserve. (The quarter-mile Morningside Trail originates at Morningside Drive in Pinole.) You soon join the Sobrante Ridge Trail on the 700-foot ridgetop and proceed a few feet east to meet the northeastern leg of the alternate trail from Coach Drive. Bear right (south) here on the wide, unpaved service road, bordered by scattered oak woodlands. Shortly you reach a clearing and picnic table, where you can see Mt. Tamalpais on the left (west) and forested San Pedro Mountain to its right. If the day is clear, Mt. Burdell, which is traversed by another Ridge Trail segment, is visible in the north. To the northeast lies Mount Wanda in John Muir National Historic Site and beyond is Suisun Bay.

As you continue south along the main trail, look to your left for the Broken Oak Trail that leads to a picnic table on a shady knoll; the trail then plunges downhill to a cluster of picnic tables in a high canopy of majestic oaks, one of which gives the area its name. This quarter-mile side trip makes a fine lunch stop on a hot day.

Side Trip on the Manzanita Trail

Sidetrack on the short Manzanita Trail loop to see the endangered Alameda manzanita. Despite the steep slope and poor soil, this manzanita thrives on this west-facing slope because of the frequent fog that blows in from the bay. Splendid specimens of native spring flowers also flourish in the Sobrante Ridge grasslands on soil that many nonnative species can't tolerate.

Sheep in Sobrante

One late spring day, when a friend and I first hiked this trail, we saw a small trailer parked here and a low, temporary, wire pen. A brownish cloud was moving slowly up the hillside above Coach Drive. At first thinking it must be dust, we realized there was no wind and looked more closely: it was a flock of sheep tended by a herder who lived in the trailer and the dogs who occupied the pen. We walked toward the flock and saw that the sheep "mowed" the tall grass as they moved ahead of the shepherd. At night, the "fire-prevention team" remained inside a movable plastic fence topped by a low-voltage electric wire.

The Sobrante Ridge Trail gently undulates over the grasslands; clearings along the way bring ever more expansive views of the North Bay, and picnic tables attest to the popularity of this ridge, despite the uphill trip to reach it. As you round the east side of the preserve's highest point (an unnamed 832-foot knoll), elderberry and toyon bushes and oak trees shade your route. Soon you will pass the Manzanita Trail, which makes for an interesting side trip.

The double summits of Mt. Diablo are visible in the east, behind the nearer Oursan Ridge, covered in tight rows of houses. The main trail trends downhill, forks, and forms a small loop. Although not marked as one-way, for safety's sake, users should take the right-hand (west) segment and return on the left-hand (east) leg. Follow the right-hand trail to a 620-foot knoll and yet another picnic table. Return to the main trail from the knoll and follow the loop trail to the right to the base of a high power-line tower. **Mountain bikers** must turn left on the east side of the loop and retrace your route north across the ridgetop to the trailhead.

Hikers and **equestrians** turn right on the final leg of this trail to Conestoga Way. Descend the narrow 0.7-mile trail across an open slope on a contoured reach, and curve into the head of a shady ravine, under a canopy of oak and bay trees. In late summer and fall, the trail surface is covered with spent leaves and can be slippery. You then round the brow of a hill and drop into the willow-filled creekbed that drains into the wildlife refuge pond on the preserve's southeast corner. Climb out of this canyon and finally drop down to the short paved trail that leads to Conestoga Way.

◆ ◆ ◆

The next leg of the Bay Area Ridge Trail starts in Kennedy Grove, on the other side of San Pablo Ridge.

Kennedy Grove to Tilden Regional Park

From the Grove to Inspiration Point

Length 4.4 miles

Accessibility Hikers, equestrians, mountain bikers, and wheelchair users

Agency East Bay Regional Park District

Regulations Kennedy Grove Regional Recreation Area, Wildcat Canyon, and Tilden regional parks are open from 5 AM to 10 PM (or as posted). Dogs must be on leash in parking lots, at picnic sites, and on lawns and under voice control on Nimitz Way. Kennedy Grove charges a fee for dogs and parking. The reservoir recreation area is open from sunrise to one hour before sunset; swimming is prohibited. Hikers and equestrians must have an East Bay Municipal Utility District use permit to hike the Eagle's Nest Trail; dogs and bikes are prohibited; and the trail is open from sunrise to one hour before sunset. Close gates behind you because of grazing cattle.

Facilities Water, restrooms, and phone at Kennedy Grove; restrooms at Inspiration Point; water and restrooms at Steam Trains on Lomas Cantadas Drive

From shady eucalyptus grove to narrow shoreline path to wide ridgetop trail, this route passes diverse landscapes and takes in far-flung views of the Bay Area. You'll climb 810 feet on wide East Bay Municipal Utility District trails through grasslands to San Pablo Ridge and then follow the paved ridgecrest trail to Inspiration Point.

Getting There

By Car

NORTH TRAILHEAD, KENNEDY GROVE: From Interstate 80 in the Richmond area, take the San Pablo Dam Road exit. Go east 4 miles to the park entrance on the left, 0.5 mile south of Castro Ranch Road.

From the Berkeley, Oakland, Orinda, and Walnut Creek area, take Highway 24 to the Orinda exit and turn north on Camino Pablo, which becomes San Pablo Dam Road. After passing San Pablo Dam Recreation Area, continue 1 mile to the Kennedy Grove entrance on the right.

SOUTHERN TRAILHEAD, INSPIRATION POINT: From Highway 24, take the Fish Ranch Road exit. Go 1 mile and turn right on Grizzly Peak Boulevard. Pass Lomas Cantadas Road and turn right on South Park Drive after 1.3 miles. Go 1.5 miles to Wildcat

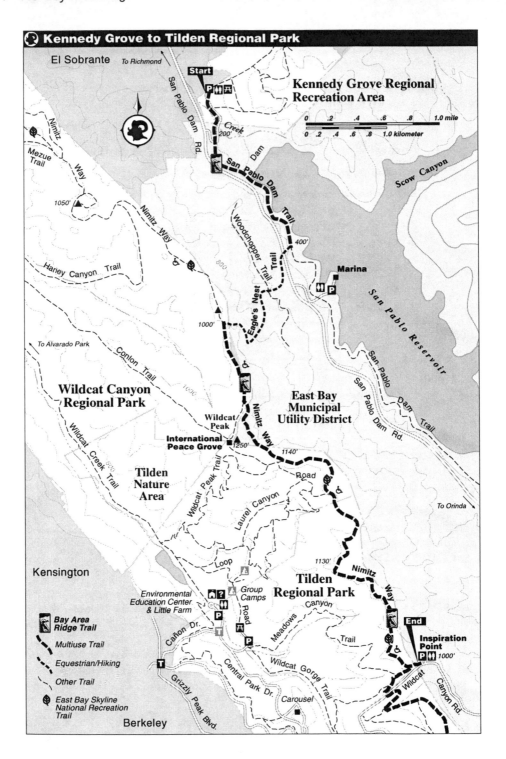

Kennedy Grove to Tilden Regional Park

El Sobrante *To Richmond*

Start

Kennedy Grove Regional Recreation Area

0 .2 .4 .6 .8 1.0 mile
0 .2 .4 .6 .8 1.0 kilometer

San Pablo Dam Rd.

Creek 200'

San Pablo Dam

Dam

San Pablo Dam Trail

400'

Marina

Nimitz Way

Mezue Trail

1050'

Woodchopper Trail

Scow Canyon

Haney Canyon Trail

800

Eagle's Nest Trail

1000'

To Alvarado Park

Conlon Trail

1000

Wildcat Canyon Regional Park

Wildcat Creek Trail

600

Nimitz Way

East Bay Municipal Utility District

San Pablo Dam Rd.

San Pablo Reservoir

Wildcat Peak

International Peace Grove 1250'

1140'

Tilden Nature Area

Wildcat Peak Trail

Road

To Orinda

Kensington

Laurel Canyon

Loop

1130'

Nimitz Way

Tilden Regional Park

Environmental Education Center & Little Farm

Group Camps

Canyon

Meadows

Cañon Dr.

Road

Trail

End

Inspiration Point 1000'

Central Park Dr.

Wildcat Gorge Trail

Grizzly Peak Blvd.

Carousel

Wildcat Canyon Rd.

Bay Area Ridge Trail

Multiuse Trail

Equestrian/Hiking

Other Trail

East Bay Skyline National Recreation Trail

Berkeley

> ## Rancho El Sobrante
>
> This trip takes you through lands that were once part of the 17,754-acre Rancho El Sobrante, granted to Juan José and Victor Castro in 1841. The rancho consisted of unclaimed lands between other established ranchos, hence its name, which translates as "the left-over place." The Castros maintained a flourishing ranch, grazed cattle on the surrounding hillsides, and shipped hides and tallow via bayside ports. By the 1870s, the Castros were beset by struggles with squatters and newly arrived settlers over legal rights to the land. A settlement granted the Castros only a small portion of the former rancho; however, they and their heirs continued operations on the land into the 1980s. Modern-day place names nearby—Castro Ranch Road, El Sobrante, and Sobrante Ridge—remind us of these early landowners.

Canyon Road and turn right. Follow it for about 1.5 miles to a large parking area on the left at Inspiration Point.

When South Park Drive is closed to motor vehicles during the salamander migration season (November to March), continue on Grizzly Peak Boulevard to Golf Course Drive. Turn right, pass the clubhouse, and turn right again on Shasta Road. Turn right on Wildcat Canyon Road, and continue about 1.6 miles to Inspiration Point.

From Interstate 80 in Berkeley, take the University Avenue exit, and head east for 2 miles to Oxford Street (border of the University of California–Berkeley campus). Turn left (north) on Oxford, and after a few blocks turn right (east) on Rose. Go one block, turn left (north) on Spruce, and continue to Grizzly Peak Boulevard. Cross Grizzly Peak and veer right (east) on Wildcat Canyon Road. Continue about 3 miles to Inspiration Point.

By Bus

An AC Transit bus serves Tilden Regional Park from downtown Berkeley; the weekend and holiday schedule and destinations are different from weekdays.

On the Trail

Hikers, equestrians, and **mountain bikers** start this trip in Kennedy Grove. Head west from the main parking area toward the spacious lawns and eucalyptus groves. Past the Senior Center, at the south edge of the next parking area, a Bay Area Ridge Trail sign marks a trail entrance on your left. Turn here and go downhill beside an intermittent stream; cross San Pablo Creek, easily forded except after heavy rains. Then bear left and reach Kennedy Grove's entrance road. Across the road, you go through a gate and enter East Bay Municipal Utility District land. Climb up the west side of San Pablo Dam to Old San Pablo Dam Road, now an unpaved trail, and follow it to the top of the dam.

Continue on Old San Pablo Dam Road, along the reservoir edge. You have glimpses of the water and Sobrante Ridge above it. Pass the road to the Oaks Picnic Area on your left and veer right, uphill. At a log gate beside San Pablo Dam Road, bear left and follow the road shoulder for 0.2 mile to a crosswalk. On the other side of the road, a gate leads into EBMUD watershed lands on the east side of San Pablo Ridge. Turn around

---

California and Nevada Railroad

Look for a boulder with a bronze plaque on the lawn just off the paved parking area. The plaque recounts the history of the California and Nevada Railroad, a wood-burning, narrow gauge train that ran through this valley in the 1890s. The train carried freight and farm products between Orinda and Oakland and introduced picnickers and vacationers to recreation sites along San Pablo Creek. Plagued by washouts in winter, dust in summer, and continual financial problems, the railroad never reached Nevada. Today's picnickers can see the wide swath of the train's former roadbed between the rows of eucalyptus trees in Kennedy Grove. The one-third-mile Kennedy Loop Trail that encircles the upper lawn passes picnic sites named for stops on this historic railroad.

---

here for a view of the reservoir's recreation complex, where visitors can enjoy picnicking, fishing, and boating.

Hikers and **equestrians** join the 0.9-mile Eagle's Nest Trail on the other side of the gate. Cross the Woodchopper Trail, veer left and then right almost immediately. From here the trip to the top of San Pablo Ridge traces a wide fire trail through eucalyptus groves and open grasslands. The eucalyptus trees were planted here and all over the Berkeley and Oakland hills around 1910. Originally planted for use as building material, the soft wood of eucalyptus proved useless for lumber, and the trees were never harvested.

Where the trail makes a wide swing to the right, you can look across the lake to identify landmarks. Sobrante Ridge rises from the east shore; little streams named for early settlers, including Sather and Dutra, flow through hillside canyons into the south end of the lake. You can see the Nunes Ranch in Scow Canyon, in operation since 1914; one of its original ranch buildings still stands.

When you reach the ridgetop, go through a gate into Wildcat Canyon Regional Park. Turn left (south) on Nimitz Way, named for World War II Admiral Chester Nimitz, who walked here daily in his retirement and scattered wildflower seeds. This paved multiuse trail is part of the 31-mile East Bay Skyline National Recreation Trail and the

---

Side Trip to Wildcat Peak

Hikers can make a short side trip to Wildcat Peak from Nimitz Way for views of the Golden Gate and a visit to the International Peace Grove. Turn left on the Conlon Trail, and climb to meet the Wildcat Peak Trail. Follow it to Wildcat Peak, where the vista point, enclosed by a double semicircle of low rock walls, and grove were established by Rotary International and East Bay Regional Park District. The grove and vista point offer the opportunity to contemplate the significance of friendship across the waters beyond the Golden Gate. Return to Nimitz Way.

Bay Area Ridge Trail. It runs for 4 miles along the crest of San Pablo Ridge, from a former Nike site northwest of here, to Inspiration Point.

You have remarkable views from this trail: San Francisco lies directly west across the bay; Mt. Tamalpais rises north of the Golden Gate; the Richmond-San Rafael Bridge crosses the northern bay, joining Marin and the East Bay; Pinole and Hercules peaks lie in the northwest; and due east, Mt. Diablo's 3849-foot summit rises above the surrounding plain.

Continue south along Nimitz Way. Pass the Conlon Trail (see "Side Trip to Wildcat Peak" on p. 142) and continue to the Laurel Canyon Trail, where another side trip leads to the Sequoia Grove, which was planted by the Berkeley Hiking Club.

On the last half mile of your trip on Nimitz Way, as you near Inspiration Point, you'll be in the company of casual walkers, hikers, bicyclists, roller-bladers, neighbors walking their dogs, and parents pushing strollers. Signs warn those on wheels to reduce their speed and call out before passing other trail users. Benches spaced conveniently along the way invite you to rest and enjoy the passing parade. Occasionally you can see Vollmer Peak, a high point on the Bay Area Ridge Trail route southeast through Tilden Regional Park.

Soon you skirt the stone pillars at the end of Nimitz Way and reach the Inspiration Point viewpoint and parking area. Below you lies San Pablo Reservoir, nestled between the rounded hills of San Pablo and Sobrante ridges. At the far north end of the lake lies Kennedy Grove; a 4.4-mile, mostly downhill trip will return you to your starting point there. The Inspiration and Lakeview trails downhill (east) connect with the Old San Pablo Dam Road for an alternate route back to Kennedy Grove.

San Pablo Dam

Built as a water supply for the growing population in Berkeley and surrounding areas, San Pablo Dam impounds the waters of San Pablo Creek. It was constructed by Anthony Chabot, who used hydraulic mining techniques to whittle away hillside rock and soil and sluice it to the dam site. The dam project began in 1916 and was completed in 1921, although the reservoir stood empty during many drought years. It wasn't until an aqueduct brought water from the Mokelumne River in 1936 that the reservoir reached capacity; it now stretches southeast for 3 miles.

In the 1970s, the reservoir was drained to rebuild the dam according to modern earthquake standards. Archaeologists found Native American artifacts in shell mounds and graves, clues to native settlements in the San Pablo Creek valley. (By 1810, most indigenous people from this area had been relocated to Mission San José; the few who remained to work on the Castro ranch died of pneumonia in 1850.)

Archaeologists also found former farm sites of early American settlers. Before the dam was built, ranchers ran both dairy and beef cattle, grew hay, and raised goats in this valley. Several dairies flourished, notably the Scow Dairy, for which Scow Canyon (due east of Kennedy Grove) is named, and the Varsity Creamery.

If you have a car shuttle waiting here, drive east down Wildcat Canyon Road for a little more history. On the northeast corner of the junction with San Pablo Dam Road remain the scant foundations of a hotel. Rancher and former army general Theodore Wagner built the hotel to serve passengers on the California and Nevada Railroad. Wagner's fine home is now the rural campus of John F. Kennedy University (southeast of this intersection). General Wagner surveyed and built Wildcat Canyon Road in 1889, though it was not paved until 1930.

◆ ◆ ◆

If you are continuing on the Bay Area Ridge Trail, see the next trail segment, which begins in Tilden Regional Park.

Tilden Regional Park to Redwood Regional Park

From Inspiration Point to Skyline Gate

Length 9.3 miles

Accessibility Hikers, equestrians, and mountain bikers

Agency East Bay Regional Park District

Regulations Tilden, Sibley, and Huckleberry are open from 5 AM to 10 PM, and dogs on leash are permitted. The East Bay Municipal Utility District, responsible for the trail between Tilden and Sibley, prohibits dogs and bikes and doesn't require a permit for this hike.

Facilities Restrooms at Inspiration Point; water, restrooms, and telephone at Steam Trains; water and restrooms at Sibley; water, restrooms, and telephone at Redwood

Climb to dramatic views from San Pablo Ridge, descend to wooded streamsides, and traverse open grasslands: This challenging trip along the spine of the East Bay Hills crosses varied landscapes on trails that range from wide and rocky service roads to duff-covered narrow paths. You'll find sheltered, tree-covered sections and exposed, breezy segments, and often encounter fog that rolls in from the Golden Gate. You'll gain and lose considerable elevation in short stretches—an 860-foot gain in Tilden Regional Park and a 600-foot loss in Robert Sibley Volcanic Regional Preserve.

Getting There

By Car

NORTH TRAILHEAD, INSPIRATION POINT: From Highway 24, take the Fish Ranch Road exit. Go 1 mile and turn right on Grizzly Peak Boulevard. Pass Lomas Cantadas Road and after 1.3 miles turn right on South Park Drive. Go 1.5 miles to Wildcat Canyon Road and turn right. Follow it for about 1.5 miles to a large parking area on the left at Inspiration Point.

When South Park Drive is closed to motor vehicles during the salamander migration season, November to March, continue on Grizzly Peak Boulevard to Golf Course Drive. Turn right, pass the clubhouse, and turn right again on Shasta Road. Turn right on Wildcat Canyon Road and continue about 1.5 miles to Inspiration Point.

From Interstate 80 in Berkeley, take the University Avenue exit and head east for 2 miles to Oxford Street (border of the University of California–Berkeley campus). Turn left (north) on Oxford, and after a few blocks turn right (east) on Rose. Go one block, turn left (north) on Spruce, and continue to Grizzly Peak Boulevard. Cross Grizzly Peak and veer right (east) on Wildcat Canyon Road. Continue about 3 miles to Inspiration Point.

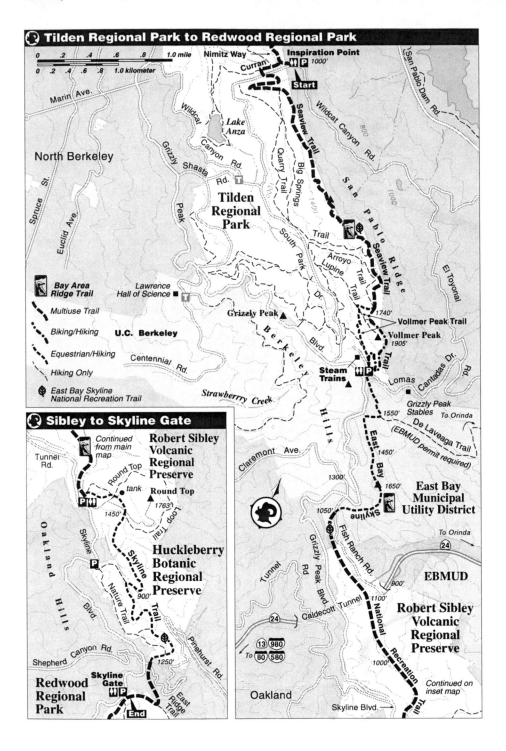

Tilden Regional Park to Redwood Regional Park

0   .2   .4   .6   .8   1.0 mile
0   .2   .4   .6   .8   1.0 kilometer

Nimitz Way
Curran
Inspiration Point
1000'
Start

Marin Ave.
North Berkeley
Spruce St.
Euclid Ave.
Wildcat Canyon Rd.
Lake Anza
Grizzly Peak
Shasta Rd.
Peak

Tilden Regional Park

Big Springs Trail
Quarry Trail
Seaview Trail
Wildcat Canyon Rd.
San Pablo Dam Rd.
San Pablo Ridge
900
1000
El Toyonal

South Park Dr.
Trail
Arroyo Lupine Trail
Seaview Trail
1740'

Bay Area Ridge Trail
Lawrence Hall of Science
Vollmer Peak Trail
Vollmer Peak 1905'

Multiuse Trail
Biking/Hiking   **U.C. Berkeley**
Equestrian/Hiking
Hiking Only
East Bay Skyline National Recreation Trail

Grizzly Peak ▲
Centennial Rd.
Blvd.
Berkeley Hills
Strawberry Creek

Steam Trains
Lomas
Cantadas Dr.
Rd.
Grizzly Peak Stables
1550'   To Orinda
De Laveaga Trail
(EBMUD permit required)

Sibley to Skyline Gate

Continued from main map
Robert Sibley Volcanic Regional Preserve
Tunnel Rd.
Round Top
tank
1450'
Round Top 1763'
Loop Trail

Oakland Hills
Skyline
Skyline Trail
900'
Nature Trail
Blvd.

Huckleberry Botanic Regional Preserve

Shepherd Canyon Rd.
1250'
Redwood Regional Park
Skyline Gate
End
East Ridge Trail
Pinehurst Rd.

Claremont Ave.
1300'
1450'
1050'
1650'
East Bay Municipal Utility District
To Orinda
24
Skyline

Grizzly Peak Blvd.
Fish Ranch Rd.
Tunnel Rd.
Caldecott Tunnel
1100'
900'
EBMUD

24
13 980
To 80 580

Robert Sibley Volcanic Regional Preserve

Oakland
National Recreation Trail
1000'
Continued on inset map
Skyline Blvd. →

SOUTH TRAILHEAD, SKYLINE GATE: From Highway 24 take the Fish Ranch Road exit. After 1 mile, turn left onto Grizzly Peak Boulevard. Continue to Skyline Boulevard and turn left. Continue 0.1 mile past Shepherd Canyon Road to Skyline Gate parking area on the left (east) side of Skyline Boulevard.

By Bus

An AC Transit bus serves Tilden Regional Park from downtown Berkeley; the weekend and holiday schedule and destinations are different from weekdays.

On the Trail

This 9.3-mile section of the Ridge Trail is part of the 31-mile East Bay Skyline National Recreation Trail (EBSNR Trail), also known as the Skyline Trail, which forms the backbone of a vast trail network in the East Bay. The Skyline Trail traverses East Bay Regional Park District and East Bay Municipal Utility District lands, from Wildcat Canyon Regional Park in Richmond to Cull Canyon Recreation Area in Castro Valley. Signposts display the Bay Area Ridge Trail logo, as well as the EBSNR Trail symbol.

Two trailheads en route make it possible to divide this 9.3-mile trip into shorter sections—at Lomas Cantadas Drive near the Steam Trains overflow parking lot (3 miles from Inspiration Point) and at the Robert Sibley Volcanic Regional Preserve parking area (3.4 miles from Lomas Cantadas Drive).

Inspiration Point to Lomas Cantadas Drive

From the trailhead at Inspiration Point, **all trail users** have impressive views of rolling hills and San Pablo and Briones reservoirs. You begin this trip from the west side of the parking area. Go around the stone gates to Nimitz Way, and immediately turn left onto the Curran Trail. Pass the Meadows Canyon Trail on the right, and then turn left on a narrow trail that leads uphill to Wildcat Canyon Road.

Cross the road and pick up the broad, multiuse Seaview Trail, which climbs steadily to reach the vistas that its name promises. Panoramic views unfold at every step (if the day is clear): through the Golden Gate to the sea; San Francisco Bay and its surrounding cities; and our tallest mountains—Tamalpais, St. Helena, and Diablo.

The Bay Area Ridge Trail route follows the Seaview Trail for 1.3 miles along San Pablo Ridge. This 1500-foot ridge was uplifted some 10 million years ago by stresses on the nearby Hayward and Moraga faults. Pass two junctions with the Big Springs Trail. At the Lupine Trail junction, **mountain bikers** split ways with both **hikers** and **equestrians**.

Mountain bikers continue straight on the Seaview Trail. You'll have splendid views of the North Bay hills as you climb; at the trail's highest point, look east across the ridges and valleys of Contra Costa County to Mt. Diablo, which dominates the landscape. Continue around the northeast side of Vollmer Peak (1913 feet) and then descend to the intersection of Lomas Cantadas and Grizzly Peak Boulevard, the end of the signed Ridge Trail route for bicyclists.

At the junction of Seaview and Lupine trails, **hikers** and **equestrians** turn right (south) on the Lupine Trail, marked bay area ridge trail and east bay skyline national recreation trail. (Be sure not to make a sharp right on the Arroyo Trail, which goes north from this junction.) Continue along a coyote bush-wild blackberry-tangled hillside below Vollmer Peak to a junction with the Vollmer Peak Trail, where you make a very

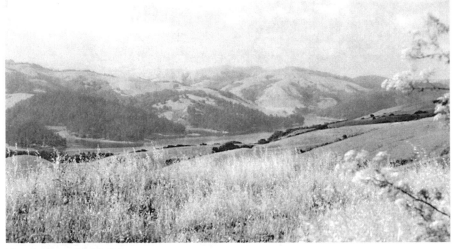

View from Inspiration Point

sharp left turn uphill (east). Climb 200 feet on this rocky path, and then veer right on the signed Bay Area Ridge Trail. (The Vollmer Peak Trail continues straight). Your narrow trail follows the contour of the steep hillside, through grasslands dotted with purple lupine and yellow mule ears in spring. Beyond a small bay-tree woods, you emerge at the Steam Trains overflow parking area. Pass through the parking area and meet the paved service road, where **bikers** rejoin the route; continue straight to reach the picnic area by the Steam Trains at Lomas Cantadas Drive.

Lomas Cantadas Drive to Sibley Preserve

The second segment of this trip, for **hikers** and **equestrians**, extends from Lomas Cantadas Drive to the Sibley preserve, a 3.4-mile trip. A narrow trail begins on the south side of the road and leads to a gate into EBMUD lands. Beyond the gate, the trail crosses a hillside carpeted with a variety of annual grasses and native perennial bunchgrasses and offers views east of the Contra Costa hills. In an oak woodland, you pass the De Laveaga Trail, which descends east to Orinda. You veer right, again in grasslands. In this peaceful scene of ranches nestled in valleys and cows grazing on hillsides, you can easily forget the proximity of nearby urban centers.

The trail soon makes a zigzag descent next to Grizzly Peak Boulevard to Fish Ranch Road. Cross the road and pass through the gate to the well-marked Skyline Trail. (Please close the gate). You have come 1.45 miles from Lomas Cantadas Drive.

Masses of poison oak and thistles border the narrow trail in some places, and fragrant sticky monkeyflower and cow parsnip blossom in spring and summer. As you head uphill to cross over the Caldecott Tunnel, you can hear the traffic on Highway 24 below, but near the top you will find a quiet, peaceful rest stop at a rustic bench in a mature oak woodland.

In an opening in these woods, proceed a few hundred yards along an old wagon road to a wooden gate on your right. Here you enter the Robert Sibley Volcanic Regional Preserve, and then continue another 2 miles on the EBSNR Trail. Keep to the north side of a creek, under a canopy of large evergreen oaks, multitrunked bays, and tall bigleaf maples. The trail crosses a bridge over the creek and turns due south, along the west side of the creek. You join a wide fire road and gain 300 feet in elevation to reach the Sibley parking area and visitor center.

Sibley Preserve to Skyline Gate

The third segment of this Ridge Trail route, 2.9 miles, starts at the entrance to the Sibley preserve. Take the narrow trail that begins just to the left (north) of the visitor center. Follow it 0.2 mile through pine forests to a junction with a gated road on your left. A side trip on the Round Top Loop Trail begins through this gate. Round Top is an extinct volcano that last erupted more than 9 million years ago. Deposits from this volcano underlie some of the ridges you traveled over along this Ridge Trail route. Pick up an explanatory brochure at the visitor center to learn about the exposed volcanic rocks in Sibley preserve.

To continue on the Ridge Trail route along the Skyline Trail, cross the Round Top Loop Trail and the paved road to the water tank, and follow a narrow trail 0.15 mile through a fragrant pine forest. Then you cross another paved road, which leads to Round Top's 1763-foot summit, and arrive at the top of a steep, rocky hillside, where the other end of the Loop Trail comes in from the east. You descend a rugged, precipitous, south-facing hillside, where you may see the brittleleaf and the pallid manzanitas, found in only two places in the world.

At the bottom, you reach San Leandro Creek Canyon and enter the East Bay Regional Park District's Huckleberry Botanic Regional Preserve. You cross San Leandro Creek on a defunct dam, under a dense cover of oak and bay trees grown spindly in their search for light. Make a sharp right turn (west) and start uphill on the north-facing slope. (A preserve gate bars an old trail along the creek, which is not recommended). Continue through this delightful, verdant section on a well-designed trail with a lush understory of ferns, ocean spray, and huckleberry. This preserve receives heavy winter rainfall and dense summer fogs. In the wet season, you may be crossing full-flowing rivulets coursing down the ravines.

At a junction about 200 yards on your uphill way, you make a sharp left turn (southeast); a gated trail goes straight, uphill, to Huckleberry's parking area on Skyline Boulevard. Your trail follows the contour of the hillside through a damp oak-and-bay forest and then climbs steeply up and around the head of a ravine. When you reach a junction with the Huckleberry Preserve Nature Trail, go left on the EBSNR Trail and cross warmer slopes in an oak-and-madrone forest.

Shortly you reach Pinehurst Road at its junction with Skyline Boulevard. Cross Pinehurst and proceed south along the east side of Skyline Boulevard, looking to your left for a trail entrance. Climb steeply through a eucalyptus grove, and continue over the hilltop to the junction with the East Ridge Trail in Redwood Regional Park. Turn right (southwest) on the East Ridge Trail, also the Skyline Trail, a broad service road. Continue about 0.25 mile to the Skyline Gate and the end of your trip. If you have a shuttle car waiting here, you can make this a one-way trip. Equestrians able to travel greater distances in a day than hikers can probably make this a round-trip.

◆ ◆ ◆

The next leg of the Bay Area Ridge Trail, an 8.3-mile trip, continues through Redwood Regional Park to Bort Meadow in Anthony Chabot Regional Park.

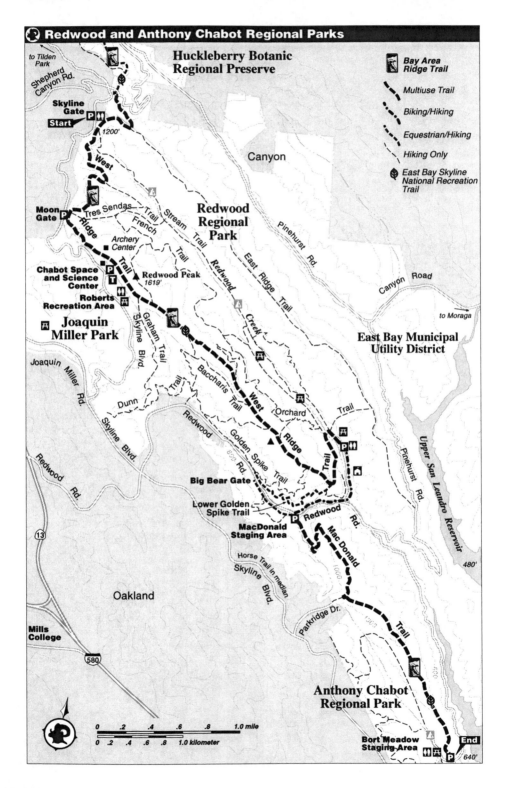

Redwood and Anthony Chabot Regional Parks

Huckleberry Botanic
Regional Preserve

to Tilden
Park

Shepherd
Canyon Rd.

Skyline
Gate
Start
1200'

West

Canyon

Redwood
Regional
Park

Moon
Gate

Tres Sendas Trail

French

Trail

Stream Trail

Archery
Center

Ridge Trail

Redwood

Redwood Peak
1619'

Chabot Space
and Science
Center

Roberts
Recreation Area

Skyline Blvd.

Graham Trail

Creek

Pinehurst Rd.

East Ridge Trail

Canyon Road

to Moraga

Joaquin
Miller Park

Joaquin Miller Rd.

Dunn Trail

Baccharis Trail

West

Orchard

Trail

East Bay Municipal
Utility District

Redwood

Ridge

Golden Spike Trail

Trail

Pinehurst Rd.

Upper San Leandro Reservoir

Skyline Blvd.

Redwood Rd.

Big Bear Gate

Lower Golden
Spike Trail

MacDonald
Staging Area

Redwood

Rd.

Mac Donald

1660

480'

Redwood Rd.

13

Horse Trail in median
Skyline Blvd.

Oakland

Parkridge Dr.

Skyline Blvd.

Trail

1560

Mills
College

580

Anthony Chabot
Regional Park

0   .2   .4   .6   .8   1.0 mile
0 .2 .4 .6 .8 1.0 kilometer

Bort Meadow
Staging Area

End
640'

Bay Area
Ridge Trail

Multiuse Trail

Biking/Hiking

Equestrian/Hiking

Hiking Only

East Bay Skyline
National Recreation
Trail

Redwood and Anthony Chabot Regional Parks

From Skyline Gate to Bort Meadow

Length	8.3 miles
Accessibility	Hikers, equestrians, and mountain bikers
Agency	East Bay Regional Park District
Regulations	Redwood and Anthony Chabot are open from 5 AM to 10 PM (or as posted). Dogs on leash are permitted.
Facilities	Water, restrooms, and telephone at Redwood; restrooms at MacDonald Staging Area; water and restrooms at Bort Meadow; group camping available at Bort Meadow and the Anthony Chabot family campgrounds by reservation

Follow the East Bay Skyline National Recreation Trail along the ridgeline of the East Bay hills to a broad valley, taking in views of rolling Contra Costa County ridges. You'll travel wide trails through second-growth redwoods, descend into a wooded canyon, and climb to open grasslands. Forested segments provide relief from warm sun or fog on open ridgetops. Elevation gain on this route is 700 feet, and loss is 1200 feet.

Getting There

By Car

NORTH TRAILHEAD, SKYLINE GATE: From Highway 24, take the Fish Ranch Road exit. After 1 mile, turn left onto Grizzly Peak Boulevard. Continue to Skyline Boulevard and turn left. Continue 0.1 mile past Shepherd Canyon Road to Skyline Gate parking area on the left (east) side of Skyline Boulevard.

SOUTH TRAILHEAD, BORT MEADOW STAGING AREA (BIG TREES): From Highway 13 in Oakland, take Redwood Road northeast. At the Pinehurst Road junction, veer right and continue on Redwood Road for 2 miles to the Bort Meadow Staging Area on the south side of the road.

By Bus

AC Transit bus buses run to Skyline Boulevard at Roberts Recreation Area on weekends only, and to Moon Gate.

On the Trail

This segment of the Bay Area Ridge Trail route continues southeast on the EBRPD's 31-mile East Bay Skyline National Recreation Trail (EBSNR Trail). **Hikers, equestrians,** and **mountain bikers** begin this trip from Skyline Gate on the West Ridge Trail. The wide, level path is frequented by a variety of trail users—strollers, bicyclists, runners, and local residents escorting their toddlers or walking their dogs. The first half mile is exposed, although oaks, madrones, pines, and eucalyptus trees fill the canyon below. After rains, a rivulet trickles down an assemblage of smooth, sandstone boulders.

Beneath the first clump of redwoods, the trail surface is sprinkled with soft duff, composed of redwood branchlets and small cones. These tall, second-growth redwoods, intermixed with luxuriant bay trees, support an understory of ferns and shade-loving white and blue wildflowers in spring.

You round a bend and pass the French Trail on the left, about a half mile from the trailhead. If the day is very hot, the French Trail offers a cool, though longer, route for hikers and equestrians; it follows the canyon wall midway between the high West Ridge Trail and the Stream Trail on the canyon floor.

After another 0.5 mile on the West Ridge Trail, you pass the Tres Sendas Trail on the left, a footpath that descends into the canyon to join the French Trail. Soon you pass a short spur on your right that leads to the Moon Gate at Skyline Boulevard and begin a steady climb around the flank of a hill dominated by communications equipment and a water tank. At the outer edge of the flank is a bench overlooking some of Redwood Regional Park's 1800 acres north and east of here.

For the next half mile the trail goes through an extensive eucalyptus forest. You may wonder about the origin of these trees: in the early 1900s, a real-estate developer planted vast eucalyptus forests in the Oakland hills, planning to use the wood for lumber; he also built Skyline Boulevard to take investors to his project. However, his timber-harvesting scheme was ill-fated, as eucalyptus wood turned out to be financially unprofitable. The trees were also ecologically disastrous: the fast-growing and invasive eucalyptus, an import from Australia, inhibits the growth of native plant species, such as redwood and oak trees.

Despite the dense, shaggy eucalyptus forests, some native plants spring up in the tangle of litter. You will see robust toyon bushes on the hillside and wild huckleberry bushes in moist ravines. You can recognize the huckleberries by their small, shiny green, oblong leaves on long, graceful branches; in late summer, you may see their blue-black

California's Biggest Redwoods

Redwood Regional Park was once the site of a magnificent redwood forest; some trees measured more than 20 feet in diameter, larger than the greatest redwood of the North Coast. Ships that entered the Golden Gate, 16 miles away, are said to have used two of the tallest trees to steer their course across San Francisco Bay.

This majestic redwood forest was part of early 19th-century Spanish land grants. Sadly, between 1840 and 1860, with the rapid growth of Bay Area cities—San Francisco, Oakland, Benicia, and Martinez—it was felled to the last tree; even the tree stumps were rooted out for firewood. After the 1906 earthquake, young redwoods that had sprouted from the remaining stumps were cut to rebuild devastated buildings. Today, all the redwoods in the park are second- or third-growth, although some trees tower above the ridges, reaching 100-foot heights. Former mill sites for the logging operations serve as picnic areas in the park.

berries, much-favored by deer and Steller's jays. You'll pass seven maple trees to the right of the trail, planted on Arbor Day in 1986, to commemorate the seven astronauts lost on the *Challenger*. A wooden plaque marks the site.

You cross the entrance road to the Chabot Space and Science Center and continue on the West Ridge Trail below the center. If you have time, stop in to see the exhibits and take a tour; if not, you will surely want to plan a visit. Cross another paved road and pass the Archery Center. Fog moisture drips from redwood trees along this wide, shady path and keeps it damp and cool. A fence lines the trail, its massive redwood posts draped with thick, green moss. About 2 miles from the trailhead, you reach inviting picnic facilities at Redwood Bowl, an open expanse on your left.

At the far end of Redwood Bowl, you meet the Graham Trail and bear left (east) to stay on the West Ridge Trail. (The Graham Trail leads off right to the swimming pool complex, children's play equipment, and picnic tables in the Roberts Recreation Area.) In 500 feet, the Peak Trail branches left on a 0.2-mile climb to 1619-foot Redwood Peak, the highest point in Redwood Regional Park. You continue on the Bay Area Ridge Trail route, still on the long ridge on the west side of the park. Following the ridgeline on a bare sandstone surface, this wide trail marks the limits of chaparral on the west and forest on the east. Best taken during the cool hours of a hot day, this trail's southwest-facing orientation is most welcome on cool but sunny winter days.

You pass the north and south ends of the Baccharis Trail on your right, as well as several trails that head into the redwood canyon on your left. The Orchard Trail drops into the canyon and meets Redwood Creek just east of the Orchard and Old Church picnic areas. In the 1920s settlers built small homes and a church and planted orchards in the cut forests. Some of their fruit trees still send out fragrant blossoms in spring.

Before long, the chaparral slopes on your left give way to a dense mixed woodland of oak, madrone, bay, and the occasional redwood. You may see deer bounding across the trail or hear them crashing in the woods. The West Ridge Trail descends steeply.

Hikers and **equestrians** leave the West Ridge Trail here and turn right (south) on a short spur trail, just before the West Ridge Trail makes a wide arc to the left (north). The spur trail joins the narrow Golden Spike Trail for a pretty trip through the woods, across a rivulet, and down the hillside to the Lower Golden Spike Trail. Here you swing left and emerge in a clearing (probably the site of a former settler's home), marked by exotic plantings, several sizable redwood trees, and a plank bridge across Redwood Creek.

Cross Redwood Road and veer left on the lovely, shady Big Bear Trail through Redwood Canyon; you are now in Anthony Chabot Regional Park. In spring, white plum blossoms glow among the dark conifers at the creekside. In summer, their deep purple leaves add contrast to the various greens of maples, sycamores, and bay laurels.

Mountain bikers stay on the West Ridge Trail, pass the hiker/equestrian spur trail, and reach the park entrance road. Cross a stone bridge at the Fishway Interpretive Site, and ride south on the entrance road. Turn right (west) on Redwood Road, and continue about 0.3 mile to the MacDonald Gate Staging Area.

Hikers, equestrians, and **bikers** meet again at the MacDonald Gate Staging Area to begin the second half of this trip, through 4927-acre Anthony Chabot Regional Park. The park was named for a pioneer Californian who built an earth-fill dam across San Leandro Creek to form Lake Chabot. Long before Chabot's time, the Ohlone people lived in these hills, fished the streams, hunted small game, gathered acorns, and dug bulbs for food.

Redwood's Native Trout

Explanatory plaques at the Fishway Interpretive Site tell the story of a unique species of rainbow trout, *Salmo iridia*. Descendants of the pure native strain of the original rainbow trout, these fish are found only in Redwood Creek. They migrate from a downstream reservoir up the creek to the park; a Denil Fishway near the park's Redwood Road entrance helps the trout reach their spawning grounds farther upstream. Because the fish are the subject of scientific studies, fishing is not permitted anywhere in Redwood Creek.

Begin your 3.2-mile trip through Anthony Chabot Park on the MacDonald Trail, another segment of the EBSNR Trail. Climb steeply on the wide, dirt park service road through oak woodlands to the park's central ridge; pause to look back northwest into wooded Redwood Canyon and over the vast public lands you have traversed. Just before the crest of the ridge, turn left on a little side trail that leads to a vista point. From a bench in this pleasant, shady spot you can see across a deep canyon to the opposite ridge where Pinehurst Road swings northwest. The town of Moraga lies beyond, and Mt. Diablo, the central survey point for Northern California, towers above the ridges and valleys of the East Bay.

Return to the MacDonald Trail, which travels just below the ridgetop, through grassland and chaparral. In 1 mile the trail arcs right and passes a junction with the Parkridge Trail; this trail begins at the park's south boundary and crosses a narrow, transverse ridge that divides two drainages—the eastern one feeds Chabot park's Grass Valley Creek.

You bear left on the MacDonald Trail and round a small knoll graced by a few oak trees and many wildflowers in spring. This trail continues for another 1.7 miles along the southwest-facing ridge with no tree cover, so plan to take it in the cool hours. On the ridgecrest above you, a fringe of oak trees grows; coyote bush (*baccharis*) gains a toehold on the grassy slope below you. Stay on the main park service road past many informal trails that branch off of the MacDonald Trail.

Before long, you begin to see the grassy valley and tall trees of Bort Meadow. Please stay on the trail to the green gate. The Bort Meadow Staging Area, the end of this Bay Area Ridge Trail segment, is about 500 yards beyond the green gate. To reach the staging area and parking lot, turn right on the trail that goes down to the valley. Then turn right again to find picnic tables, barbecues, water, and restrooms in Bort Meadow.

You can have a shuttle car waiting here to return to the Skyline Gate or to drive east on Redwood Road to family campsites in Anthony Chabot Park. (Use the Marciel Gate entrance to reach camping areas.) Group camping can be arranged for Bort Meadow; make reservations online at www.ebparks.org/activities/camping or by calling 1-888-EBPARKS.

◆ ◆ ◆

If you are continuing on the Ridge Trail route another 3.5 miles to Anthony Chabot campsites, head east on the Grass Valley Trail or the Brandon Trail.

Anthony Chabot Regional Park

From Bort Meadow to Chabot Staging Area

Length	6.1 miles
Accessibility	Hikers, equestrians, and mountain bikers
Agency	East Bay Regional Park District
Regulations	Park is open from 5 AM to 10 PM (or as posted). Dogs on leash are permitted.
Facilities	Water and restrooms at Bort Meadow; water and restrooms at Chabot Staging Area; group camping available at Bort Meadow by reservation

Explore the little-traveled lands of Chabot Regional Park. Your trail runs through a long, grassy valley beside a willow-lined creek and climbs gradually through eucalyptus forests to the ridgetop, a 340-foot elevation gain. Take in sweeping views to the east and then zigzag down 620 feet in the last 1.2 miles. Mostly on wide service trails, this route offers half sun and half shade.

Getting There

NORTH TRAILHEAD, BORT MEADOW STAGING AREA (BIG TREES): From Highway 13 in Oakland, take Redwood Road northeast. At the Pinehurst Road junction, veer right and continue on Redwood Road for 2 miles to Bort Meadow Staging Area on the south side of the road.

SOUTH TRAILHEAD, CHABOT STAGING AREA: From Interstate 580 eastbound, take the Redwood Road exit and turn left (north), passing under the freeway. Continue on Redwood Road about 3 miles. After the road narrows, pass the Willow Park Golf Course on your left. Where Redwood Road makes a hairpin turn to the left, the entrance to the Chabot Staging Area is on your right.

From Interstate 580 westbound take the Castro Valley Boulevard exit and continue west on it to Redwood Road. Turn right (north) and follow directions above.

MOUNTAIN BIKER TRAILHEAD, PROCTOR STAGING AREA: Follow directions for the Chabot Staging Area above, but after going 2 miles on Redwood Road, watch for the Proctor Staging Area on the left.

On the Trail

From the Bort Meadow Staging Area, **hikers, equestrians,** and **mountain bikers** take the gated service road that descends from the parking area (hikers can take the foot trail west of the parking area to the trail junction). At the bottom of the paved road, you can go right (north) about a quarter mile to visit Bort Meadow, a picnic and

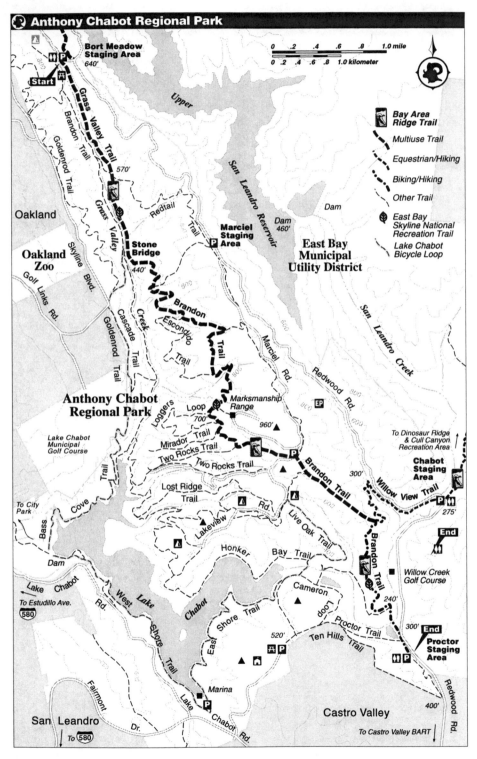

Anthony Chabot Regional Park

Bort Meadow
Staging Area
640'

Start

Upper

0 .2 .4 .6 .8 1.0 mile
0 .2 .4 .6 .8 1.0 kilometer

Grass Valley Trail

Brandon Trail

Goldenrod Trail

570'

Oakland

Grass Valley

Redtail
Trail

San Leandro Reservoir

Dam

Bay Area
Ridge Trail

Multiuse Trail

Equestrian/Hiking

Biking/Hiking

Other Trail

East Bay
Skyline National
Recreation Trail

Lake Chabot
Bicycle Loop

Oakland
Zoo

Oakland

Golf Links Rd.

Skyline Blvd.

Stone
Bridge
440'

Cascade Trail

Goldenrod Trail

Creek

Brandon

Escondido

Trail

Marciel
Staging
Area

Dam
460'

East Bay
Municipal
Utility District

San Leandro Creek

Marciel Rd.

Redwood Rd.

EP

Anthony Chabot
Regional Park

Loggers

Loop

Marksmanship
Range

960'

Lake Chabot
Municipal
Golf Course

Mirador
Trail

Two Rocks Trail

Two Rocks Trail

To Dinosaur Ridge
& Cull Canyon
Recreation Area

Chabot
Staging
Area

Willow View Trail

Brandon Trail

300'

275'

To City
Park

Cove

Lost Ridge
Trail

Rd.

Lakeview

Bass

Dam

Live Oak Trail

Honker Bay Trail

End

Brandon Trail

Willow Creek
Golf Course

Lake Chabot

To Estudillo Ave.
580

West

Lake

Chabot

East

Shore Trail

Shore Trail

Cameron

Loop

240'

520'

Proctor Trail

Ten Hills Trail

300' End

Proctor
Staging
Area

Fairmont

San Leandro

Marina

Lake

Chabot Rd.

Castro Valley

Dr.

To 580

To Castro Valley BART

400'

Redwood Rd.

From Ranchland to Parkland

Once the 525-acre Grass Valley Ranch, this area was purchased by the East Bay Regional Park District in 1951 and called Grass Valley Park. Today it is part of 4,927-acre Anthony Chabot Regional Park. Later additions to today's park included the lands of Don Luis Maria Peralta and Don Guillermo Castro, who raised cattle to sell the hides for leather. In the 1860s, Don Castro's accumulated gambling debts led to the sale of his lands, which were later subdivided and sold to American beef cattle ranchers. As the Bay Area population grew, these lands became valuable watershed and were eventually consolidated into the East Bay Municipal Utility District. The EBRPD now leases the Lake Chabot area from EBMUD and makes it available for public recreation.

group camping area enclosed by high ridges and rimmed by tall eucalyptus and young redwood trees.

The Bay Area Ridge Trail route goes left (south) through Grass Valley on the Grass Valley Trail, a segment of the East Bay Skyline National Recreation Trail. For the next mile, the trail traverses the east side of the valley, bordered by the willow-lined Grass Valley Creek and chaparral slopes. Across the creek, the Brandon Trail runs parallel to the Grass Valley Trail. The trails converge at the stone bridge at the south end of the valley. Cattle often graze on or near the trail; even if you don't see them, heed the signs asking you to close gates. On the eastern ridge, power-line towers are perches for indigenous creatures—red-tailed hawks, which search the grasslands for rodents on broad, flat wings, and turkey vultures, whose wide, V-shaped wings and wobbly flight distinguish them from the hawks.

You pass the Redtail Trail on the left, just 1 mile from the trailhead. Then the valley narrows and your trail edges closer to the creek; you enter a eucalyptus grove, where coyote bush and young redwoods grow among the trees. The eucalyptus forests in this park were planted in the 1910s by the People's Water Company of Oakland; they spread rapidly and greatly altered the ecology of the hills. Severe freezes in the last 30 years turned the eucalyptus brown, but these hardy trees still survive. If you pass through eucalyptus groves on a foggy or rainy day, you will probably notice the trees' characteristic menthol fragrance.

Soon the Grass Valley and Brandon trails meet at the stone bridge, where the Grass Valley Trail terminates and the Brandon Trail crosses to the east side of the valley. Take a moment to walk out on the bridge to admire its huge sandstone block construction. Downstream from the bridge, Grass Valley Creek courses southeast through a tight canyon to reach Lake Chabot.

Now Ridge Trail users follow the Brandon Trail uphill as it gently climbs into the heads of ravines and around bends. This wide park service road is part of the well-traveled Lake Chabot Bicycle Loop. In about a quarter mile, you pass an old trail that takes off left, but you continue on the broad Brandon Trail through the eucalyptus forest. In spite of the eucalyptus's dominance, the trail is edged with blackberries, ferns, and seasonal blossoms—inconspicuous creamy white miner's lettuce and white, four-petaled milkmaids early in spring. In sunny areas, you may see the white clusters of Fremont lilies atop their long stalks and the vibrant orange hues of California poppies. Ubiquitous poison oak plants explode each spring with shiny green, three-lobed leaves. In fall, you can easily recognize poison oak by its brilliant red and orange leaves. At any time of the year, this plant should be avoided.

Almost a mile from the stone bridge, you pass the right-branching Escondido Trail and continue straight (east) on the Brandon Trail as it curves into canyons and rounds shoulders of the hillside. The prints of many trail users mark the sandy surface of the trail—the corrugated tread of athletic shoes, the continuous pattern of bicycle tires, U-shaped prints of equestrians' steeds, spindly, three-toed bird prints, and the paw prints of many animals. If you look closely, you may see the sinuous track of a snake's passage. After you pass the other end of the Escondido Trail and make a deep sweep into the back of a ravine, you begin to hear rifles cracking in the forest. Unnerving as the noise may be, these weapons are contained in a marksmanship range.

You emerge from the shade of the eucalyptus groves to a south-facing, sloping grassland. Continue through grasslands on the Brandon Trail, past the Logger's Loop, Mirador, and Two Rocks trails to Marciel Road. Across Marciel Road, you'll find a parking area and restrooms. (If you plan to camp in the park, take the Towhee Trail right [south] to reach the campground kiosk.)

Continue on the Bay Area Ridge Trail route; after less than a quarter mile, you will find some trailside boulders—good perches for lunch or views northeast across two canyons to Dinosaur Ridge, the highest point of the next Ridge Trail segment. On clear days, the ridge's distinctive white rock is visible from here, almost 2 miles away. Beyond is an impressive vista of the East Bay's seemingly endless succession of rugged ridges.

When it's time to move on, start down the ridgetop trail flanked by evergreen oaks, toyon, and coyote bush. On the Brandon Trail, immediately past the Willow View Trail,

Poppy and fossils on Dinosaur Ridge

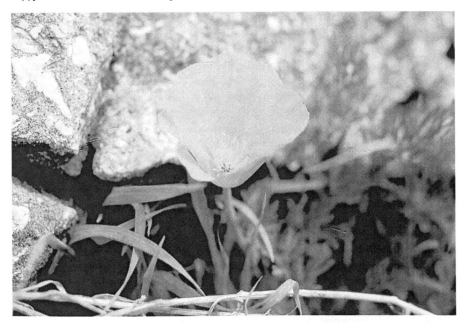

bicyclists curve right sharply. Continue downhill on the Brandon Trail for another 1.6 miles to the Proctor Staging Area, the end of the Ridge Trail route for bicyclists.

On the left, the Willow View Trail begins beside a bench in the shade of a beautiful evergreen oak tree. **Hikers** and **equestrians** descend this trail into the woods on the east side of the ridge. You wind along the canyonside under oaks and madrones and pass huge sandstone outcrops decorated with feathery moss and high trail banks festooned with ferns. The trail drops more than 200 feet in 0.3 mile and then travels upstream along a little tributary of San Leandro Creek. You cross the tributary and then follow it downstream for another 0.3 mile. This trail, delightfully cool on a hot day, might be muddy after heavy winter rains.

A canopy of bushes and trees shields the trail from Redwood Road, which runs along the bank above this section of the Willow View Trail. An old fence post entwined with wild cucumber vines, a remnant of former ranching days, is on the right side of the trail. A little farther down the trail lies a jumble of smooth-edged, lichen-encrusted boulders under overarching oak and bay trees, from which you can watch the golfers on adjacent Willow Park Golf Course.

Continue on the Willow View Trail north, through a damp, woodsy flat; in early spring, a fabulous garden of three-petaled trillium flowers blossom in shades of pink, mauve, and burgundy. These plants are worth a special trip to see. In the midst of this garden, the Bay Area Ridge Trail arcs right at a fork in the trail; it then crosses the creek and goes under Redwood Road. (After heavy rains, take the left trail out to Redwood Road.) The Chabot Staging Area, on the other side of the road, is the end of this Bay Area Ridge Trail segment for **hikers** and **equestrians**.

◆ ◆ ◆

The Bay Area Ridge Trail continues from the Chabot Staging Area on to Independent School.

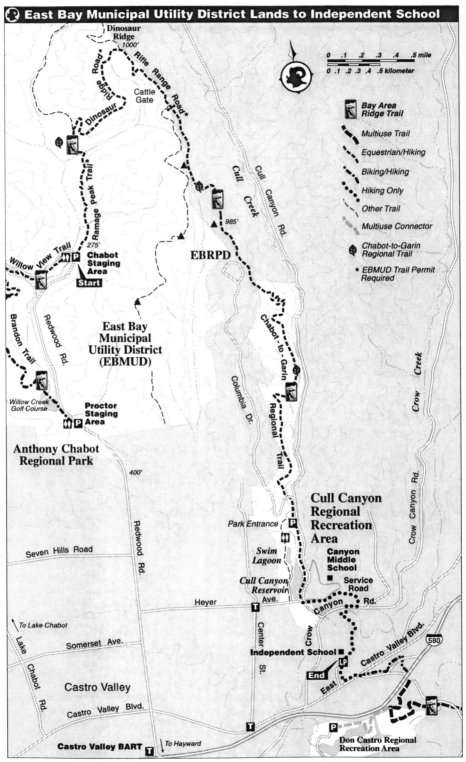

East Bay Municipal Utility District Lands to Independent School

Dinosaur
Ridge
1000'

Rifle Range Road*

Ridge Road*

Cattle
Gate

Dinosaur

Ramage Peak Trail*

275'

Cull Creek

Cull Canyon Rd.

985'

EBRPD

Willow View Trail

Chabot
Staging
Area

Start

Brandon Trail

Redwood Rd.

**East Bay
Municipal
Utility District
(EBMUD)**

Chabot - to - Garin

Regional Trail

Columbia Dr.

Crow Creek

Willow Creek
Golf Course

**Proctor
Staging
Area**

**Anthony Chabot
Regional Park**

400'

0   .1   .2   .3   .4   .5 mile
0 .1 .2 .3 .4 .5 kilometer

Bay Area
Ridge Trail

Multiuse Trail

Equestrian/Hiking

Biking/Hiking

Hiking Only

Other Trail

Multiuse Connector

Chabot-to-Garin
Regional Trail

* EBMUD Trail Permit
Required

**Cull Canyon
Regional
Recreation
Area**

Park Entrance

Swim
Lagoon

**Canyon
Middle
School**

Service
Road

Cull Canyon
Reservoir
Ave.

Seven Hills Road

Redwood Rd.

Heyer

Canyon   Rd.

To Lake Chabot

Somerset Ave.

Center St.

Crow

Independent School

End

Castro Valley Blvd.

580

Castro Valley

Lake Chabot Rd.

Castro Valley Blvd.

East

Crow Canyon Rd.

Castro Valley BART

To Hayward

**Don Castro Regional
Recreation Area**

East Bay Municipal Utility District Lands to Independent School

From Chabot Staging Area and Cull Canyon Regional Recreation Area to Independent School

Length	8.4 miles (7.2 miles from Chabot Staging Area to Cull Canyon Recreation Area and 1.2 miles from Cull Canyon to Independent School)
Accessibility	Hikers and equestrians
Agencies	East Bay Regional Park District and East Bay Municipal Utility District
Regulations	Dogs and bikes are prohibited on the East Bay Municipal Utility District trails from Chabot Staging Area to the water-tank clearing, and an EBMUD permit is required. The EBRPD trail through Cull Canyon Regional Recreation Area to Independent School is open from dawn to dusk, permits dogs, prohibits bikes, and doesn't require a permit.
Facilities	Restrooms at Chabot Staging Area and restrooms and water at Cull Canyon Regional Recreation Area

A long ramble through rolling grasslands arrives at a popular swimming, fishing, and picnicking site. This exposed route begins with a steady, 2-mile, 920-foot ascent on a path through oak woodlands. You arrive at Dinosaur Ridge and its 360-degree views, follow wide service roads along a rolling ridgetop, pass through cattle-grazed lands with little shade, and then descend to Cull Creek. From Cull Canyon Regional Recreation Area, hikers can continue on a shadier trail past residential areas.

Getting There

NORTH TRAILHEAD, CHABOT STAGING AREA: From Interstate 580 eastbound, take the Redwood Road exit and turn left (north), passing under the freeway. Continue on Redwood Road about 3 miles. After the road narrows, pass the Willow Park Golf Course on your left. Where Redwood Road makes a hairpin turn to the left, the entrance to the Chabot Staging Area is on your right. From I-580 westbound take the Castro Valley Boulevard exit, continue west on it to Redwood Road Turn right (north), and follow directions above.

SOUTH TRAILHEAD, CULL CANYON RECREATION AREA: From Interstate 580 eastbound, take the Center Street exit, and go north on Center Street. Turn right (east) on Heyer Avenue, turn left (north) on Cull Canyon Road, and then turn left into the recreation area parking lots. From I-580 westbound, take the Castro Valley exit, turn left (west) on East Castro Valley Boulevard, and then go right (north) on Crow Canyon Road. After 0.6 mile, turn left (northwest) onto Cull Canyon Road and proceed to the recreation area.

SOUTH TRAILHEAD, INDEPENDENT SCHOOL: From Interstate 580 eastbound, take the Crow Canyon Road exit, cross over the freeway, turn right on East Castro Valley Boulevard, cross Crow Canyon Road, and turn left on Independent School Road Park outside school gates on a cul-de-sac. From I-580 westbound, take the East Castro Valley Boulevard exit, turn right on it, and then turn left on Independent School Road.

On the Trail

With your East Bay Regional Park District permit in hand, **hikers** and **equestrians** leave the east side of the Chabot Staging Area and go a few paces along a graveled road to the East Bay Municipal Utility District's Ramage Peak Trail entrance on your right. Also well-marked as the Bay Area Ridge Trail, this path leads into a shady glade and then winds uphill through oak woodlands on the east side of San Leandro Creek canyon.

About 0.75 mile from the trail entrance, you drop into the Tamler Memorial Redwood Grove, dedicated to the father of Lou Tamler. Lou supervised the Civilian Conservation Corps crew that built this trail.

In another 0.25 mile the Bay Area Ridge Trail route veers right (east) on Dinosaur Ridge Road, a wide ranch road. After a couple of zigzags under the power lines, the trail heads straight up the nose of a bare hillside. An elevation gain of 480 feet in less than a half mile promotes frequent stops to enjoy views back across San Leandro Creek canyon and the forested ridges of Anthony Chabot Regional Park and out to San Francisco Bay.

Partway up, the trail curves around a knoll and levels off a little; it then dips into a saddle before beginning another ascent. Looking ahead to the heights of Dinosaur Ridge, you see large white protrusions on the rounded mountaintop; regularly spaced and jagged, they stretch across the summit. From here it's unclear what they might be.

About 2 miles from your start, at a trail junction just below the summit, a Bay Area Ridge Trail sign points east, and wisely avoids an old ranch road that leads directly uphill; you follow the Ridge Trail route around to the east flank.

The Ridge Trail turns right (south) on Rifle Range Road, which you follow for about a mile, passing grazing cattle. Although oak and bay trees fill the canyons below the trail, only a few offer shelter on this west-facing slope. However, wildflowers, including lupine, wild cucumber, and Indian paintbrush, bloom in an extravagant display of color in springtime.

Turn left (east) where the Bay Area Ridge Trail leaves Rifle Range Road, and follow a short connector trail uphill to a green cattle gate. (Be sure to close the gate.) Beyond this gate turn right (south) beside an electric cattle fence. For a little more than a mile you are on an easement through private land. (Please stay on the trail and respect private property rights.) Your views open up eastward: steep-sided ridges clothed in spring green or summer gold, canyons filled with dark green oak and bay trees, and Mt. Diablo's pyramid in the distance.

You pass through two more green gates, with shy cattle clustered nearby at watering troughs and salt licks, and enter a broad clearing behind a subdivision surmounted by a

Side Trip to Dinosaur Ridge

The 0.2-mile side trip to the summit of Dinosaur Ridge is a worthwhile detour that reveals the derivation of the ridge's name. Turn left where the Bay Area Ridge Trail turns right (south) to join Rifle Range Road and climb gently on a short path to the ridge. The jagged protrusions indeed look like the protective plates or fins of a giant dinosaur; a closer look discloses white seashell fossils embedded in the rocks. Probably uplifted from the ocean floor during some ancient folding/faulting process, these rocks remained when softer materials eroded away.

From the top of Dinosaur Ridge you have around-the-compass views of the Bay Area—west to the Golden Gate guarded by Mt. Tamalpais, north to Mt. Street Helena, east to ridge after ridge of open space lands capped by Mt. Diablo, and south to Mt. Umunhum and Loma Prieta. To the southeast, your trail undulates along the ridgetops toward Cull Canyon.

water tank. This is the EBMUD/EBRPD boundary and the north end of the Cull Canyon Regional Recreation Area; you have come 4 miles from Chabot Staging Area. Cross the clearing and descend into a beautiful forest on the Chabot-to-Garin Regional Trail. Wide-branched, symmetrically shaped specimen oaks stand at several switchbacks, immense bay trees grow around sandstone boulders, and shady stream canyons indent the steep hillside. On warm days, you will be pleased to plunge into these east-facing woods. Trailside gardens of blue hounds' tongue, blood-red trillium, and white milkmaids are early spring treats. Later in the year wild roses show their pink blossoms, and in the fall, white snowberries hang on bare-branched shrubs.

About halfway through this trip, you step out onto a knoll with views over Cull Canyon. Here the trail becomes a wide, bare path through a pygmy forest of coyote bush. On a grassy shoulder between two forested canyons, you can find sunny picnic places or sheltered rest stops under wide-spreading oaks. You'll also find yellow suncups, blue-eyed grass, and blue brodiaea blooming beside and along the trail when in season. You then plunge back into the forest and zigzag down the mountain to steep-sided Cull Creek and the sounds of frogs croaking and birds singing. The creek is easily forded on rocks at low water, but it may be more difficult to cross in the wet season.

A surprise awaits on the other side of the creek—fluffy-furred, thin-legged, steely-eyed llamas grazing in a pasture. A charming Victorian house across the pasture brings reality to a momentary illusion of the high Andes. These sure-footed Andean creatures are sometimes used as pack animals for local mountains too.

The trail gently undulates along Cull Creek for about a mile, up and down its high, fern-draped banks, back into ravines to cross intermittent streambeds, through a flowery meadow, and again into the woods. The creek is diverted through a huge culvert under Columbia Drive; **hikers** and **equestrians** follow a path through the culvert as well, to enter Cull Canyon Regional Recreation Area.

Just over 7 miles from Chabot Staging Area, Cull Canyon provides opportunities to swim and fish in the lake and to picnic at tables beside it. This popular recreation area is an attractive place to spend a few hours with friends who could meet you here after your trip.

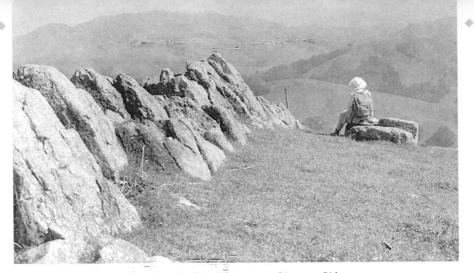

Uplifted rocks with embedded fossilized shells surmount Dinosaur Ridge.

The Bay Area Ridge Trail continues a short distance south to Independent School, for **hikers** only. **Equestrians** can ride back to the Chabot Staging Area from Cull Canyon Regional Recreation Area, for an approximately 14-mile round-trip. Or they can have a horse trailer waiting in the unpaved parking area at Cull Canyon Regional Recreation Area.

To continue to Independent School, **hikers** follow the lake's east shore for about a half mile on a path bordered by tall willow trees. To the tune of ducks quacking and red-winged blackbirds singing in the dense rushes, you continue until the trail rises to the side of Cull Canyon Road. At Heyer Avenue you cross Cull Canyon Road at the stoplight and then proceed uphill along the south side of Canyon School Road.

The Bay Area Ridge Trail route stays on the road's unpaved shoulder to the crest of the hill and then descends on an asphalt service road to Crow Canyon Road. Turn right on Crow Canyon Road and head downhill to a stoplight. Cross the road and bear right; cross a side street on your left and in a few paces enter a woodland trail on your left. Under arching oaks, this trail ascends the sheer side of the fern-draped canyon of Cull Creek.

As the trail climbs steadily, the woodland thins out. Now you see straight down to homes along the creek and above to fences, some quite elaborate, enclosing manicured gardens of an adjoining subdivision. After a last little rise, the trail edges Independent School's fenced playground and emerges at a cul-de-sac, the trail's end.

Since the trip back to Chabot Staging Area is more than 8 miles, hikers might prefer to avoid the long round-trip by having a shuttle car waiting at the cul-de-sac near Independent School.

The next dedicated segment of the Ridge Trail begins here at Independent School.

Independent School to Five Canyons

From Independent School through Don Castro Regional Recreation Area to Five Canyons

Length	5.4 miles round-trip from Independent School; 4 miles round-trip from Don Castro Regional Recreation Area
Accessibility	Hikers, equestrians, and mountain bikers
Agency	East Bay Regional Park District
Regulations	Dogs on leash are permitted. Respect private property.
Facilities	Restrooms, water, and telephone at Don Castro Regional Recreation Area

Follow city streets, a creekside path under a shady canopy, and trails through gently contoured grasslands to high meadows with 360-degree views of East Bay ridges and canyons. Most of this trip is in full sun.

Getting There

By Car

INDEPENDENT SCHOOL: From Interstate 580 eastbound, take the Crow Canyon Road exit, cross over the freeway, and turn right on East Castro Valley Boulevard. Cross Crow Canyon Road and turn left on Independent School Road to limited parking outside school gates on street.

From I-580 westbound, take the East Castro Valley Boulevard exit, turn right on it, and then left on Independent School Road.

DON CASTRO REGIONAL RECREATION AREA: From Interstate 580 eastbound, take the Center Street exit in Castro Valley. Go right on Center, left on Kelly Street, and then left on Woodroe Avenue to park entrance. Park at Ridgetop Picnic Area. From I-580 westbound, take the Castro Valley exit and go west on East Castro Valley Boulevard. Turn left on Grove Way, left on Center, left on Kelly, and then left on Woodroe to park entrance. Park at Ridgetop Picnic Area.

By Bus

Trailhead is accessible from BART daily and an AC Transit bus hourly.

On the Trail

Hikers and **mountain bikers** can begin this 2.7-mile (one-way) trip near the gate to Independent School and follow city streets east to Five Canyons Parkway, or do a 2-mile (one-way) trip that starts at the Ridgetop Picnic Area in Don Castro Regional Recreation Area. **Equestrians** begin this segment at the recreation area.

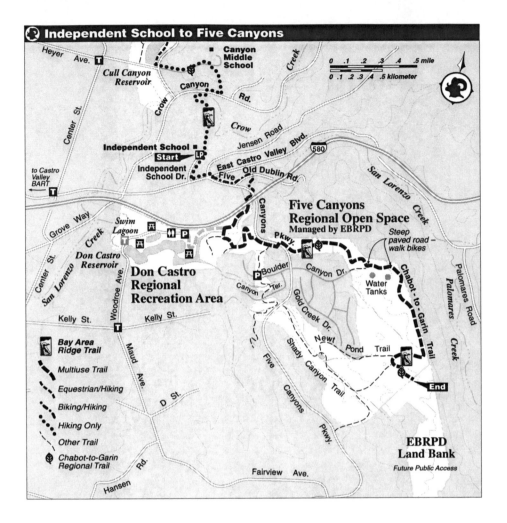

Independent School to Five Canyons

Independent School to Don Castro Regional Recreation Area

As you leave the Independent School gate, **hikers** and **mountain bikers** turn left (east) on East Castro Valley Boulevard. Stay on the north sidewalk until after crossing Jensen Road; then cross East Castro Valley Boulevard at the stoplight and entrance to Five Canyons Parkway. Cross Five Canyons Parkway at the crosswalk, and shortly veer left onto Old Dublin Road. On a short descent along this narrow paved road, look for a trail on the right, which drops down to the first of three bridges over San Lorenzo Creek that you will cross on this trip. Swollen by Eden and Palomares creeks, this stream flows full and swift in winter but becomes a gentle trickle in summer. Turn right (west) on the other side of the bridge and go under the high, arched span of I-580. Continue above the creek on a narrow paved road under the shade of willows and oaks to a second bridge, beyond which your quiet route runs adjacent to, but below I-580.

At the third and last bridge, the trail and creek widen as they approach the lake at Don Castro Regional Recreation Area. Beyond this bridge, a spur trail goes right (uphill) to parking, picnic tables, barbecues, water, a telephone, restrooms, fishing, and swimming at Don Castro Recreation Area.

Don Castro Regional Recreation Area to Five Canyons Regional Open Space

From Don Castro, **hikers, equestrians,** and **mountain bikers** descend a wide, steep trail that bends northeast along San Lorenzo Creek. Cross a bridge over the creek and go left uphill on a wide, rocky trail under a canopy of oaks, bays, and eucalyptus. When you reach a paved road, go left on it and watch for a trail entrance on the right, which is just beyond a rest area on the left. Framed by a semicircle of large boulders and shaded by a canopy of live oaks, it is a pleasant place to listen to birdsong while enjoying a little rest.

This narrow trail climbs switchbacks up a steep, grassy hillside dotted with spring wildflowers. At Five Canyons Parkway, continue right and uphill on the sidewalk (equestrians use the gravel path next to the sidewalk) to a crossing that leads to a trail along the south side of a swale and drainage area below the houses in the Five Canyons development. After crossing a concrete drainage ditch, your ascent becomes steeper and quite rocky but in springtime is festooned with blossoms of deep purple lupines and bright orange poppies.

Shortly you go through an East Bay Regional Park District gate and traverse a hillside trail to a very steep paved road that leads to two immense East Bay Municipal Utility District water storage tanks. Pass through another EBRPD gate and take in ridgetop views: the Bay Area Ridge Trail route through Contra Costa County lies to the north and west and a future route to Garin Park lies to the southeast.

You now wander southeast on the ridge above Palomares Creek Canyon, through gentle, open grasslands with 360-degree views of East Bay hills, canyons, forested ridges, and burgeoning subdivisions. Past isolated trees sprouting from jumbled outcrops and stock ponds for thirsty cattle and local wildlife, you turn right and make a short descent to end your trip at another green gate. Retrace your steps to your starting point, either Independent School or Don Castro Recreation Area. Someday this Ridge Trail trip will be extended across the intervening hills and valleys to Garin Park.

◆ ◆ ◆

The next segment of the Ridge Trail visits Mission Peak Regional Preserve and Ed R. Levin County Park.

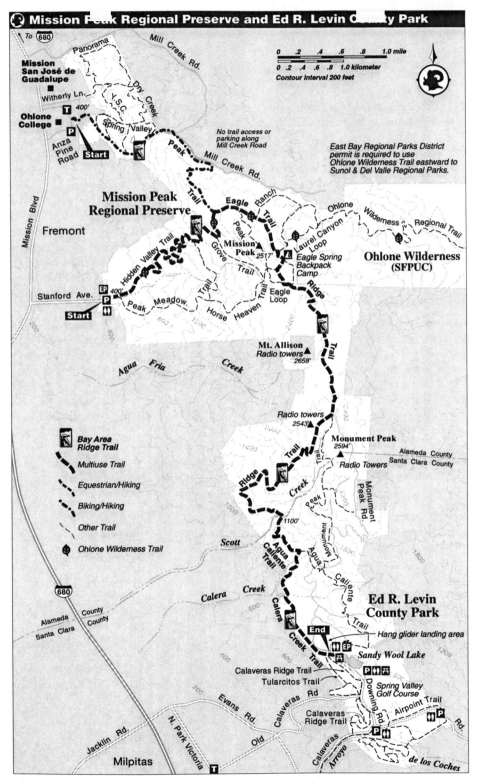

Mission Peak Regional Preserve and Ed R. Levin County Park

From Ohlone College to Sandy Wool Lake

Length   10.4 miles

Accessibility Hikers, equestrians, and mountain bikers

Agency   East Bay Regional Park District

Regulations   Mission Peak Regional Preserve is open from 5 AM to 10 PM (or as posted) but may be closed during extreme fire-danger periods; dogs must be under voice control in open space areas. Ed R. Levin County Park is open from 8 AM to dusk, charges an entrance fee on weekends, prohibits dogs on trails but allows them on a 6-foot leash in designated areas. Cattle graze along the entire trail; close gates behind you.

Facilities   No drinking water at all; water, restrooms, and telephone at Ohlone College and Stanford Avenue Staging Area; chemical toilet at junction of Hidden Valley and Peak trails; water, restrooms, and telephone in Ed Levin Park

Climb through high grasslands past three lofty peaks that top a rugged ridgeline. You'll have views of rippling hills, tree-filled canyons, and bayshore marshlands from these exposed and often windy trails. Get an early start to do the bulk of the 2220-foot elevation gain before the day warms and to watch the sun rise above the fog-shrouded peaks, illuminating the landscape with an ethereal glow. With a 1920-foot elevation loss, you'll encounter some very steep segments in the final 4-mile descent to a pretty lake in a quiet valley. The side trip to Mission Peak's summit is on a narrow, steep, and rocky trail.

Getting There

By Car

NORTH TRAILHEAD, OHLONE COLLEGE: From Interstate 680 in Fremont, take the Washington Boulevard exit and turn east. Go right (south) on Mission Boulevard and turn left on Anza Pine Road to Ohlone College parking. On weekends and holidays, parking is free in the college lots. When college is in session, obtain a parking permit for a small fee at the vending machines in Lot D or H, and park in any lot.

ALTERNATE NORTH TRAILHEAD AND EQUESTRIAN STAGING AREA: In Fremont, take Mission Boulevard to Stanford Avenue. Turn east and continue to parking at the end of the road.

SOUTH TRAILHEAD, ED LEVIN PARK: From Interstate 680 in Milpitas, take the Calaveras Road exit and continue east to park entrance. Turn left on Downing Road and continue to parking at Sandy Wool Lake. The trailhead is near the hang-glider landing zone across from the parking area. The equestrian staging area is near Sandy Wool Lake.

By Bus

AC Transit lines run to Ohlone College daily. Separate lines run daily to the intersection of Mission Boulevard and Stanford Avenue.

On the Trail

Hikers and **mountain bikers** begin this trip from the parking area at Ohlone College on the southern leg of Anza Pine Road. Cross the road and pick up the adjoining, paved Ohlone Trail. Follow it uphill, turn right (east), and go past the swimming pool, where a dirt service road leads to the green gate into Mission Peak Regional Preserve. (There are many gates on this hike, each of which should be shut after you.)

Take the Peak Trail, the wide service road on your right (south), where a signpost bears a Bay Area Ridge Trail logo. The trail heads uphill under a string of power lines, and views of the South Bay and its urban fringe unfold as you climb steadily around the west side of a 1000-foot hill.

Continue uphill past a small cave carved into the limestone bank, and bend north around the shoulder of the hill above a tree-canopied creek canyon. For the next half mile, you climb through a narrow pass between high, rounded hills; in early spring, masses of shiny, yellow-faced buttercups and luminous, purple lupines cover these grasslands. In a basin at the top of the rise, a seasonal cattle pond sits among three hills; you might see swallows and red-winged blackbirds here also.

Bear right under evergreen oak and bay trees to follow the Peak Trail. As you pass through this shady glen, small rabbits may dart across the trail and tiny quail skitter into the bushes while a sentinel parent cries its warning call from a nearby fence post. When you emerge from the woods, your vista northeast takes in the grassy hills and tree-filled canyons that form the drainage of Mission Creek, which once powered the grist mill at Mission San José.

Now on a graveled service road, you begin a gradual climb up the north shoulder of Mission Peak. Young trees crowd into little clefts in the north-facing hillside, promising future shade on these open slopes. In springtime, watch for the hairy, curled necks of white phacelia peeking out of narrow crevices in a jumble of lichen-splashed rocks. Masses of yellow fiddlenecks crowd the surrounding fields. The shear, scarred west face of Mission Peak appears above you, dropping abruptly to the valley below.

Equestrians join **hikers** and **mountain bikers** in a sometimes windy saddle, where the Hidden Valley Trail meets the Peak Trail. The 2.7-mile Hidden Valley Trail begins from the Warm Springs Staging Area at the preserve's Stanford Avenue entrance and is the official equestrian route for this segment of the Ridge Trail; part of the Ohlone Wilderness Trail, it is a good hiker and mountain biker route as well. Drainage from Mission Peak and the surrounding high plateau flows into Agua Caliente Creek, which runs down the west side of Hidden Valley. In the Spanish era, an aqueduct carried warm water from this creek to Mission San José for laundering and bathing.

Mission San José de Guadalupe

This entire trip takes place on lands once part of Mission San José de Guadalupe. In 1797, Spanish colonizers established the mission at the base of Mission Peak, near the site of a Native American village, Oroysom. At its height, the mission held lands from Oakland to Coyote Hills and from the bay to Mt. Diablo.

Originally built of wood with thatched roofs, the mission church and out-buildings were later reconstructed with adobe walls and tile-covered, hewn redwood roof beams. Orchards, vegetable gardens, and promenades surrounded the mission, and extensive vineyards flourished at 400 to 500 feet on the rolling hills. On the upper hills, large herds of cattle ranged, said to number some 12,000 head. After the Mexican government took over Alta California and following the arrival of the Anglos in 1849, the mission complex fell into disrepair; the buildings were further damaged by an earthquake in 1868.

Today, the refurbished mission church and a museum lie just north of Ohlone College, and the campus occupies some of the former mission gardens, promenades, and orchards. Mission Boulevard, which you followed to reach the college, approximates the trail that the Spanish explorers and mission padres traveled between the Santa Clara and San José missions. Some of the gnarled, gray-leafed olive trees lining the route remain from the mission plantings.

When the advance guard of mission founders chose this site, they noted it was "beside a perennial stream, found good tillable soil . . . lime deposits and a rock formation called hewing stone, suitable for construction." You can still see these features today along the Bay Area Ridge Trail route.

Veer left (east) at the junction of the Hidden Valley and Peak trails and go a quarter mile to the Eagle Trail. Veer right to follow the Eagle Trail around the peak's east side; from a high, grassy plateau filled with spring wildflowers, the Laurel Canyon Trail branches off to the park boundary. (Trail users with East Bay Municipal Utility District permits can follow the Ohlone Wilderness Trail 25 miles east to Del Valle Regional Park, across San Francisco Watershed lands and the beautiful, rugged Sunol and Ohlone Regional Wilderness preserves.)

Follow the fence line across high grasslands to a green gate. Pass through the gate to a wide trail that heads southeast toward an array of antennae on the distant peaks. On a gradual climb, the trail passes remnants of ancient rock walls of uncertain origin, possibly predating the Ohlone period. The Spanish recorded that the hills "abounded in rocks which could be easily transported" to building sites. Here too are some of the springs the Spanish reported.

Beyond a private road on the right, you curve around the east side of 2658-foot Mt. Allison, the highest point on this three-peak trip. To the east you may see the Ohlone Wilderness Trail on the west face of 3817-foot Rose Peak on Valpe Ridge.

Shortly you enter the land acquired in 1992 from the Wool family, whose ranch lies off to the left. Mr. E. O. (Sandy) Wool, a prominent 1900s rancher, once farmed the valley in present-day Ed Levin Park, where the lake now bears his name. This 400-acre acquisition provided the link between Mission Peak Regional Preserve and Ed Levin Park in Santa Clara County.

For more than a mile you travel through a high valley between Mt. Allison and Monument Peak, both bristling with tall radio and TV towers—a veritable communications village or giant pincushion. Ignore all roads leading to these towers and head due south. The trail then trends west and surmounts a small rise, where a view of the bay unfolds below you. In the South Bay, you'll see the salt ponds, tinged shades of blue-green to rosy lavender, and the marshes, sloughs, mud flats, and open waters of Don Edward's San Francisco Bay National Wildlife Refuge. Due west, Jarvis Landing, an important grain and hide shipping port in the 1800s, was located on the shoreline. Now, the expanding communities of Fremont, Milpitas, and Newark stretch from the foothills to the bay, yet more than 4000 mountainside acres through which the Bay Area Ridge Trail travels remain in public open space.

Over the next 4 miles, you lose 2000 feet in elevation as you descend a wide ranch road on the steep prow of the East Bay hills. Caught between the Hayward and Calaveras faults, these hills were uplifted through the eons by fault movement. Rocky knobs dotting the hillsides are remains of sedimentary deposits formed as the Pacific Plate slid northward along the edge of North America some 15 million years ago.

A multitrunked bay tree grows in a heap of boulders at a wide switchback, casting welcome shade on a southwest-facing slope. Although the steepness of the trail requires your close attention, pause occasionally to glance skyward for turkey vultures and red-tailed hawks wheeling on the updrafts, or for the golden eagles known to soar over these still-wild lands.

Spring wildflowers bloom in rainbow hues, from magenta redmaids and frilly pink checkerblooms to yellow buttercups, tiny baby blue eyes, and tall purple brodiaea. Great swaths of orange California poppies glow on south-facing hillsides. By early summer, the

Hiker Side Trip to Mission Peak

Hikers have two options for a short detour to the summit of 2517-foot Mission Peak; whichever one you choose, do not fail to make the less-than-a-half-mile ascent. From the junction of the Eagle and Peak trails, hikers can stay right (south) on the Peak Trail to climb the eroded, rocky flank of Mission Peak. The other option is to follow the Eagle Trail around the peak's east side and veer right at the second junction of the Eagle and Peak trails to ascend the peak's south flank.

If the day is clear, you'll have views of prominent peaks around the Bay Area—west from Loma Prieta and Black Mountain to Mt. Tamalpais, north to Mt. Diablo, and south to Mt. Hamilton. On a tall post a few feet north of the summit, directional sighting holes point to other important Bay Area landmarks. Just below you, on Mission Peak's craggy face, you occasionally see a herd of feral goats leaping from rock to rock.

Rejoin mountain bikers and equestrians on the main Bay Area Ridge Trail route to Ed Levin Park.

drying grasses turn golden, contrasting with the dark green oaks that fill the lower canyons, nourished by Agua Fria, Toroges, Scott, Calera, and other small, unnamed creeks.

You continue to descend the rounded shoulders of the hills and reach the wooded banks of Scott Creek, the Alameda/Santa Clara County boundary and the entrance to Ed R. Levin Park. In Levin Park, the Bay Area Ridge Trail follows the Agua Caliente Trail past a catch basin for watering cattle and reaches Calera Creek in about a half mile. Lofty sycamore trees line the creekside, their gray-and-white-patterned bark mimicking the shades of the limestone deposits for which this creek is named. The Spaniards, and later the Mexican settlers, burned this stone in kilns to make mortar and whitewash for their adobes.

Go straight to follow the wide Calera Creek Trail to Sandy Wool Lake, 2.1 miles ahead. Now on a less-precipitous route, you cross Calera Creek and stay close enough to its banks to hear the rushing water and to appreciate the afternoon shade from trees along the trail.

You leave the main creek and ford a tributary of Calera Creek in a meadow filled with brilliant yellow mustard in spring. An early settler remarked that the mustard stalks were so strong that "ground squirrels climbed them to get a better view."

The trail hugs a fence surrounding former Minnis Ranch fields, which Santa Clara County purchased in 1967 for Ed Levin Park. These lands were once part of the Tularcitos Ranch ("little rules"), granted to José Higuera in 1821 by Pablo Vicente de Sola, the last Spanish governor of Alta California.

After passing a fenced, private development of homes surrounding a golf course and a pond, continue to a paved road heading left. Continue on the Calera Creek Trail across this road, and go through a gate to an unpaved path that follows the fence line for 0.25 mile. At the next gate, you turn left and descend to yet another gate at the park road.

You have skirted a landing field where, especially on weekends, brightly colored hang-gliders alight after their flight from Monument Peak. Just beyond are the picnic tables and greensward beside the blue waters of Sandy Wool Lake, a cool, refreshing finishing point. It was at this pretty picnic area on April 24, 1993, that Bay Area Ridge Trail volunteers celebrated the completion of this long-planned regional trail.

As you plan your trip, you might arrange with friends to meet you here for a picnic and a car shuttle after your exhilarating ridgetop trek. Although hikers would probably eschew a round-trip, stalwart bicyclists and equestrians with an early start could make this a 20-mile trip. The return entails considerable elevation gain.

◆ ◆ ◆

The next Bay Area Ridge Trail segment begins about 8 miles south at Alum Rock Park in San Jose.

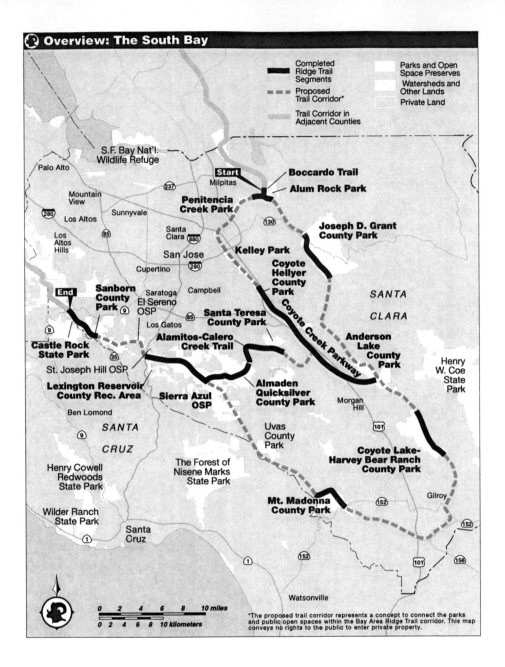

Overview: The South Bay

Legend:
- Completed Ridge Trail Segments
- Proposed Trail Corridor*
- Trail Corridor in Adjacent Counties
- Parks and Open Space Preserves
- Watersheds and Other Lands
- Private Land

Palo Alto
S.F. Bay Nat'l. Wildlife Refuge
Mountain View
Sunnyvale
Los Altos
Los Altos Hills
280
85
Santa Clara
880
237
Milpitas
Start
Boccardo Trail
Alum Rock Park
Penitencia Creek Park
130
Joseph D. Grant County Park
Kelley Park
San Jose
Cupertino
280
Coyote Hellyer County Park
SANTA CLARA
End
Sanborn County Park
9
Saratoga
El Sereno OSP
Campbell
Los Gatos
85
Santa Teresa County Park
Coyote Creek Parkway
Anderson Lake County Park
Henry W. Coe State Park
9
Castle Rock State Park
35
St. Joseph Hill OSP
Alamitos-Calero Creek Trail
Lexington Reservoir County Rec. Area
Sierra Azul OSP
Almaden Quicksilver County Park
Morgan Hill
101
Ben Lomond
SANTA CRUZ
9
Uvas County Park
Coyote Lake-Harvey Bear Ranch County Park
Gilroy
Henry Cowell Redwoods State Park
The Forest of Nisene Marks State Park
Mt. Madonna County Park
152
152
Wilder Ranch State Park
1
Santa Cruz
1
152
101
156
152

Watsonville

0 2 4 6 8 10 miles
0 2 4 6 8 10 kilometers

*The proposed trail corridor represents a concept to connect the parks and public open spaces within the Bay Area Ridge Trail corridor. This map conveys no rights to the public to enter private property.

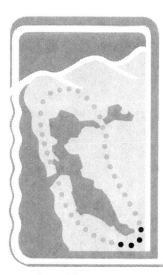

THE SOUTH BAY

Alum Rock Park and Boccardo Trail Corridor...................177

Joseph D. Grant County Park.................................181

Coyote Lake-Harvey Bear Ranch Trail 185

Mount Madonna County Park 188

Sierra Azul Open Space Preserve............................193

Coyote Creek Parkway North................................195

Coyote Creek Parkway South................................199

Santa Teresa County Park and Los Alamitos/Calero Creek Trail ..201

Almaden Quicksilver County Park 207

Sanborn County Park and Castle Rock State Park..............211

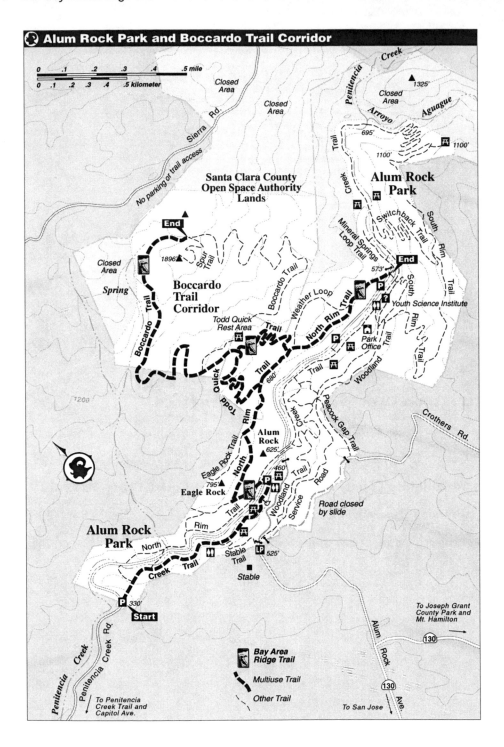

Alum Rock Park and Boccardo Trail Corridor

0   .1   .2   .3   .4   .5 mile
0   .1   .2   .3   .4   .5 kilometer

Penitencia Creek

1325'

Closed Area

Closed Area

Closed Area

Sierra Rd.

No parking of trail access

Arroyo Aguague

695'

1100'

1100'

Santa Clara County Open Space Authority Lands

Trail

Creek

Alum Rock Park

Switchback Trail

South Rim Trail

End

1896'

Spur Trail

Boccardo Trail

Weather Loop

Mineral Springs Loop Trail

573'

End

Youth Science Institute

South Rim Trail

Closed Area

Spring

Boccardo Trail Corridor

Todd Quick Rest Area

Trail

North Rim Trail

Park Office

Boccardo Trail

680'

Trail

Trail

Woodland

Crothers Rd.

1200

Quick

Todd

North Rim

Creek

Peacock Gap Trail

Alum Rock 625'

Eagle Rock Trail

460'

Trail

Road

Road closed by slide

795'

Eagle Rock

Trail

Woodland

Service

North

Rim

525'

Alum Rock Park

North

Creek Trail

Stable Trail

LP

Stable

To Joseph Grant County Park and Mt. Hamilton

330'

Start

130

Penitencia Creek

Penitencia Creek Rd.

Alum Rock Ave.

130

To Penitencia Creek Trail and Capitol Ave.

To San Jose

Bay Area Ridge Trail

Multiuse Trail

Other Trail

Alum Rock Park and Boccardo Trail Corridor

From Alum Rock's West Entrance to a High Valley

Length	6 miles round-trip, including 3 miles round-trip to Todd Quick Rest Area, 2.4 miles round-trip to end of trail, and 0.6 mile round-trip extension to summit
Accessibility	Hikers, equestrians, and mountain bikers; wheelchair users on Creek Trail only
Agencies	City of San Jose and Santa Clara County Open Space Authority
Regulations	Park is open from 8 AM to a half hour after sunset daily, charges an entrance fee, and prohibits dogs.
Facilities	Water, restrooms, and telephone

Climb to a secluded valley surmounted by a high, rounded hill on the east side of the Santa Clara Valley for a bird's-eye view of nearby San Jose that expands to include all the South Bay and the Peninsula. The trail winds up a southwest-facing, grassy hillside, gaining about 1000 feet in elevation. This round-trip is best done with an early start on cool spring days or midday in winter when skies are clear after rains.

Getting There

By Car

At this writing, the only access to the trail is from Alum Rock Park's Penitencia Creek Road entrance. From Interstate 680 in east San Jose, take McKee Road east, turn left (north) on White Road and then right (east) on Penitencia Creek Road. Continue past Dorel Drive on the left and go 0.2 mile to an unpaved parking area.

By Bicycle

Take Mabury Road east, turn left (north) on White Road, and then turn right (east) on Penitencia Creek Road, where there are bike lanes and an off-road path. Follow directions for cars to parking but continue to the paved road entrance and watch for a concrete and rock bridge, take it through the former quarry, and join the Creek Trail.

By Bus

Valley Transit Agency buses run to Piedmont and Penitencia Creek Road and to Penitencia Creek Road and Toyon entrance on Alum Rock Avenue.

On the Trail

The Boccardo Trail Corridor is the first Santa Clara County Open Space Authority site to open to the public and its first Bay Area Ridge Trail segment. The property is adjacent to the north side of Alum Rock Park at the Todd Quick Loop Trail rest area. Since there is no outlet on the north side of Boccardo, this is a 6-mile round-trip that combines the Alum Rock Park trip with a round-trip on the Boccardo Trail.

All trail users start on the Creek Trail in Alum Rock Park, then cross Penitencia Creek, and continue on the North Rim Trail to the first turnoff for the Todd Quick Trail. Follow this trail uphill to the Todd Quick rest area, a one-way trip of 1.5 miles. After pausing here, perhaps to enjoy a snack at the picnic table under the eucalyptus trees, go through the green gate on your right and step onto the wide Boccardo Trail.

Here you'll find explanatory panels and a map on the information boards. Note the sandstone boulder that is embedded with a dedication to the Boccardo family, who helped fund the purchase of this beautiful, open ranchland. Take a few steps beyond to glimpse the high, grassy hill that shields the secluded valley on its north side. (Its rounded, 1896-foot summit affords fabulous views of the mountains, valleys, and cities of the South Bay and Peninsula, as well as some prominent peaks of the North Bay.)

The trail swings left and quickly bears right on a short, but steep climb. You reach a level area on your right, probably a slump from the side of the high hill, long since settled; note the hill's concave face. A horse watering trough sits beside the trail and a dense grove of oaks lies off-limits to the right. As a friend and I approached this flat, a doe and her fawn appeared, pausing to assess our potential threat. Then, sedately and gracefully, they disappeared among the trees.

After a pause here to appraise your uphill route, bear right (northeast) on the wide service road and continue past lush stands of tall, yellow-flowered mustard. In spring, you may hear the cheery, lilting song of red-winged blackbirds calling to their mates from perches on the mustard. These glossy black birds with brilliant red shoulder patches will accompany you most of the way uphill, flitting across your path to nests in the oak trees. Listen, too, for the meadowlarks' trilling song from their nests hidden in the grass.

After rounding a bend, you traverse a south-facing shoulder of the hill to reach a small, grassy promontory. Here you have your first view of the South Bay scene, growing more extensive as you quickly gain altitude. A patch of oaks, both coast live oak and deciduous blue oak, graces the hillside to your left as you curve around the top of a west-facing prominence on a long, rounded ridge (sometimes called a hogback).

On an eastern reach, you begin a steady, uphill climb. On your right, the hill rises abruptly; on your left, a sheer bank clothed with trees drops into a tight ravine. Spring

Alum Rock Steam Railroad

At a sharp bend in the Creek Trail, note the remnants of large concrete pillars that once supported the Alum Rock Steam Railroad. From 1890 until it was destroyed by heavy floods in 1911, the railroad ferried passengers between downtown San Jose and Alum Rock Park, then a popular health spa and recreation area. Mount the steep steps on your right to a platform on the former roadbed, where a plaque commemorates Richard H. Quincy, a San Jose wood and coal dealer who promoted the railroad. You'll also have a view of Eagle and Alum rocks, two large volcanic outcrops, and be able to trace the verdant, tree-lined path of Penitencia Creek through the canyon.

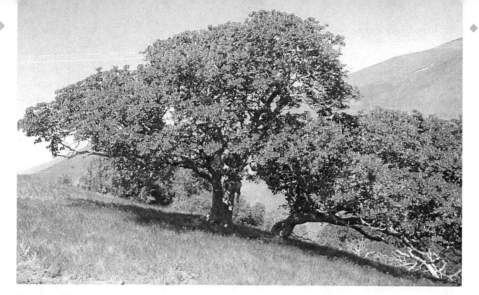

Boccardo Trail

wildflowers bloom in abundance on either side of the trail. Golden poppies and yellow mule ears stand tall and bright, but you may need to search for the reddish-purple tomcat clover among the grasses; lupine and blue-eyed grass complete the show. Later in spring, you may find yellow mariposa lilies waving on tall stems, intermixed with deep blue brodiaea. In summer and fall, this route is redolent with the fragrance of California sagebrush, the 2- to 3-foot gray bush commonly found here and on many west- and south-facing California hills.

A few openings in the cluster of trees reveal a tiny, unnamed stream in the ravine, a tributary of Penitencia Creek and no doubt the water source for the deer and other wildlife that make their homes in these hills. (Thanks to Santa Clara County Open Space Authority for preserving their terrain.)

Soon the oak, bay, and buckeye forest becomes more dense and covers both sides of the trail, forming a veritable tunnel for a brief stretch. Look for small, white-petaled woodland stars waving on tall, slender stems and red shooting stars clustered among the ferns and mosses on the high, moist right bank. Shortly, you bear east and leave the canopy of trees to emerge in a valley where, in early spring, shiny buttercups paint the hills yellow. Off to your left, a carpet of brilliant orange poppies covers a west-facing slope. In summer and fall, these hills take on the California "golden" hue of drying oat grass.

About 100 yards ahead is the end of the Ridge Trail segment in the Boccardo Trail Corridor. Before you start back, however, be sure to take the new, well-designed trail on your right for a 0.3-mile trip to the summit. It heads due east and then makes a switchback west above a clump of venerable buckeye trees. At the next switchback stands another majestic buckeye whose bare limbs seem stained by rusty lichen. Beyond this turn, you round the east side of the hill, climbing gradually southwest to reach the summit. Fierce spring winds can blast Bay Area summits, so hang on to your hats and bring a warm jacket.

Interpretive plaques at the trail's end point out what you can see from the top: north to San Francisco with Mt. Tamalpais rising beyond it, and south to Mt. Hamilton topped by its observatories. West lie the Santa Cruz Mountains surmounted by Loma Prieta and Mt. Umunhum. At your feet is the trail you just climbed and the tree-filled canyon of

Alum Rock Park. On the broad Bay plain, the sprawling metropolis of San Jose stretches south to Coyote Valley and north to the edge of San Francisco Bay. If the day is very clear, you can discern the salt ponds at bay's edge and watch their color change from blue to pink as the brine is pumped from the west to the east side of the bay.

The strong winds that often sweep this hill offer challenges to raptors. I have seen red-tailed hawks here soaring overhead in search of small rodents and snakes. Updrafts provide the loft these big birds need to glide on their 3- to 6-foot wingspan. You can identify a red-tailed hawk by its rusty-red tail feathers. Other "frequent flyers" include turkey vultures and red-shouldered hawks; an occasional golden eagle also soars here.

After savoring the summit views, stop often on your descent to look into the steep, rugged canyons of Penitencia Creek and Arroyo Aguague. The Penitencia rises in the hills east of Alum Rock Park and the Arroyo Aguague flows north from the heights of Joseph Grant County Park to join the Penitencia at the northeast end of Alum Rock's Creek Trail.

It's all downhill from here to the junction with the Todd Quick Trail through grass-lands dotted with clusters of wind-gnarled buckeye trees. The east side of the loop trail crisscrosses a small arroyo that nourishes these buckeyes and the nearby tall light blue ceanothus shrubs (the very fragrant California lilac). At the first trail junction, you could bear right to return to the parking area on the North Rim Trail; to make a loop, bear left and circle the east side of the Weather Loop. (Rangers use this area to take weather measurements.) At the next junction, veer left (east) on the North Rim Trail, go 0.45 mile, and then descend to the large parking area at the eastern terminus of the park road. There are many picnic sites along the creek, both up and down the canyon of Penitencia Creek, where friends might meet you for lunch or supper.

To return to the park entrance, cross the creek on one of the park's ornate 1930s bridges, its balustrades faced with fossil rocks taken from the creek bed. You can visit other remnants of the park's early days, such as the mineral baths upstream and the classic structure that encloses the park's only potable spring, just downstream.

Following the Creek Trail you could stop at the visitor center to see photos of the park's heyday: mineral baths, an indoor swimming pool, a tea garden, a grand restaurant, and even a dance pavilion made this a popular recreation area in the early 20th century. Continuing west on the sycamore-shaded Creek Trail, you pass several picnic areas and a children's playground and then reach the park's western end at Penitencia Creek Road.

◆ ◆ ◆

The next Ridge Trail segment begins in Joseph D. Grant County Park, just 10 miles south of Alum Rock Park on the Mt. Hamilton Road.

Joseph D. Grant County Park

From Edwards Trail Gate on Mount Hamilton Road to Dutch Flat Trail Gate at Park's Southwest Boundary

Length	8.4 miles (5.6 miles to southern boundary of park and 2.8 miles from southern boundary to main parking area)
Accessibility	Hikers, equestrians, and mountain bikers
Agency	Santa Clara County Parks and Recreation Department
Regulations	Park is open from 8 AM to sunset year-round and charges an entrance fee on weekends and holidays and on weekdays from one week before Memorial Day until the day after Labor Day. Dogs are prohibited from trails and must be on a 6-foot leash in limited areas. Park charges fees for camping and group picnic areas. Helmets are mandatory for mountain bikers.
Facilities	Water, restrooms, and telephone

Traverse remote oak woodlands and an ancient bay-tree forest to reach a 2457-foot vista point with outstanding views of the high peaks of the Coast Range. This segment traces the western boundary of 9522-acre Joseph D. Grant County Park on a broad trail, at times rocky and dusty, and gains 700 feet. Most of the route is in full sun, so plan for an early start and carry plenty of water.

Getting There

From Highway 101 or Interstate 680 in San Jose, take the Alum Rock Avenue exit east. Go 2.5 miles and turn right on Mt. Hamilton Road. Look for the Edwards Trail on the west side of the road after 6.5 miles, with a small roadside pullout for three or four cars on the east side. Do not block the gated entrance to a private road and the Washburn Trail. If you leave a car here, you will need to walk or ride 1.5 miles back to it after your trip. For additional parking, or to leave a shuttle car, continue 1.5 miles to the main park entrance, on the right. Park at any of several designated areas, and return to the trailhead on Mt. Hamilton Road.

On the Trail

From the trailhead on Mt. Hamilton Road, **hikers, equestrians**, and **mountain bikers** begin a fairly steady climb on the Edwards Trail, an old ranch road. In spring, you may meet grazing cattle along this trail, still used to tend cattle. Occasional monarch live oaks shade your route, and blue lupine and large yellow mule ears bloom in spring. At one of several wide switchbacks you can look back over Hall's Valley to the buildings of Joseph D. Grant's former ranch house complex. Beyond, the park's steep eastern

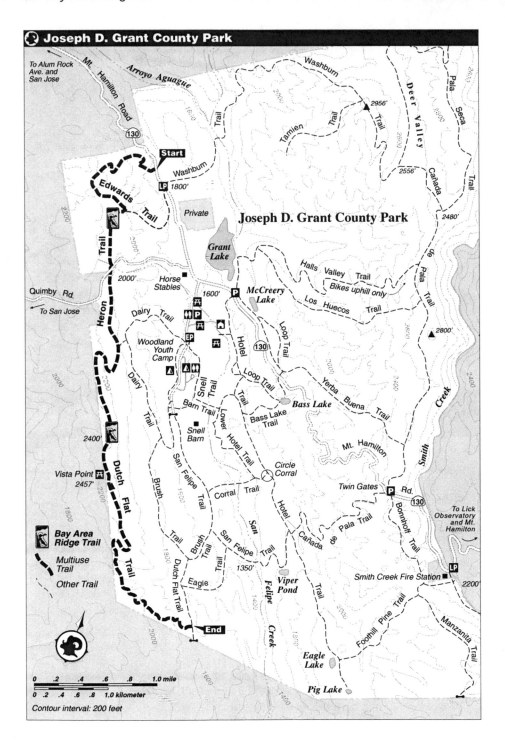

Joseph D. Grant County Park

To Alum Rock Ave. and San Jose

Mt. Hamilton Road

Arroyo Aguague

130

Washburn

Deer Valley

Pala Seca

Tamien Trail

2956'

2556'

Start

Washburn

LP 1800'

Edwards Trail

Private

Grant Lake

Joseph D. Grant County Park

2480'

Trail

Quimby Rd.

To San Jose

Heron

2000'

Horse Stables

1600'

McCreery Lake

Halls Valley Trail

Bikes uphill only

de Pala Trail

2800'

Los Huecos Trail

Dairy Trail

P

Hotel

130

Loop Trail

Woodland Youth Camp

EP

Snell Trail

Loop Trail

Trail

Yerba Buena Trail

Smith Creek

2400'

Dairy Trail

Barn Trail

Lower Hotel Trail

Bass Lake Trail

Bass Lake

Snell Barn

Mt. Hamilton

Trail

Vista Point 2457'

Dutch Flat

Brush Trail

San Felipe Trail

Corral Trail

Circle Corral

Twin Gates

P Rd.

130

Hotel

de Pala Trail

To Lick Observatory and Mt. Hamilton

Bonhoff Trail

Bay Area Ridge Trail

Multiuse Trail

Other Trail

Brush Trail

San Felipe Trail

San Felipe Trail

1350'

Eagle

Viper Pond

Cañada

Smith Creek Fire Station

LP

2200'

Dutch Flat Trail

Felipe Creek

Trail

Foothill Pine Trail

Manzanita Trail

End

Eagle Lake

0   .2   .4   .6   .8   1.0 mile
0 .2 .4 .6 .8 1.0 kilometer

Pig Lake

Contour interval: 200 feet

hills rise from the valley, and the domes of Lick Observatory on Mt. Hamilton glisten in the sun.

You soon pass a spring where cattle have trimmed the wide-spreading branches of a huge live oak. When you reach the highest point of this first 1-mile leg of your trip, you turn south, intersect the other leg of the Edwards Trail, and pass a small pond shaded by a stand of black oaks. Shortly, you turn right onto the Heron Trail and proceed under the power lines for 0.6 mile to the green-gated crossing of Quimby Road and reassuring Ridge Trail signs. You will follow high power lines for a good part of this trip.

Continue south on the undulating Heron Trail beyond Quimby Road; huge white oaks arch over the trail, and bay trees and willows grow in shaded ravines. Quite unexpectedly, you dip into a dense, cool grove of very large and mature bay trees—one has 14 trunks growing from its central bole.

The Heron Trail ends at a junction with the Dairy Trail on your left, and you continue your route to the south end of the park on the Dutch Flat Trail. After a wide swing to the right, your climb begins in earnest through a fine stand of black oaks—deciduous in winter, bronze-red in spring when they get their new leaves, and tawny-gold and orange in fall. You may find fox, bobcat, or snake tracks in the dust, and through openings in the woods, you see vast Hall's Valley, the centerpiece of this park. Grant Lake shimmers in the sunlight, and the park's many trails meander down the valley and up grassy hillsides indented by streamlets that nourish stands of oaks and sycamores.

On a steady climb toward the vista point, you pass through a couple of cattle gates and follow the fenced park boundary for the next few miles. Ducks swim in several water impoundments for cattle, and birds swoop down for a drink. In this remote area, the dominant sounds are birds singing, hawks calling, and the wind in the trees. Lovely pinkish-white buckeye blossoms fill the spring air with their sweet scent.

Hikers on Dutch Flat Trail on a sunny winter day

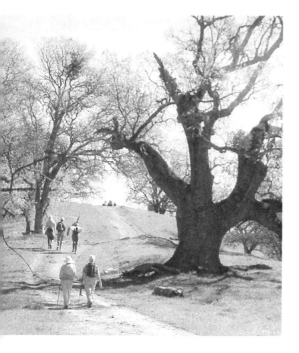

From the 2457-foot vista point, Mt. Umunhum and Loma Prieta in the Sierra Azul, the southern portion of the Santa Cruz Mountains, dominate the western skyline, their summits often backed or obscured by fog. If you have lunch in your pack, sit at the picnic table here and note how well the two arms of the Coast Range mountains enclose the Santa Clara Valley. Look north from the dominant southern peaks in the outer Coast Range to Black Mountain, San Bruno Mountain, and Mt. Tamalpais.

You begin your descent on the Dutch Flat Trail through an avenue of deciduous black and valley oaks. In fall, the spent oak leaves carpet the trail and hillsides, their acorns crunch underfoot, and mistletoe hangs from branches. These magnificent trees are long-lived, but you may see a fallen giant lying beside the trail, its bark riddled with woodpecker holes and its undersides inhabited by ground-burrowing creatures. The trail descends steeply through a live oak-madrone woodland with a tangled understory of toyon, poison oak, and wild rose.

The vegetation changes to chaparral, and you soon reach the park's southern boundary. You are now at 1660 feet, almost 800 feet lower than the vista point. The Ridge Trail segment through Joseph D. Grant Park officially ends here. For an alternate route back to the park entrance, turn left on the Dutch Flat Trail and head due north. Continue through rolling grasslands past the Eagle Trail to the Brush Trail; bear right and then left on the San Felipe Trail.

Hikers and **equestrians** can follow the San Felipe Trail all the way back to the parking areas. **Mountain bikers,** however, turn right (east) on the Corral Trail and cross San Felipe Creek to either the Lower Hotel Trail or the Hotel Trail to return to the parking area. From the junction of Dutch Flat and Brush trails to the parking areas, the route drops another 150 feet in elevation with small gains and losses en route.

This last leg of the trip is quite spectacular in spring when the grasslands put on a brilliant display of yellow, purple, pink, and orange wildflowers. Hawks circle overhead in their never-ending search for rodents. You may see their favorite prey—a plentiful supply of ground squirrels—scurrying through the grasses or sounding their warning calls from upright positions by their burrows.

◆ ◆ ◆

The next Bay Area Ridge Trail segment begins about 13 miles south at the Harvey Bear Ranch entrance to Coyote Lake-Harvey Bear Ranch County Park in San Martin.

Coyote Lake-Harvey Bear Ranch Trail

From Harvey Bear Ranch Entrance South to Mendoza Ranch

Length	7.2 miles, which is 4.6 miles on north-south route, plus 2.6 miles on Harvey Bear Trail from San Martin Avenue to its junction with north end of Coyote Ridge Trail
Accessibility	Hikers, equestrians, and mountain bikers
Agency	Santa Clara County Parks and Recreation Department
Regulations	Dogs must be on leash. A camping and picnicking fee is required at the Mendoza Ranch area.
Facilities	Parking, camping, picnic tables, and restrooms available at the campground on Lakeside Trail (there's a 0.4-mile connector trail to Coyote Ridge Trail); parking, restrooms, and picnic tables near Harvey Bear Ranch Entrance

After a vigorous climb on the 2.6-mile link to the trail's north entrance, this trip heads south on a relatively level trail with views of the lake, the surrounding foothills, and the coastal mountains.

Getting There

HARVEY BEAR RANCH ENTRANCE: From Highway 101 in San Martin, take the San Martin Avenue exit. Proceed east on San Martin Avenue for 2 miles. The entrance to the park is on the left, 0.25 mile east of Foothill Avenue.

MENDOZA RANCH ENTRANCE: From Highway 101 in Gilroy, take the Leavesley Road exit. Proceed east on Leavesley Road 2 miles to New Avenue. Go north on New Avenue for 0.5 mile, and turn right (east) on Roop Road. Continue on this road (east) toward the foothills for 3.5 miles. Turn left into the parking area at the Mendoza Ranch Entrance. If you are going camping or picnicking, continue a third mile past the Mendoza Ranch entrance to the Coyote Lake entrance, and go 1 mile north to the entrance station, parking, and trail access.

On the Trail

After turning off Highway 101 onto San Martin Avenue, you go through former ranching country, now gradually being subdivided into smaller parcels. However, as of this writing there are still working farms in the park's vicinity, and land conservation organizations are trying to save farmlands.

From the north end of the parking area on San Martin Avenue, take the park road going east, pass an old barn and farmhouse, go through a couple of park gates and emerge into typical, coastal foothills country. In spring the hills are a vibrant green, the birds

Coyote Lake-Harvey Bear Ranch Trail

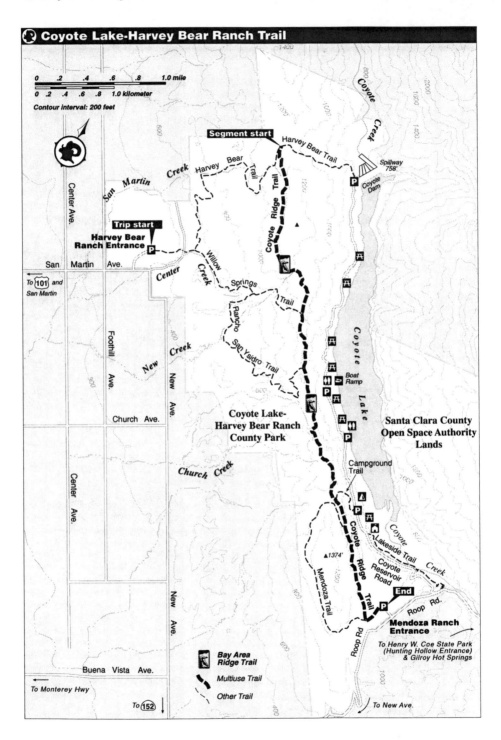

0 .2 .4 .6 .8 1.0 mile
0 .2 .4 .6 .8 1.0 kilometer
Contour interval: 200 feet

Center Ave.

San Martin Creek

Harvey Bear Trail

Segment start

Coyote Creek

Spillway
758'

Coyote Dam

Harvey Bear Trail

Coyote Ridge Trail

Trip start
Harvey Bear
Ranch Entrance

San Martin Ave.

To 101 and
San Martin

Willow Creek

Center Creek

Springs Trail

Rancho San Ysidro Trail

New Creek

New Ave.

Foothill Ave.

Church Ave.

Coyote Lake-
Harvey Bear Ranch
County Park

Coyote Lake

Boat Ramp

Santa Clara County
Open Space Authority
Lands

Center Ave.

Church Creek

Campground Trail

Coyote Creek

Coyote Ridge Trail

Lakeside Trail

▲1374'

Coyote Reservoir Road

Mendoza Trail

End

New Ave.

Roop Rd.

Mendoza Ranch
Entrance

To Henry W. Coe State Park
(Hunting Hollow Entrance)
& Gilroy Hot Springs

Buena Vista Ave.

To Monterey Hwy

Bay Area
Ridge Trail

Multiuse Trail

Other Trail

To 152

To New Ave.

are singing in the trees, hawks call out en route to unwary prey, and wildflowers extravagantly clothe the trailside with rainbow hues. This is the ideal time to visit this park.

After the second gate and just 0.2 mile from the entrance station, take the left-hand trail going north, the Harvey Bear Trail. The first half mile is fairly level, but after making a sharp turn east the trail begins to climb in earnest. You pass a cattle pond on the right and make a sharp swing south before climbing seriously northeast to the Coyote Ridge Trail junction. Here, at 1150 feet, you can see back across the Santa Clara Valley to the foothills where other parks in Santa Clara County lie—Almaden Quicksilver, Sierra Azul Open Space Preserve, and Mt. Madonna—pockets of meadows and woodlands in an urban metropolis.

You turn right (south) onto the Coyote Ridge Trail and begin the actual Ridge Trail route that traverses the length of the Harvey Bear and Mendoza ranches, now Santa Clara County parkland. For most of the way you have views of Coyote Lake, generally placid, except when large numbers of motorboats are plying the waters. You can see them as they follow park rules that prescribe a set route and certain maximum speeds on the lake.

Just 1.6 miles down the trail you reach the Willow Springs Trail junction, a turnoff you could take northwest for a 1.3-mile return to the parking area. However, to continue on the Ridge Trail route, go straight ahead (south) on the Coyote Ridge Trail, gradually getting closer to the lake and views of the campsites near the lake. At the Rancho San Ysidro Trail junction on your right is another opportunity to do a loop trip back to the parking area by following this trail to its junction with the Willow Springs Trail and thence west to the parking area on San Martin Avenue.

However, continuing south on the Coyote Ridge Trail, you have fine views of the lake as you amble up and down over small hills for the next 1.4 miles. If you are camping in the park, look for the Campground Trail cut-off toward the lake. Here you may have family members and friends waiting for you with lunch at a nearby picnic table. Then, some of them could join you for the last mile of the trip south to the Mendoza Ranch entrance.

This last section of the Coyote Ridge Trail goes through rolling grasslands on the east side of a high, longitudinal ridge clothed with an oak and madrone forest that casts a shadow on the trail in late afternoon—quite welcome after your lengthy trip in the sun. If you have spotted a car here or someone is meeting you, the route back to Highway 101 is on adjacent Roop Road west. Or if you left a car at the San Martin Avenue parking area, turn around and retrace your steps via the route described until you reach the Willow Springs Trail turnoff, and then go left (northwest) to the parking area on San Martin Avenue.

◆ ◆ ◆

The next leg of the Ridge Trail lies in Mt. Madonna County Park, about 15 miles as the crow flies across the Santa Clara Valley in the Outer Coast Range.

Mount Madonna County Park

From Sprig Recreation Area Entrance to Old Mt. Madonna Road

Length	3.1 miles
Accessibility	Hikers and equestrians
Agency	Santa Clara County Parks and Recreation Department
Regulations	Park is open from sunrise to a half hour after sunset, charges an entrance fee, and prohibits bicycles. Dogs are prohibited on trails, must be on a 6-foot or shorter leash in campground, and must be in confined areas overnight.
Facilities	Water, restrooms, and telephone; overnight camping by reservation through the parks department at http://gooutsideandplay.org

On an uphill trip from Sprig Recreation Area trailhead to redwood summit, you'll gain 1230 feet and take in excellent views of southern Santa Clara County and the inner Coast Range mountains. The wide service road skirts an intermittent creek, crosses boulder-strewn grasslands, swings through chaparral and scrub-oak forest, and finishes in a cool, steep-sided redwood canyon. Before you reach the redwood-forested Loop Trail, the southeast-facing trail is mostly in sun.

Getting There

SPRIG RECREATION AREA, FROM THE EAST: From Highway 101, take the Highway 152 (Hecker Pass) west exit and follow signs through Gilroy. About 7 miles east of Highway 101, watch for the Sprig trailhead on the right.

SPRIG RECREATION AREA, FROM THE WEST: From Highway 1 in Watsonville, take Highway 152 (Hecker Pass). Pass Pole Line Road at the summit and continue 3 more miles to the Sprig Recreation Area entrance on left.

MAIN PARK ENTRANCE, FROM THE EAST: From Highway 101, take the Highway 152 (Hecker Pass) west exit and follow signs through Gilroy. Go 10 miles to Pole Line Road at Highway 152 summit. Turn right (north) and proceed to the park entrance.

MAIN PARK ENTRANCE, FROM THE WEST: From Highway 1 in Watsonville, take Highway 152 (Hecker Pass) to Pole Line Road at summit. Turn left (north) on Pole Line Road and proceed to the park entrance gate.

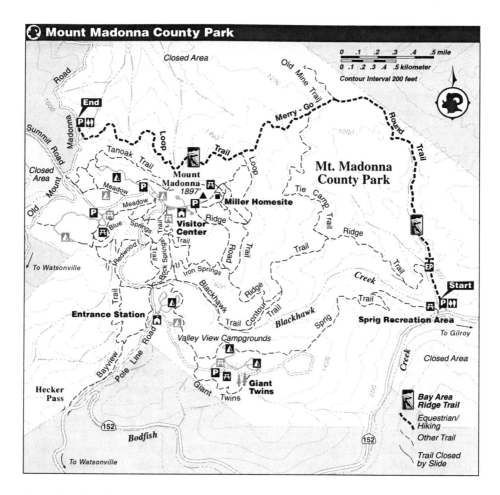

On the Trail

Starting from the Sprig Recreation Area (the former Sprig Lake now silted in), **hikers** and **equestrians** head up the Merry-Go-Round Trail, a wide dirt road, beside an unnamed tributary to Blackhawk Creek. Under a shady canopy of tall oaks, buckeyes, and bigleaf maples you can glimpse the small creek bouncing over its rocky bed through the tangled undergrowth well below the left side of the trail. On the right, perennial streams have cut deep canyons on a forested ridge.

After 0.3 mile, you come to a fork in the road where you go right on the Merry-Go-Round Trail; the Blackhawk/Ridge Trail takes off left. A staging area offers a turn-around for horse trailers, a horse watering-trough, and a picnic table or two.

Go around the barrier to vehicle traffic on the Merry-Go-Round Trail, and continue on the Ridge Trail route through a leafy corridor. Oaks and buckeyes predominate, but tall madrones search for sunlight and offer climbing posts for persistent poison oak and occasional native honeysuckle vines. After 0.1 mile on this trail, you reach a small grove of tall, second-growth redwoods; moss-covered rocks, old tree stumps, and lush redwood sorrel complete this patch of coastal redwood community.

After a short climb, you emerge in a bare opening between high banks, perhaps a borrow-pit for road repairs. You pass through grasslands below a west-facing ridge topped by mixed conifer forest. Back in a woodland of oak and willows, note two side trails on the right—one to a horse trough and another to a small meadow dominated by an ancient live oak. Early spring wildflowers at trail's edge—buttercups, some milkmaids, and lupine—will cheer you on this uphill leg; in summer and fall, bushy, yellow sticky monkeyflower and magenta clarkia brighten the trailside.

As the Merry-Go-Round Trail swings northwest and enters open grasslands, you may see a gate on the right that leads out of the park. Continue past the gate and then pass the right-branching Old Mine Trail. Large boulders dot the grasslands, accented by a springtime riot of orange poppies, yellow mule ears, and blue lupine. To the west, near the terminus of the Ridge Trail, rises the Mt. Madonna summit, the southernmost high point of the Santa Cruz Mountains.

After 1.4 miles on the Merry-Go-Round Trail, the Tie Camp Trail branches left. A cut log under an oak of promising stature offers a shaded seat at the junction. Indeed, there was a tie camp along this trail, where redwoods were cut and shaped to form railroad ties. You continue on the Merry-Go-Round Trail's pebbly, fine black-gravel surface. As you ascend steadily with little shade, you'll realize the importance of starting early on a summer day. Your chances of garnering shade along the trail's edge are hampered by a drainage ditch, a vital ingredient in maintaining a good roadbed for service vehicles. In winter, the exposure to full sun is most welcome.

The chaparral plants found here—artemesia, sticky monkeyflower, toyon, and honeysuckle—offer good forage for the birds whose calls you may hear. Before long the trail narrows a little, and live oaks reach over manzanita, toyon, and other chaparral plants. Less than a half mile beyond the last junction, the Merry-Go-Round Trail ends and the Loop Trail forks straight ahead and left. To continue on the Ridge Trail route, you go straight on the Loop Trail.

Beneath the shade of oaks, tanoaks, bays, and madrones, this old logging road is pleasantly cool. The trail levels off and then, in a dramatic change of terrain and vegetation, descends slightly into a second-growth redwood forest. Note the horizontal ax cuts on huge redwood stumps. Loggers inserted boards into these cuts and then placed cross boards on top. Two hardy men stood on the cross boards, 8 to 10 feet aboveground, and used a long, two-handled saw to cut through the gigantic trees. They always felled the tree uphill because it might have splintered in the longer fall.

As you follow the trail along a shelf that is cut into a high, steep, north-facing mountainside, you'll hear the sound of water, sometimes just rivulets, falling over sandstone boulders in the still forest. The moisture from rain and fog-drip promotes the growth of these second- and third-growth redwoods into a healthy forest. The forest exists today as a park for all to appreciate because of Santa Clara County's foresight in purchasing this land.

Recent rains and high winds may clutter the trail with fallen limbs and twigs of redwood. Scattered eucalyptus trees, grown exceedingly tall in the forest's dense shade, yet accustomed to sunshine, are more likely to lose limbs and even topple.

The trail heads into deep ravines cut by intermittent streams and then swings out around the shoulders of the mountain. Drooping branches of wild roses and several kinds of ferns grace the hillsides above the trail. A few immense sandstone boulders accent the steep hillside, and others form jumbled streambeds for tumbling, intermittent creeks.

Shortly, look for a small shed on your left, backed by a 15-foot-high, moss-covered rock wall; another lower wall is on the other side of a lively stream. Henry Miller, a 19th-century cattle baron and former owner of today's parkland, built these walls to protect his underground water tank and pumphouse; a steam engine pumped water hundreds of feet uphill to his mountaintop home. Today, the water serves as a backup supply for fire suppression.

A few minutes beyond the water tank you reach a gate that bars vehicle entry to this beautiful trail. Beyond the gate, Old Mt. Madonna Road, formerly the Old Watsonville Road, ends this segment of the Ridge Trail.

If you have a car shuttle waiting for you, there is some room to park beside this old road for a return to the Sprig Recreation Area trailhead. Better still, have your friends meet you at one of the beautiful picnic sites in this 3500-acre mountaintop retreat. You can walk up this old mountain road through redwood groves of impressive girth and height with a thick carpet of pink-blossomed, three-leafed redwood sorrel. At the corner of Old Mt. Madonna and Pole Line roads, the Meadow Trail parallels Pole Line Road, heading south to picnic areas among the redwoods. The Tanoak Trail branches left from the Meadow Trail and wanders through the woods to park headquarters, picnic areas, and the old Miller homesite.

To return to the Sprig Recreation Area parking by trail, take the Bay Area Ridge Trail in reverse (downhill all the way), or try the well-designed, shady Sprig Trail by following the Tanoak and Rock or Blue Springs trails to a wide opening in the woods about 1 mile south, just off Pole Line Road. The Sprig Trail **(hikers only)** leads right and the Ridge and Blackhawk trails **(hikers** and **equestrians)** go straight. The Sprig Trail returns to the west side of the former Sprig Lake, which is easily accessible to the east side parking where you started this trip.

If you take the Blackhawk Trail, you must go left at the Contour Trail and then take the right turnoff onto the Ridge Trail, which reaches the last leg of the Blackhawk Trail and then on to the parking area. (As of this writing, the Blackhawk Trail is closed, due to serious storm damage, from its junction with the Contour Trail to its junction with the Ridge Trail.)

◆ ◆ ◆

The next segment of the Ridge Trail lies about 20 miles north in Sierra Azul Open Space Preserve on the west side of the Santa Cruz Mountains.

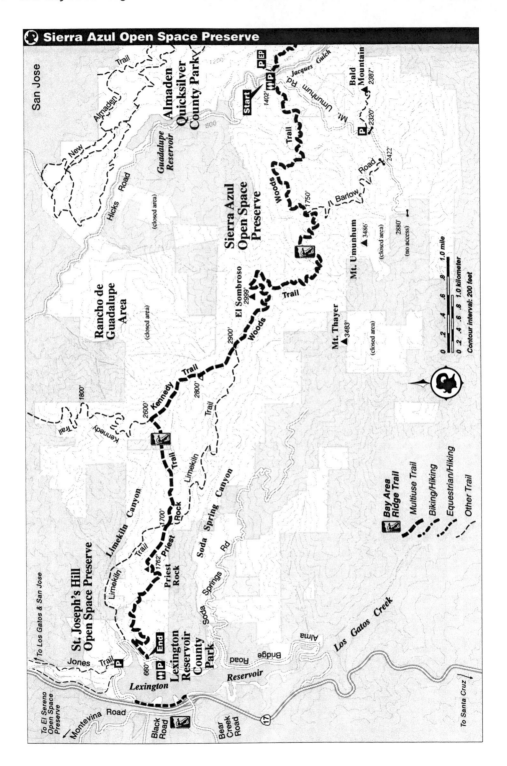

Sierra Azul Open Space Preserve

San Jose

Almaden Quicksilver County Park

Trail

Almaden

New

Hicks Road

Guadalupe Reservoir

(closed area)

Rancho de Guadalupe Area

(closed area)

Sierra Azul Open Space Preserve

Start

P EP

P 1402'

Jacques Gulch

Mt. Umunhum Rd.

Bald Mountain 2387'

2320'

P

2422

Barlow Road

V

Woods Trail

1750'

Mt. Umunhum ▲ 3486'

(closed area)

2880'

(no access)

El Sombroso 2999'

▲

Woods

Trail

2900'

Mt. Thayer ▲ 3483'

(closed area)

Kennedy Trail

Trail

1800'

2600'

2800'

Kennedy

Trail

Limekiln

1700'

Priest Rock Trail

1762'

Priest Rock

Limekiln Canyon

Soda Spring Canyon

Soda Springs Rd

St. Joseph's Hill Open Space Preserve

Limekiln Trail

660'

End

P

Jones Trail

Lexington Reservoir County Park

Lexington Reservoir

Alma Bridge Road

Los Gatos Creek

To Los Gatos & San Jose

To El Sereno Open Space Preserve

Montevina Road

Black Road

Bear Creek Road

17

To Santa Cruz

Bay Area Ridge Trail

Multiuse Trail

Biking/Hiking

Equestrian/Hiking

Other Trail

0 .2 .4 .6 .8 1.0 mile

0 .2 .4 .6 .8 1.0 kilometer

Contour interval: 200 feet

N

Sierra Azul Open Space Preserve

Length 11.8 miles

Accessibility Hikers, mountain bikers, and equestrians

Agency Midpeninsula Regional Open Space District

Regulations Preserve is open from sunrise to a half hour after sunset. Mt. Umunhum Road is closed to public traffic from its intersection with Hicks Road from a half hour after sunset to a half hour before sunrise. Dogs are prohibited on the Woods Trail segment but are allowed on the Priest Rock, Kennedy, and Limekiln trails.

Facilities Water, restroom, and horse hitch racks at Hicks Road entrance

Views from high points on the trail, which includes an elevation gain of 1800 feet and a loss of 2200 feet, give an aerial view of Santa Clara County from Mt. Umunhum to the peaks of the Diablo Range.

Getting There

In southwest San Jose take Highway 85 to Camden Avenue (if you were southbound, turn left on Camden Avenue; if you were northbound, turn left on Branham Avenue and then turn left on Camden Avenue). Go about 1.6 miles and turn right on Hicks Road. Travel about 6 miles on Hicks Road, passing the Guadalupe Reservoir on your left; turn right on Mt. Umunhum Road, and immediately turn right into a Midpeninsula Regional Open Space District parking area. Equestrian parking is on the other side of Hicks Road at the Jacques Ridge lot.

Conversely, all trail users can reach the trail's upper entrance by starting in Almaden Quicksilver County Park on the Virl O. Norton Trail (see trail description on pp. 209–210). When this trail was dedicated as a segment of the Bay Area Ridge Trail, sturdy hikers and mountain bikers joined equestrians on the Virl O. Norton, Mine Hill, and the Woods trails in Almaden Quicksilver County Park to reach this trail in Sierra Azul Open Space Preserve.

As described here, this trip requires a car shuttle from the Priest Rock Trail exit on Alma Bridge Road on the south side of the Lexington Reservoir in Los Gatos.

On the Trail

Prepare for this trip with plenty of water, lunch, snacks, weather-wise clothes, gear for your mode of travel, and an early start. Go through the gate at the Woods Trail entrance on Mt. Umunhum Road and begin an uphill leg around several switchbacks. As you move higher, Mt. Umunhum (3486 feet) comes into view with its battery of fire, radio, and TV towers. Also on this mountain is an immense structure built for a U.S. Air Force base, part of an early-warning radar network during World War II and in continual

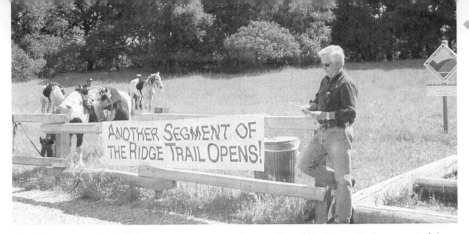

General manager Craig Britton greets guests at the opening of the Sierra Azul segment of the Ridge Trail.

use into the 1970s. Along with 1700 surrounding acres it is now part of the Midpeninsula Regional Open Space District.

You cross several small creek drainages and contour around the upper reaches of Guadalupe Creek. When you pass the Barlow Road cut-off going uphill on the left, you are still gaining elevation gradually, but now you begin to climb seriously around many turns toward the flanks of El Sombroso. This 3.7-mile leg of the trip is in oak and madrone forest and passes lovely Rincon Creek, which with Guadalupe and several smaller watercourses, flow downhill to fill the Guadalupe Reservoir. These creeks are in deep canyons with Douglas firs and bay trees growing on their north-facing slopes. Chaparral covers the high, south-facing ridges, and in spring orange sticky monkeyflower and pink wild currant brighten the trailside.

From occasional openings in the forest you can see the towers supporting the transmission lines that cross the deep canyons. In a shady nook at one of the trail's zigzags you may encounter a large basin full of water, especially for horses. Now heading north you gain elevation and go up, around, and over El Sombroso, with an elevation of 2999 feet. On clear days you can see Monterey Bay glistening in the sunshine.

After 6.5 miles you reach the Limekiln Trail going left, but the Ridge Trail route follows the Kennedy Trail, which cuts off to the right. Gradually you lose altitude as you work your way 1.4 miles toward the junction where you join the Priest Rock Trail. (The Kennedy Trail takes off north on a downhill route to the lower reaches of Los Gatos.)

Now you are losing altitude quickly and the going can be tricky—so pause for views across the canyon to the upper reaches of Bear Creek Road. There, MROSD has yet another large acreage preserved in the Bear Creek Redwoods area.

At the "four corners" area where you join the Priest Rock Trail, the Limekiln Trail goes off to the right, a pleasant and slightly longer route for a hot day. However, the Ridge Trail route stays left, continues downhill and meets Priest Rock at 1700 feet. From there you make your way 1.2 miles to the shores of Lexington Reservoir.

If you have spotted a second car here, you can drive back to the Hicks Road parking area, or friends with a car can join you for a late picnic lunch or snack at the nearby lakeside rest area and then take you to the Hicks Road parking area before sunset to pick up your car.

◆ ◆ ◆

The next Ridge Trail segment begins in Coyote Hellyer County Park.

Coyote Creek Parkway North

From Coyote Hellyer Park North to Stonegate Park and South to Metcalf City Park

Length 8.1 miles (1.8 north of and 6.3 south of Coyote Hellyer Park)

Accessibility Hikers and bicyclists; wheelchair users on most of trail

Agencies Santa Clara County Parks Department and the City of San Jose

Regulations Coyote Hellyer Park is open from 8 AM to dusk and charges an entrance fee. Dogs must be on a 6-foot or shorter leash. Horses are prohibited. All City of San Jose parks are open during daylight hours. Stonegate Park is closed when school is in session; the tiny tots playground is open during daylight hours with adult supervision.

Coyote Creek travels 31 miles from the Diablo Range to San Francisco Bay. On this 8.1-mile segment, you follow the creekbed beneath shady riparian cover and beside remnants of the Santa Clara Valley's agricultural history to freshwater lagoons at Metcalf Park, habitat for many year-round and migratory bird species. The wide, paved trail travels a nearly level course.

Getting There

COYOTE HELLYER PARK TRAILHEAD: From Highway 101 in San Jose south of Interstate 280, take the Hellyer Avenue exit to the west side of Highway 101 and then bear right (north). At the park stop sign, continue straight ahead to parking beyond the ranger station, or go left at the park sign and then turn left to parking at Cottonwood Lake

STONEGATE PARK: From Highway 101 in San Jose take Capital Expressway west, turn north on Tuers Road and go a half mile to limited on-street parking near Stonegate Park at Sherlock and Shilsone Streets.

SOUTH TRAILHEAD, METCALF PARK: From Highway 101 in southeast San Jose, take the Bernal Road exit. After a quarter mile on Bernal Road, take the Monterey Road exit, and turn left (southeast) on Monterey Road. At Metcalf Road make a **U**-turn and go a half mile northwest to Metcalf Park staging area on the right.

On the Trail

North to Stonegate Park

From the northernmost parking areas in Coyote Hellyer Park, find the wide, paved trail that goes under Yerba Buena Road and then zigzags uphill to the west side of the

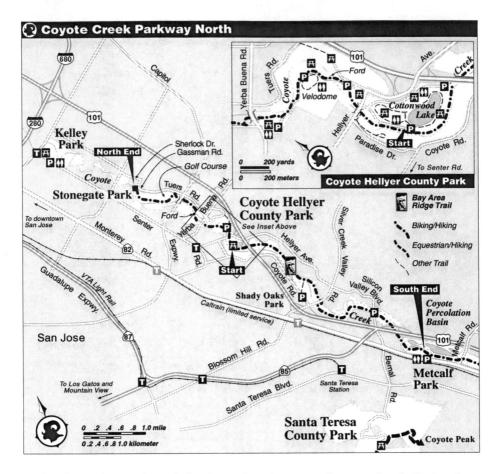

Coyote Creek Parkway North

Coyote Hellyer County Park

Legend:
- Bay Area Ridge Trail
- Biking/Hiking
- Equestrian/Hiking
- Other Trail

creek. This trail is popular with families on bicycles, especially on weekends. During the week, trail users would be wise to travel with a friend.

Shortly after passing the Los Lagos driving range and golf course, the trail switches to the east side of the creek, passing just above creek level on a low concrete apron. (Most of the year the creek flows through culverts beneath the trail; after heavy winter rains it may cover the trail—if it does turn back and take an alternate route.) On the other side of the creek, look for the trail in the woods. From here the trail rises to the top of a high creek bank; in some sections 50 feet above the creek. A dense forest of red ironwood eucalyptus, cottonwood, and live oak trees shade the creek and ubiquitous poison oak is there as well. Although chain-link fencing runs along the top of the bank, you can see the creek and hear it, especially after heavy rains.

You might like to stop for lunch at one of several small picnic sites, watch the children play on swings and slides, and watch skateboarders try daring leaps at a skateboard park. Then, after skirting the west and north sides of the playing fields at Stonegate School and Park, you pass large stables surrounded by a sturdy white fence—the San Jose Mounted Patrol grounds. The trail ends here at Sherlock and Shilsone streets. Now retrace your way to Coyote Hellyer County Park and the southern leg to Metcalf Park as described below.

Coyote Creek

The longest creek in Santa Clara County, Coyote Creek begins in the steep, rugged ridges of Henry W. Coe State Park and flows north through the eastern foothills into Santa Clara Valley. It is joined and enlarged by many tributaries, including Silver, Penitencia, and Berryessa creeks, as it makes its way through a corridor of riparian vegetation to the salty waters of San Francisco Bay. The creek's fresh water empties into the complex system of sloughs and marshes in the Don Edwards San Francisco Bay National Wildlife Refuge.

Before European settlers arrived in the Santa Clara Valley, the Ohlone used trails along Coyote and other creeks to reach settlements of other tribes, with whom they traded shells, salt, cinnabar, arrowheads, and stone knife blades. Spanish explorers also followed the creek along Ohlone routes, keeping to high ground above the water's edge. Early settlers in the valley built houses along Coyote Creek and used its water for their homes, farms, and orchards. Periodic floods destroyed many settlers' homes and inundated their crop lands. In the 1930s, the Santa Clara Valley Water District dammed the valley's major streams—Guadalupe, Los Gatos, Stevens, Calero, Los Alamitos, and Coyote—to provide drinking and irrigation water and reduce ground subsidence, and they built percolation ponds along some watercourses to recharge the groundwater supply. Today, Coyote Creek's broad, tree-lined course provides a recreation corridor for the residents of urbanized Santa Clara Valley, as well as food, shelter, and a travel route for wildlife.

South to Metcalf Park

Begin at any of several parking areas in Coyote Hellyer County Park, and take the paved hiking and bicycle trail under a leafy canopy of cottonwood, sycamore, and oak trees. A veil of poison oak vines and elderberry bushes shields the creek here, but you can frequently peak through the vegetation to see the creekbed. In summer, very little water flows through the creekbed, but during winter storms it can be a raging torrent.

In Coyote Hellyer Park you pass picnic tables, lawns, and pretty Cottonwood Lake. When this section of the Ridge Trail was dedicated in October 1990, children lined up along the lakeshore to vie for its stocked trout and bluegill.

The trail follows the creek upstream as it curves east to dip under the Highway 101 bridge. Under tall cottonwoods, the creek flows through a wide, gravelly flat tangled with berry vines and reeds. Soon the trail rises to the bluffs high above the creek, where venerable oaks shade the way. These ancient oaks send their roots deep to tap the creek's underground moisture. White-barked, big-leafed sycamore trees and the cottonwoods, whose roots prefer a streamside location, grow closer to the water.

The trees, along with an understory of shrubs, grasses, and flowers, make a hospitable environment for trail users, as well as for birds, mammals, and reptiles. You will probably see swallows and blue jays flitting in and out of the trees and hear mourning doves and quail calling. At dusk you may see deer or smaller animals searching for food or going to the creek for a drink.

On your right, about 2 miles south from Coyote Hellyer Park, a wide, wooden plank bridge arches over the creek. Cross it to the City of San Jose's Shady Oaks Park, a pleasant place under the oak and pepper trees for your backpack lunch. In this neighborhood park you'll find acres of invitingly green turf, basketball courts, and young children's play equipment.

Return to the trail to meander for another mile under wide-spreading oaks, past a few truck gardens and unkempt walnut orchards. When you go under the large Silver Creek Valley Road bridge leading to an industrial park and new housing developments, you turn sharply right onto a former vehicular bridge. Now closed to motor vehicles, this bridge is the trail route to the creek's west side.

A staging area on the south side of Silver Creek Valley Road is another entrance to the Coyote Creek Trail. A paved path descends from the staging area to creek level, flanked by rangy sycamore trees whose mottled white trunks grow at odd angles. In the creekbed, tall reeds, cattails, and grassy thickets make good nesting sites for migratory and resident ducks and grebes.

You veer away from the creek, pass through an old prune orchard, and then travel beside widely spaced oaks and tall black walnut trees. On the low eastern foothills across the creek there are still a few truck gardens and greenhouses. The trail follows the creek as it swings left, past acres of percolation ponds. During drought years, these ponds, which depend upon water from upstream reservoirs, may be dry.

Between the trail and the freeway to the west, a large floodplain is planted with orchards and bordered by a few houses. This still semipastoral setting is particularly delightful on a summer evening when sunset casts its slanting, golden light.

Before you reach Silicon Valley Boulevard, new commercial and industrial development fills the land between the Coyote Creek Trail and the freeway. Cross the road and continue south along the wide, shallow creekbed. A Caltrans riparian-habitat planting project was installed here to mitigate for wetlands lost during completion of the Highway 85 extension. Just beyond, the trail, protected by cyclone fencing, comes close to the freeway and then passes beneath it.

Soon you see the first Parkway Lakes percolation pond on your left. These ponds are the largest freshwater lagoons in the county, harboring many year-round and migratory bird species. Look for white egrets and terns, black cormorants, and blue-gray kingfishers as you travel the last part of this trail. A large new subdivision on your right fills once-open land, but you can still look west to Santa Clara County's high peaks, Mt. Umunhum and Loma Prieta. You will find some magnificent ancient oak trees that still border the lakes and shade the Coyote Creek Trail as it meanders through Metcalf Park.

◆ ◆ ◆

The next Bay Area Ridge Trail segment, Coyote Creek Parkway South, continues another 7.7 miles south from Metcalf Road to the Anderson/Burnett Ranger Station. The Bay Area Ridge Trail will someday lead south from Alum Rock Park along the ridges higher up on the eastern hills and cross over to a completed segment in Mt. Madonna County Park. But for now, the Ridge Trail route encompasses the entire Coyote Creek Trail, one to treasure and travel often. Another segment of the Ridge Trail begins 3.5 miles west of Metcalf Road in Santa Teresa County Park at the end of Bernal Road.

Coyote Creek Parkway South

From Metcalf Park to Burnett Avenue Ranger Station

Length 7.7 miles

Accessibility Hikers, bicyclists, equestrians, and wheelchair users

Agencies Santa Clara County Parks and Recreation Department and City of San Jose

Regulations Dogs must be on a 6-foot or shorter leash.

Facilities Water and restrooms at Burnett Avenue; water, restrooms, and telephone at model airplane site

Take a short, creekside stroll through the broad Coyote Creek floodplain. You'll enjoy pleasant rest stops under large shade trees and awesome views of the nearby Coast Range. The entire route follows a level paved trail (with an unpaved path for horses).

Getting There

NORTH TRAILHEAD, METCALF PARK: From Highway 101 in southeast San Jose, take the Bernal Road exit. After 0.25 mile on Bernal Road, take the Monterey Road exit, and turn left (southeast) on Monterey Road. At Metcalf Road make a **U**-turn and go 0.5 mile northwest to the Metcalf Park staging area on the right.

Coyote Creek Parkway South

SOUTH TRAILHEAD, BURNETT RANGER STATION: From Highway 101 in Morgan Hill, take the Cochrane Road exit west, continue 0.9 mile to Highway 82 (Monterey Highway) and then bear right. Go north less than 0.8 mile and turn right (east) on Burnett Avenue. Continue to creekside parking at the end of the road. Alternatively, from Metcalf Park travel south on Highway 82 to Burnett Avenue and turn left.

SOUTH TRAILHEAD, COCHRANE ROAD: From Metcalf Road, continue south on Highway 82 to Cochrane Road, cross the freeway, and continue to parking on the east side of the creek.

On the Trail

All trail users head south from the parking area to the Metcalf Road pedestrian and bicycle bridge. Cross the bridge and turn right (south) onto the Creek Trail. This trail follows the willow- and blackberry-bordered creek closely, shifting back and forth between the east and west banks. At Coyote Ranch Road, you bear east, and just before the Coyote Ranch picnic area, the equestrian and hiker/mountain biker/wheelchair trails split and take separate routes on opposite sides of the creek.

You reach the Sycamore Rest Area midway through your trip, the first of three shady, attractive stops with picnic tables. This is a delightful lunch place where you can enjoy the lush creekside environment. As the name implies, tall, white-barked, big-leaved sycamores provide welcome shade on a hot summer day. These deciduous trees are shorn of their leaves in fall offering dappled sunlight as the weather cools.

Farther on, at a mini-airport for model airplanes, you might enjoy watching the planes take off and land but perhaps not the buzz of their little motors. Beyond the airport, the trail skirts the golf course, often just below a landscaped, high berm. Shortly you pass under Highway 101 and reach the Burnett Avenue Ranger Station parking area. Across the creek, the Walnut Rest Area provides barbecues and picnic tables under a canopy of oak trees and is a popular spot for anglers who try their luck in the rushing waters below the Anderson Dam outflow. If you have hiked or ridden your bike to this place, you might arrange for friends to meet you here for an evening barbecue beside the creek.

◆ ◆ ◆

From here you have the choice of two segments of the Ridge Trail: Northwest is the Santa Teresa/Los Alamitos Creek Trail, and southwest is the Mt. Madonna County Park leg. The former is about 10 miles north, the latter about 16 miles south.

Santa Teresa County Park
and Los Alamitos/Calero Creek Trail

From Pueblo Group Picnic Area
to Junction of McKean Road and Harry Road

Length 6.3 miles, including 2.0 miles round-trip to Coyote Peak and 4.3 miles to junction of McKean Road and Harry Road

Accessibility Hikers, equestrians, mountain bikers, and wheelchair users

Agency Santa Clara County Parks

Regulations Trail is open during daylight hours, and dogs on leash are permitted.

Facilities Water and restrooms at Pueblo Group Picnic Area

The Ridge Trail route branches east and west through Santa Teresa County Park. Take a round-trip trail east through high, oak-studded grasslands to Coyote Peak. Then head west on well-graded, exposed paths, past spring wildflower displays, serpentine outcrops, and Coast Range views; listen to the sound of running water on tree-lined, creekside trails. Finish on the wide, paved Los Alamitos/Calero Creek Trail through San Jose, partially shaded in late afternoon.

Getting There

By Car

EAST TRAILHEAD, SANTA TERESA COUNTY PARK: Take Highway 101 to the Bernal Road exit, turn south and go 1.6 miles to the park entrance. Continue 1 mile uphill on Bernal Road, and turn left to the Pueblo Group Picnic Area and parking.

WEST TRAILHEAD, LOS ALAMITOS/CALERO CREEK TRAIL: In south San Jose, take the Almaden Expressway to Harry Road, and turn right (south). In the next 300 yards look for street parking on Harry Road or on adjacent McKean Road.

To reach limited parking at the west end of Stile Ranch Trail, go south from Harry Road on McKean Road for 1.1 miles. Turn left (east) on Fortini Road and continue to its end.

By Bus

Santa Clara County Transit buses stop at the intersection of Santa Teresa Boulevard and Bernal Road daily and at Harry Road daily.

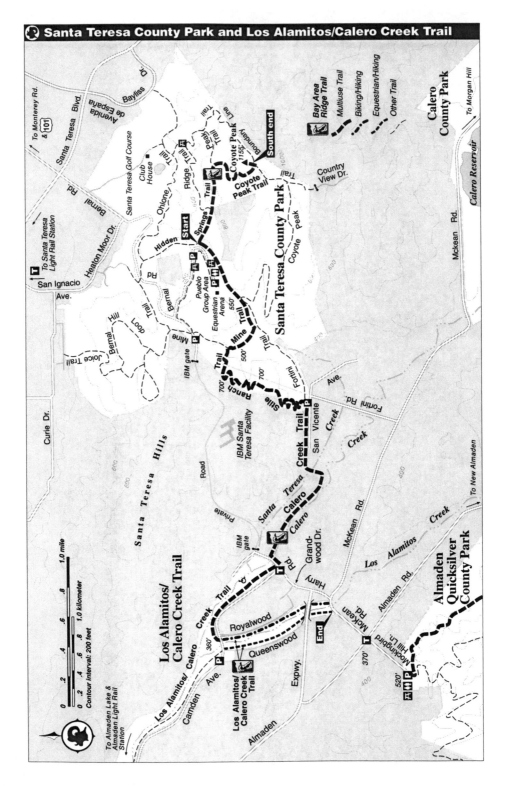

Santa Teresa County Park and Los Alamitos/Calero Creek Trail

On the Trail

The 2-mile round-trip to 1155-foot Coyote Peak, the highest point in the park, begins at the Pueblo Group Picnic Area. A few yards uphill from the picnic area, turn left (east) on the Pueblo Trail. You soon turn right on the Hidden Springs Trail, and cross a bridge over an unnamed creek. For a short while, lovely, broad-branched oaks and spring-flowering buckeye trees shade your route. As you climb, however, the shade trees disappear. Pass the park's own Ridge Trail coming in on the left and very shortly turn right on the Coyote Peak Trail.

For the next half mile, you follow the hillside up to and around the peak, with westward views to the wooded heights of the Santa Cruz Mountains. When the trail swings around to the south slope of the peak, take the left (northwest) turn to reach the summit, which offers sweeping panoramas of the Santa Clara Valley. This fertile land, once known as the Valley of Heart's Delight, the fruit bowl of America, has been developed with industrial plants, shopping malls and subdivisions. Yet, thanks to far-sighted citizens who many years ago voted funds for park acquisition, the county's foothill and mountain parks and its creekside and baylands parks preserve some of the valley's former characteristic environment. Now retrace your steps to the Pueblo Group Picnic Area, and begin the next leg of your Ridge Trail trip.

Follow the Pueblo Trail west along the base of the rocky slope above the picnic area. Continue through the equestrian arena, unless some activity is in progress. On the far side of the arena, bear left (south) on the Mine Trail, which descends gently to Santa Teresa Creek, the small stream that drains the park's lush central meadow, now closed for wildlife habitat protection.

Descend through a little valley, along the west side of the stream, bordered by a few oaks and many bay trees. The south-facing hillsides, punctuated by lichen-encrusted igneous rocks interspersed with gray sage bushes, come alive with blue brodiaea, orange poppies, and magenta clarkia after winter rains. Among the rocks you may see gray-green serpentine, the California state rock. According to the geologic maps, a small fault runs through this valley.

You curve north, away from the creek, and climb to a ridgetop where a clump of gnarled oak trees with small, leathery, dull-green leaves stands beyond the fence on your left. This native California tree, mostly found on serpentine soil, is known as the leather oak. You will see other specimens of leather oak as you traverse sections of this trail cut through serpentine rock.

The trail descends into a quiet, grassy swale, sprinkled with fine old valley oak trees and pierced by an intermittent stream. After you cross the stream, go left on the Stile Ranch Trail; the Mine Trail continues right. The Stile Ranch Trail weaves through the sloping grasslands at a very manageable grade. Then you follow well-graded switchbacks uphill through tall grasses, ungrazed for several years. In early morning or late afternoon, you may see deer going to drink from the stream in a little notch in the hills.

As you zigzag up an east-facing ridge on a trail cut through solid rock and lined with chunks of serpentine, you can appreciate the persistent, indefatigable volunteer trail-builders' work. With the combined efforts of the County Parks Department, which funded the trail construction and now maintains it; the Trail Center, which directed the trail crews; and International Business Machines (IBM), which granted an easement over its land, this 1.6-mile Stile Ranch Trail was completed in 1991.

As you dip into another valley among clumps of bunchgrass, light-pink-flowered buckwheat, and tall stalks of white yarrow, a couple of switchbacks take you to a plank

Santa Clara Valley Parks

Santa Teresa Park is one of a cluster of three Santa Clara County parks in south San Jose—Santa Teresa, Almaden Quicksilver, and Calero Reservoir parks—which encompass 7400 acres in the narrowest part of the Santa Clara Valley. This Bay Area Ridge Trail trip begins in 1677-acre Santa Teresa County Park, at the southern end of the Santa Teresa Hills. Portions of these hills and some of the adjacent valleys were part of Joaquin Bernal's vast Rancho Santa Teresa. Bernal received the 9646-acre land grant as compensation for investigating mineral deposits in California. There were no productive mines in present-day park land, but Bernal and his family lived near here and ran cattle on these hills for many years.

bridge across a wash (dry in summer). Then you begin ascending an east-facing ridge, a veritable Persian carpet of multicolored wildflowers in spring. Even in July this hillside glows with the magenta haze of Clarkia blossoms. A few oaks and an occasional bay tree offer shade in the late afternoon. When you reach a switchback, look east to see the white domes of the Lick Observatories atop Mt. Hamilton in the Diablo Range.

The trail levels at the top of the ridge and passes a couple of 6-foot-high sentinel rocks splashed with orange and red lichen. One rock set farther back from the trail could serve as a traveler's bench and rest stop to enjoy this remote oak-dotted grassland. You have a panoramic vista west of the Santa Cruz Mountains: Loma Prieta, the tallest mountain in this range, lies south of Mt. Umunhum, which you can identify by the tall structure on its summit. In the valley below, subdivisions and ranchettes are replacing the vineyards and orchards of yesteryear. Feeder roads in the valley bear former ranchers' names—Fortini and Rakstad, among others.

As you descend rapidly down numerous switchbacks, note a fine old rock wall that undulates uphill and down, defining an early boundary, which is now also delineated by a barbed-wire fence. Bluebird boxes hang from tall posts on the far side of the wall. This open, oak-studded grassland is typical habitat for the rusty-breasted Western bluebird, but rapid urbanization has decreased its natural nesting sites and reduced this beautiful bird's numbers. Yet it is known that bluebirds can be lured to nest in bird boxes.

When you reach the bottom of the hill, follow the trail between a double row of live oaks and go right (west). On the City of San Jose's Calero Creek Trail between the road and the fence, you head west for less than a quarter mile, and cross a log barrier. Proceed along the base of the slope past wide fields, planted or plowed according to the season. Signs request that you stay out of these fields. (There is no outlet on the other side.)

Carry on for a half mile, and then angle left (south) between two barbed-wire fences. The trail dips down into the channel of intermittent Santa Teresa Creek, which drains the terrain through which you just traveled. This streamcourse is a cool, damp place under a tall canopy of trees—delightful on a hot day but potentially difficult to cross after heavy rains.

On the other side of the stream, you pass a well-kept, fenced walnut orchard on the right and a small model-plane landing strip on the left. When you reach the next line of trees, veer right (west) and follow a wide track for a half mile beside Calero Creek.

Accompanied by the sounds of running water, leaves rustling in the breeze, and birds singing in the trees, you wander along the creek bank sheltered by tall, white-barked sycamores and broad-branched oaks. Through openings in the understory of elderberry, poison oak, and wild roses, you can see the creek flowing toward its confluence with Los Alamitos Creek.

Your creekside ramble continues to Harry Road, where you cross the road, jog left on the bridge over the creek, and then turn right on the paved trail that meanders through a wide easement between the creek and Camden Avenue. Although the creek is completely hidden from view, its wooded corridor adds charm to the neighboring community.

Wheelchair users can join others on the paved Los Alamitos/Calero Creek Trail. About 1 mile from Harry Road, Camden Avenue crosses Los Alamitos Creek, which joins Calero Creek just beyond. Here, at the confluence of the two creeks, in a wide half-moon-shaped easement, is a parking area on the site of a proposed park. Beyond here the City of San Jose's Los Alamitos/Calero Creek Trail extends 2.7 miles to Almaden Lake, a water sports and picnic park, from which a trail will someday follow the Guadalupe River to San Francisco Bay.

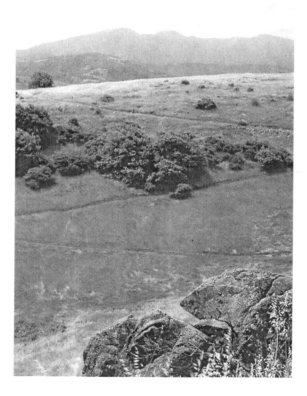

Loma Prieta from Stile Ranch Trail

However, to continue on the Bay Area Ridge Trail from Camden Avenue south to the junction of McKean Road and Harry Road, take one of the paths on either side of Los Alamitos Creek. These wide paths are built on raised levees between the generous creekbed and the adjoining subdivision roads and meander upstream for a mile, shaded by oaks, sycamores, and cottonwoods. Choose the paved trail on the east side of the creek for shade in the afternoon on a hot day. **Equestrians** use the unpaved trail on the west side.

Continue on the creek trail as it dips under the broad span of the Almaden Expressway bridge. You will be joined on this last leg of the trip by children on bicycles, neighbors strolling or walking their dogs (on leash), runners, and parents teaching youngsters to ride bikes. For the time being, the Ridge Trail segment terminates at the intersection

Quicksilver Mining

Los Alamitos Creek originates in Almaden Quicksilver County Park, west of Santa Teresa Park in Santa Clara Valley. Long before Europeans settled in this valley, Native Americans traveled upstream along Los Alamitos Creek to gather cinnabar in the hills of today's Almaden Quicksilver Park. They crushed the rock to make the red pigment with which they decorated their bodies. Cinnabar, also known as quicksilver, came under high demand during the Gold Rush, and the park was the site of a large mining operation.

Cinnabar contains mercury, and residual mercury in the soil and streams is highly toxic. Some areas of the abandoned Almaden Quicksilver mines are closed to the public, and prominent signs along the trails warn that fish in the creek are contaminated with mercury and should not be eaten.

of McKean Road and Harry roads. You can retrace your route to Santa Teresa Park or have a shuttle car waiting at one of two parking areas along the route, Camden Avenue or a limited-parking place at the foot of the Stile Ranch Trail on parklands off Fortini Road.

◆ ◆ ◆

The next segment of the Bay Area Ridge Trail climbs to the crest of the Santa Cruz Mountains in southern Santa Clara County. See Almaden Quicksilver County Park.

Almaden Quicksilver County Park

From Mockingbird Trail Entrance to Hicks Road

Length	4.5 miles
Accessibility	Hikers, mountain bikers, equestrians, and horsecart drivers
Agency	Santa Clara County Parks Department
Regulations	Park is open from 8 AM to a half hour after sunset. Dogs must be on a 6-foot or shorter leash at all times. Mountain bikers are allowed on certain marked trails but must wear helmets.
Facilities	Park office, water, and restrooms at main entrance on Almaden Road (La Hacienda); picnic areas, restrooms, potable water, equestrian staging area, and horse trough at Mockingbird Hill Lane entrance

A steady climb to the slopes of Mt. Umunhum takes you through lands once trod by miners searching for gold.

Getting There

By Car

MOCKINGBIRD HILL TRAIL ENTRANCE: From Almaden Expressway, turn south on Almaden Road, go 0.7 mile, and turn right on Mockingbird Hill Lane to lower park entrance.

HICKS ROAD ENTRANCE: From Almaden Expressway, turn right on Camden Avenue. Turn right on Hicks Road and follow it to the park entrance.

By Bicycle

An off-road bike path runs south beside Alamitos Creek from Almaden Lake to McKean Road, on which you turn right and then continue on Mockingbird Hill Lane to park entrance.

By Bus

A Valley Transit Authority bus serves the main park entrance.

On the Trail

In these parklands was once the most productive quicksilver mine in the western world. Miles of tunnels pierced the hills and more than 500 houses clustered on the

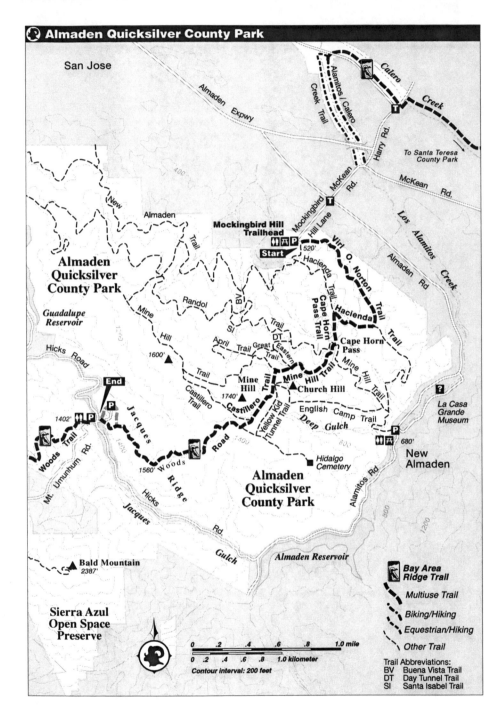

Almaden Quicksilver County Park

San Jose

Almaden Expwy

Alamitos / Calero Creek Trail

Calero Creek

Harry Rd.

McKean Rd.

To Santa Teresa County Park

McKean Rd.

Los Alamitos Creek

Almaden Rd

New

Almaden

Almaden Trail

Mockingbird Hill Trailhead

Start 520'

Hacienda Trail

Mockingbird Hill Lane

Virl O. Norton Trail

Almaden Quicksilver County Park

Guadalupe Reservoir

Randol Trail

Mine Hill

BV

SI

Trail

April Trail

Great Eastern Trail

DT

Cape Horn Pass Trail

Hacienda Trail

Cape Horn Pass

Mine Hill Trail

Hicks Road

1600' ▲

Trail

Mine Hill Trail

End

P

1402' **P**

Castillero Trail

Castillero Trail

Mine Hill ▲ 1740'

Church Hill

Mine Hill Trail

Church Hill

English Camp Trail

?

La Casa Grande Museum

Woods Trail

Mt. Umunhum Rd.

Jacques Road

Yellow Kid Tunnel Trail

Deep Gulch

P

680'

New Almaden

1560' Woods Ridge

Hicks

Hidalgo Cemetery

Jacques Rd.

Gulch

Alamitos Rd.

Almaden Quicksilver County Park

▲ **Bald Mountain** 2387'

Almaden Reservoir

Sierra Azul Open Space Preserve

0 .2 .4 .6 .8 1.0 mile
0 .2 .4 .6 .8 1.0 kilometer

Contour interval: 200 feet

Bay Area Ridge Trail

Multiuse Trail

Biking/Hiking

Equestrian/Hiking

Other Trail

Trail Abbreviations:
BV   Buena Vista Trail
DT   Day Tunnel Trail
SI   Santa Isabel Trail

ridge. Today, the Ridge Trail follows old mining roads that lead over these hills, where you can imagine New Almaden Mine's heyday.

The mine tunnels and shafts are now closed off, and the furnaces of the New Almaden Quicksilver Mining Company have long since been dismantled. English Town, Spanish Town, and a Chinese Camp where miners lived are gone. The ore they sought, known as quicksilver, gives its name to this spacious county park. Highly valued for its use in the reduction of gold, this mercury-producing cinnabar was important to the miners after they discovered that precious metal in the California hills.

In 1845 a Mexican cavalry officer and engineer, Andres Castillero, filed a mining claim to this deposit, and later Alexander Forbes acquired an interest in the mine. He named the mine "New Almaden" after the famous quicksilver mine in Spain and formed the New Almaden Quicksilver Mining Company.

By 1851 two mines were in operation in addition to the New Almaden—the Enriquita and the Guadalupe, northeast along the ridge. A village of cottages for the staff was built along Alamitos Creek. A Spanish Town for Mexicans and an English Town for Cornish miners were perched high on the hill near the mines. For a short time there was also a Chinese Camp.

New Almaden became a tourist attraction, bringing eminent visitors, including an emissary from the emperor of China, who came seeking purchases of quicksilver. By 1870 production at the mine had peaked, but under a new manager, James Randol, mining methods were improved, and some new bodies of ore were found. After Randol left in 1892, the fortunes of the company declined and by 1912 it was in bankruptcy.

The Senador Mine at the north end of the ridge produced from 1990 through 1926. Then, in an effort to reduce hazards from the mercury-producing process, the Army Corps of Engineers demolished nearly all the early structures, the miners' cottages, and two churches on Mine Hill. All mine shafts and tunnels have been sealed. However, the entrance to the San Cristobal Mine has been reconstructed so that visitors can look into the tunnel. New Almaden, listed as a Historic District in the National Register of Historic Places, and the community of New Almaden, now known as a County Historic Zoning District, retain the integrity of this more-than-a-century-old village.

At present, historical markers and interpretive plaques tell the story of cinnabar, a term derived from an ancient Persian word meaning "dragon's blood." The county's New Almaden Mercury Mining Museum is located at La Casa Grande at 21570 Almaden Road, which has displays of mining equipment, models, maps, and photographs, all of which give you some grasp of the astounding scale of mining operations at New Almaden. The New Almaden Quicksilver County Park Association supports the protection, restoration, and development of this unique site.

In 1994 Santa Clara County, jointly with the Midpeninsula Regional Open Space District, acquired 907 acres on Jacques Ridge near Hicks Road. This important purchase connects Almaden Quicksilver Park with the Mt. Umunhum Area of Sierra Azul Open Space Preserve and provides a valuable wildlife corridor connecting 18,000 acres of open space and a vital link in the Bay Area Ridge Trail.

On Saturday April 17, 2004, the Bay Area Ridge Trail Council dedicated this 4.5-mile segment of the Ridge Trail, which connects on the west to the 6.4-mile Wood Trail in the Sierra Azul Open Space Preserve, also a section of the Bay Area Ridge Trail.

Hikers, equestrians, and **mountain bikers** start up the steep hill on the Virl O. Norton Trail, a wide, power line service road that roughly follows the northeastern boundary of the park. It skirts close to the fences of neighboring houses in a series of

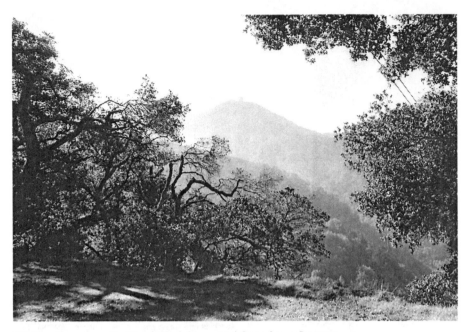

Mt. Umunhum from the Woods Trail, Sierra Azul Open Space Preserve

steep rises, broken by short, almost level stretches and then repeats this mode for 1.2 miles. Your route then turns right (west) on the Hacienda Trail and heads for Cape Horn Pass, which you reach in about a half mile. At this three-way junction turn west on the middle trail—the Mine Hill Trail—and continue uphill to the site of settlements where Cornish, Mexican, and Chinese miners once lived. A few buildings remain, boarded up and off-limits, but a plaque tells the story of these hardy men and women living so far from their native lands.

Just past English Town, pick up the Castillero Trail, follow it for a little more than a half mile, and then watch for the left turnoff to the Wood Trail. On this trail you cross Jacques Ridge on a long reach through oak woodland to the grasslands that border Hicks Road.

◆ ◆ ◆

This marks the end of the Almaden Quicksilver Park segment and the beginning of the next long trip. See Sierra Azul Open Space Preserve on p. 193.

Sanborn County Park and Castle Rock State Park

From Sunnyvale Mountain Picnic Area to Saratoga Gap

Length 6.0 miles

Accessibility Hikers, equestrians, and mountain bikers can ride on the shoulder of Skyline Boulevard and then take the Service Road Trail to Castle Rock and the Saratoga Gap Trail to Saratoga Gap.

Agencies Santa Clara County Parks Department and California Department of Parks and Recreation

Regulations Parks are open from 8 AM to dusk. Dogs and bicycles are prohibited on trails.

Facilities Small parking area, picnic tables, and restroom at Sunnyvale Mountain; no water or telephone; large parking area at Saratoga Gap

Follow the Skyline Trail along the ridgeline of two vast parks—Sanborn County Park and Castle Rock State Park. On the route of old Summit Road, you'll wind along the protected east side of the crest of the Santa Cruz Mountains through forests of Douglas fir, oak, and madrone; you'll pass immense sandstone outcrops and vestiges of early homesteaders' orchards and dwellings. This fairly level trip is ideal for warm days, entirely in shade on a trail that varies in width from wide to narrow.

Getting There

SOUTH TRAILHEAD, SUNNYVALE MOUNTAIN PICNIC AREA: Take Skyline Boulevard (Highway 35) to Sunnyvale Mountain Picnic Area, 4.7 miles south of Saratoga Gap (junction of Highway 35 and Highway 9) on east side of road.

NORTH TRAILHEAD, SARATOGA GAP: Take Skyline Boulevard (Highway 35) to Saratoga Gap, at the junction with Highway 9. There is a parking area 500 feet south of Saratoga Gap on the east side of Skyline Boulevard; some spaces are available at the trailhead on the northeast side of Highway 9.

On the Trail

From the north side of the Sunnyvale Mountain Picnic Area, **hikers** and **equestrians** follow the Bay Area Ridge Trail as it skirts the edge of an overgrown orchard and heads northward on a wide, old farm road. Stay left at a fork in the trail and climb gently under a canopy of mature Douglas firs. In a forest clearing, fragments of a sea captain's garden mark the former Seagraves' residence; beyond, on a clear day, you may see south across Monterey Bay to the Monterey Peninsula and its mountains.

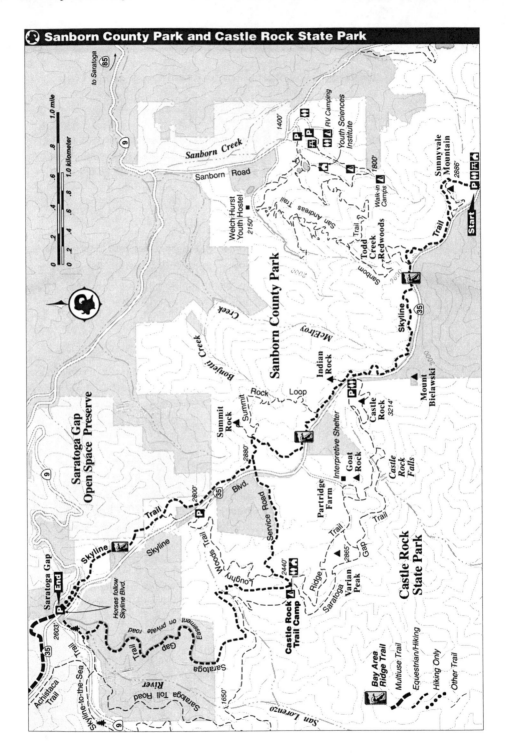

Sanborn County Park and Castle Rock State Park

Back in forest, the trail descends to a shady redwood grove with a picnic table beside a stone wall that flanked the now-closed entrance to the former Seagraves' homestead. Beyond here the trail narrows and continues through a dense forest, into and around steep-sided canyons, the headwaters of streams named for early settlers—Todd, McElroy, and Bonjetti.

You soon pass the first of several wind- and water-eroded sandstone outcrops, uplifted over the millennia by folding and faulting along the San Andreas Rift Zone.

Keep left at the next junction where many deer tracks in the dust of the trail, the sharp call of blue jays, and the chatter of squirrels in the trees attest to the presence of others who enjoy this ridgetop forest.

On a wide swing east around the shoulder of a ridge, you meet the Sanborn Trail, 1.2 miles from your starting point This trail ascends 700 feet from Sanborn County Park where you will find camping and picnic sites, a youth hostel and RV parking.

Your route on the Skyline Trail, however, continues northwest, cut into the steep sides of Todd Creek Canyon. Madrones and tanoaks intersperse the Douglas-fir forest, and you have occasional glimpses of the Santa Clara Valley. As the trail bends north, look uphill on your right for a cluster of sandstone outcrops, the largest known as Indian Rock. Some are easily climbed and make fine perches for enjoying your backpack lunch.

Just past Indian Rock, you see a sign for Castle Rock State Park, 3000 acres of semi-wilderness mostly east of Skyline Boulevard on the steep west face of the Santa Cruz Mountains. Here are hiking trails that lead to waterfalls, shady forests, extensive sandstone outcrops, and a backpack trail camp (2.7 miles from the Skyline Boulevard parking area).

The Bay Area Ridge Trail route continues north on the Skyline Trail. You pass the south end of the Summit Rock Loop Trail, which descends into Bonjetti Creek Canyon. Then, the north end of the loop trail, after curving around yet another settler's homesite, joins the main trail. A side trip on this 1.2-mile loop takes you to huge sandstone outcrops, one of which lures climbers to the top. However, a peek around the base of this outcrop also offers a sweeping view of the South Bay.

Continuing north, bear left at the second junction of the Summit Rock Loop Trail, and follow the wide, old roadbed northwest past some big mahogany-barked, broad-branched madrones. In about a half mile the Loughry Woods Trail from Castle Rock

Early Skyline Settlers

In the late 1800s, immigrants from mountainous regions of Europe settled these hillsides, set out orchards and vineyards, and built wineries. But the 1906 earthquake struck hard here, causing landslides and severe property damage. Eventually most of the hillside farms were abandoned. After Santa Clara County bought the parklands in the 1970s, the dwellings were removed, but some exotic plantings remain. As you follow the route of the old road joining their farms, imagine the hard work and tenacity required to carve out an existence on these steep hillsides far from the fertile Santa Clara Valley.

Side Trips

Todd Redwood Grove

Follow the Sanborn Trail to Todd Redwood Grove (0.3 mile) where a few venerable giants remain after the logging of the late 1800s. Farther along the Sanborn Trail, you'll find backpack campsites, 1.6 miles downhill in Sanborn Park, and the Sanborn Hostel, set in a grove of majestic redwoods off the San Andreas Trail. The hostel, known as Welch Hurst, was built as a mountain retreat by former Santa Clara County Judge James Welch in the early 1900s. It is now on the National Register of Historic Places.

Indian Rock

The best views are from Indian Rock, 1.2 gentle uphill miles from the Sanborn Trail intersection and 0.2 mile from the main trail. Rock climbers and casual hikers clamber up on these exposed sandstone rocks, set among gnarled oaks and madrones, for east and south views over the Santa Clara Valley to the high points of the South Bay—Mt. Hamilton and Mission Peak. The dramatic drop-off on the east side of the rocks is a breathtaking 150 feet.

Summit Rock

A short (0.2-mile) side trip takes you to Summit Rock, another huge sandstone outcrop. Veer right at the second junction of the loop trail. From perches some 20 feet off the ground, you'll have a hawk's-eye view of Sanborn County Park and Monte Bello Ridge to the north.

State Park joins the Skyline Trail. Shortly, when you pass between two boulders marking the trail entrance from a parking area near Skyline Boulevard, **hikers** veer right, staying on a narrow ridge until you join the old Summit Road going north. **Equestrians** must go left staying close to Skyline Boulevard before rejoining hikers 0.6 mile north.

Here you leave Sanborn County Park and enter the 120 acres of Castle Rock State Park that lie on the east side of the Skyline Ridge, formerly known as Loughry Woods. The Skyline Trail, now a narrow footpath, continues through mixed woodland, swinging around the east side of a 2920-foot ridge.

Then, skirting a fenced, private inholding, you once again pick up old Summit Road, with tall, fragrant firs overhead, soft forest duff underfoot, and trailside moss-covered rocks. Fern fronds and clumps of iris edge the trail, while fine-leafed ocean spray and hazelnut bushes often overhang it. In spring you may find blue hound's tongue blooming on tall stalks.

Continue on the narrow path, but 0.3 mile before the end of the route, you must descend to Skyline Boulevard on a cut-off to the left in order to circumnavigate one impassable stretch. For the last 0.3 mile of this trip, **hikers** traverse a very steep hillside on a narrow footpath for hikers only. After crossing a couple of sturdy wooden bridges over gullies and passing some sizable sandstone boulders, you come to the Saratoga Gap parking area.

For those who left cars at the Sunny-vale Mountain Picnic Area, it's time to turn around and make the trip southeast to your starting point or have a shuttle car waiting here for you. **Hikers, equestri-ans,** and **mountain bikers** meet at the Saratoga Gap parking area.

◆ ◆ ◆

From there **all trail users** can pick up the next leg of the Bay Area Ridge Trail on the northeast side of Highway 9. **Hik-ers** and **equestrians** may follow the Skyline-to-the-Sea Trail southwest along the east side of Highway 9 to a marked crossing of this highway that leads to the Achistaca Trail in Long Ridge Open Space Preserve.

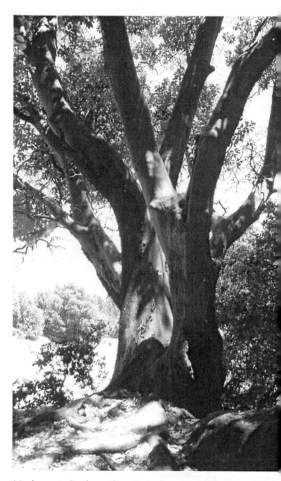

Madrone in Sanborn County Park

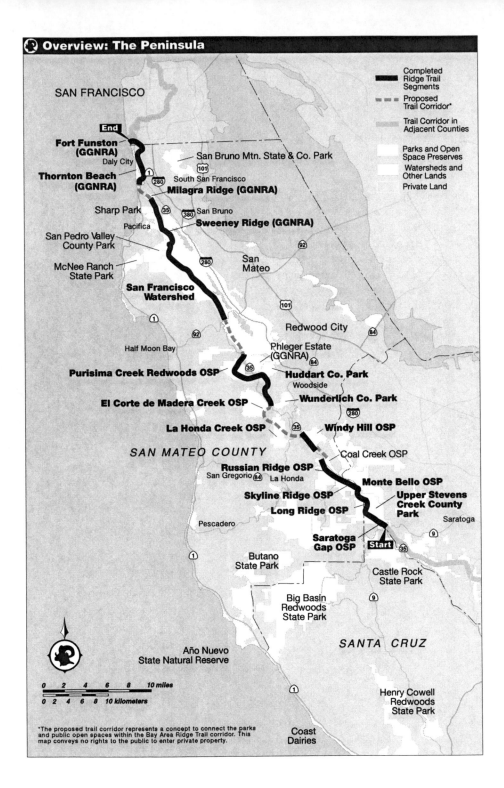

SAN FRANCISCO

End

Fort Funston (GGNRA)
Daly City

Thornton Beach (GGNRA)

Sharp Park

Pacifica

San Pedro Valley County Park

McNee Ranch State Park

San Francisco Watershed

Half Moon Bay

Purisima Creek Redwoods OSP

El Corte de Madera Creek OSP

La Honda Creek OSP

SAN MATEO COUNTY

San Gregorio   La Honda

Russian Ridge OSP

Skyline Ridge OSP

Long Ridge OSP

Pescadero

Saratoga Gap OSP

Butano State Park

Big Basin Redwoods State Park

SANTA CRUZ

Año Nuevo State Natural Reserve

San Bruno Mtn. State & Co. Park

South San Francisco

Milagra Ridge (GGNRA)

San Bruno

Sweeney Ridge (GGNRA)

San Mateo

Redwood City

Phleger Estate (GGNRA)

Huddart Co. Park
Woodside

Wunderlich Co. Park

Windy Hill OSP

Coal Creek OSP

Monte Bello OSP

Upper Stevens Creek County Park
Saratoga

Start

Castle Rock State Park

Henry Cowell Redwoods State Park

Coast Dairies

Completed Ridge Trail Segments

Proposed Trail Corridor*

Trail Corridor in Adjacent Counties

Parks and Open Space Preserves

Watersheds and Other Lands

Private Land

0   2   4   6   8   10 miles
0   2   4   6   8   10 kilometers

*The proposed trail corridor represents a concept to connect the parks and public open spaces within the Bay Area Ridge Trail corridor. This map conveys no rights to the public to enter private property.

216

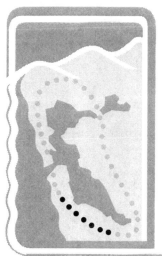

THE PENINSULA

Saratoga Gap Open Space Preserve to Skyline Ridge
Open Space Preserve. 219

Skyline Ridge and Russian Ridge Open Space Preserves 223

Windy Hill Open Space Preserve 227

Wunderlich County Park to Huddart County Park. 231

Purisima Creek Redwoods Open Space Preserve. 235

San Francisco Watershed Trail. 239

Golden Gate National Recreation Area:
Sweeney Ridge to Milagra Ridge 243

Mussel Rock to Fort Funston 249

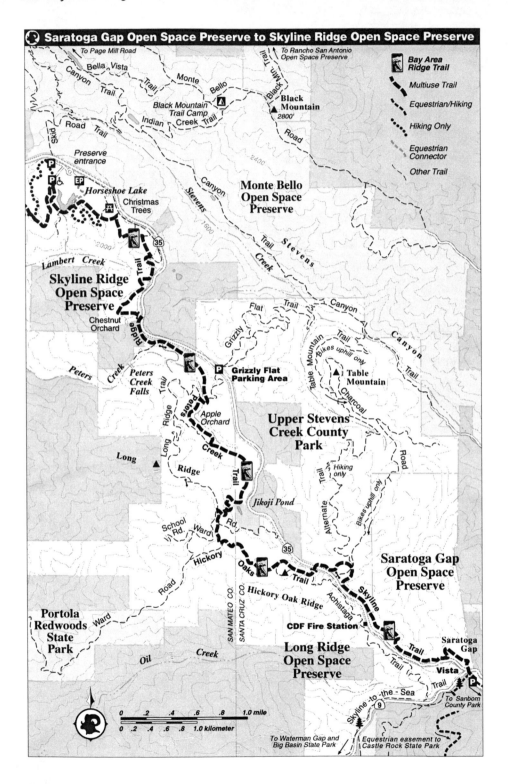

Saratoga Gap Open Space Preserve to Skyline Ridge Open Space Preserve

Saratoga Gap Open Space Preserve to Skyline Ridge Open Space Preserve

From Saratoga Gap to Horseshoe Lake

Length 7.8 miles

Accessibility Hikers, equestrians, mountain bikers, and wheelchair users

Agency Midpeninsula Regional Open Space District

Regulations Preserves are open from dawn to a half hour after sunset. Dogs on leash are permitted in a designated area of Long Ridge Open Space Preserve just north of Grizzly Flat parking area; maps are available from MROSD office. Mountain bikers must observe 15 MPH speed limit and wear helmets. Upper Stevens Creek County Park is open from 8 AM to sunset. Dogs are prohibited. Helmets are required for mountain bikers.

Facilities No water on route; restrooms at Horseshoe Lake parking area in Skyline Ridge OSP; water and telephone at Saratoga Summit Fire Station (0.7 mile north of Saratoga Gap on west side of Skyline Boulevard)

Travel through moist evergreen forests, oak-madrone woodlands, and high grasslands along the crest of the Santa Cruz Mountains. Stunning coast and bay views greet you on this Ridge Trail route through three Midpeninsula Regional Open Space District preserves and one county park. The trail roughly follows old Summit Road, a wagon route used by early settlers before Skyline Boulevard was built. Trail width and surface varies from a narrow path to a wide patrol road, soft in forests and along creekbeds, and firm and bare through grasslands. You'll gain and lose 400 feet in elevation, plus experience several ups and downs en route of 100 to 300 feet. Be prepared for wind and fog on exposed ridgetops, and for heat on protected west- and south-facing slopes. The Hickory Oak gate on Skyline Boulevard makes it easy to break this route into two trips—a shady, moderately level, 2-mile trip from Saratoga Gap to Long Ridge Open Space Preserve, and a 5.8-mile trip from there to the Horseshoe Lake parking area in Skyline Ridge Open Space Preserve.

Getting There

SOUTH TRAILHEAD, SARATOGA GAP: Take Skyline Boulevard (Highway 35) to its intersection with Highway 9 at Saratoga Gap. The parking area is 500 feet south of Saratoga Gap on the east side of Skyline Boulevard.

NORTH TRAILHEAD, SKYLINE RIDGE OPEN SPACE PRESERVE, HORSESHOE LAKE:
Take Page Mill Road to Skyline Boulevard (Highway 35), turn left (south), and go 0.75 mile to the preserve entrance on the west side of the road.

On the Trail

Hikers, equestrians, and **mountain bikers** enter Saratoga Gap Open Space Preserve under a canopy of great oaks on the Skyline Trail. For the next 1.7 miles, you meander around bends and into hollows above a steep-sided canyon. With Douglas firs towering overhead, you skirt massive wind- and rain-pocked sandstone outcrops. These rocks were probably uplifted when the Pacific Plate dipped under the North American Plate in the geologic processes that built the Santa Cruz Mountains eons ago.

Because the drop-off on your right is too sheer for farming or cattle-grazing, this mountainside has remained relatively untouched. The rather unusual California nutmeg tree, which you can recognize by its flat, prickly needles that distinguish it from Douglas-fir needles, is taking hold here. An old springhouse remains in a steep ravine below the trail. Fallen leaves from ancient madrones carpet the ground with shades of mauve, yellow, and gold.

After reaching Upper Stevens Creek County Park, you swing east into a clearing and meet unpaved Charcoal Road. This historic road, once used for hauling charcoal that was made from trees here, descends through second-growth forests to Stevens Creek in Monte Bello Open Space Preserve. However, your trail continues northwest toward Skyline Boulevard, through an oak-madrone woodland.

Cross Skyline Boulevard to the Hickory Oak gate of Long Ridge Open Space Preserve. After a short rise to the ridgetop, you head north on the Hickory Oaks Trail, part of old Summit Road and now a MROSD patrol road, through a forest of the area's namesake—mature, widely-spaced hickory oaks, also called canyon live oaks, some at

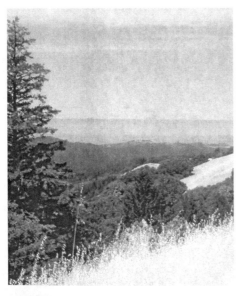

Long Ridge Open Space Preserve

least 5 feet in diameter. The canyon live oak bears dark green, prickly leaves that are powdery tan or gray underneath. Its acorns have a furry golden ruff around the cup, giving it yet another name, the golden cup oak. Regardless of your name preference, you will surely notice how well this species grows along the west side of the Skyline ridge.

Beyond the woods, the main Bay Area Ridge Trail route continues on the patrol road, but you can veer left on a narrow trail to the preserve's 2693-foot high point. Here more sandstone outcrops, lichen-splotched and weather-etched, stand near the lip of an abrupt decline into tree-filled Oil Creek canyon. From this vantage point, the panorama of successive forested ridges creased by wooded stream canyons is an uncluttered, pastoral scene to nourish your spirit.

Achistaga Trail: An Alternate Hiker and Equestrian Route

From the southeast corner of Skyline Boulevard and Highway 9 at Saratoga Gap, **hikers** and **equestrians** can follow the Skyline-to-the-Sea Trail west for about a mile and then carefully cross to the north side of Highway 9 at the Achistaga Trail entrance to Long Ridge Open Space Preserve. This 1-mile trail ambles along the west side of the Santa Cruz Mountains below the ridgetop under the shade of fine old oak and madrone trees. It passes below the Skyline California Department of Forestry Fire Station and then veers a little west before joining the main Ridge Trail route at the Hickory Oaks Trail entrance in Long Ridge Open Space Preserve.

Continue on the narrow trail around the shoulder of the knoll and zigzag downhill through the hickory and live-oak woods to loop back to the main Bay Area Ridge Trail route on the Hickory Oaks Trail. You make several descents into broad swales and subsequent climbs to hilltop viewpoints. In spring and summer bright orange poppies nestle against boulders, and pink checkerblooms peek out from the grasses; in fall vinegary-smelling blue curls add trailside touches of color to this spectacular trip.

At the next junction, you ascend right, around a shoulder of the ridge, and the Hickory Oaks Trail descends west to Portola Redwoods State Park on Pescadero Creek. You follow the ridgetop Long Ridge Trail to a junction with the Peters Creek Trail, the multiuse Bay Area Ridge Trail route for the next 1.7 miles, and turn right (east). An alternate, 2.1-mile route continues along the ridge and down the Peters Creek Loop Trail; it meets the Ridge Trail route at the last Peters Creek crossing. Your trail, the Peters Creek Trail, descends switchbacks through an oak forest to cross the earthen dam that holds back the waters of Peters Creek. On the dam's east side, turn left and follow the former wagon road, an avenue of welcome shade in summer and a moist trail under leafy arches in winter.

Past homesteaders' moss-covered fence posts and remnants of an apple orchard, you traverse a secluded valley where willow thickets mark the creek's course. Soon you and the creek arc right into a tight little canyon with delicate fern fronds draping the hillsides and exposed, gnarled tree roots growing around moss-covered boulders. After crossing the Peters Creek bridge, the Ridge Trail follows a connector trail between the Peters Creek crossing and the southern entrance to Skyline Ridge Open Space Preserve. Parts of this 1-mile trail, open to hikers, mountain bikers, and equestrians, adjoin private lands. Please respect fences, close gates, and observe trail directions. After the Peters Creek bridge, you could make a gentle, 0.5-mile ascent to Long Ridge Open Space Preserve's Grizzly Flat entrance on Skyline Boulevard; leave a second car here to shorten this trip.

The connector trail terminates in Skyline Ridge Open Space Preserve on a knoll overlooking a hillside orchard of widely spaced chestnut and walnut trees. If you come here in fall, you can buy harvested nuts from the orchard's former owners. The next leg of the Ridge Trail meanders downhill through the orchard, above a tributary of Lambert Creek under a canopy of overhanging trees. In spring, fronds of creamy Solomon's seal drape over moist, fern-clad banks, and heavenly blue and light yellow irises bloom on erect stalks.

You pass ancient oaks and are again on old Summit Road until you leave the woods. Then turn sharply left and watch for Bay Area Ridge Trail signs that guide you up and down hills on a graveled road bordering a Christmas tree farm. There are straight, tight rows of conically pruned conifers on one side and a graceful, untamed native forest on the other. Beginning in early November, this farm, leased from MROSD, draws eager urbanites searching for the perfect Christmas tree. After a final uphill pitch on the graveled surface, pause to look east across Stevens Creek canyon and the San Andreas Rift Zone to Monte Bello Ridge. Creased by tree-filled canyons, the rounded, grassy ridge is surmounted by 2800-foot Black Mountain, its summit marked by tall antennae.

From this viewpoint, the 0.6-mile **hikers-only route** angles left up to a ridgetop crowned by venerable, 3-foot-diameter Douglas firs. Wend your way along the ridge under these magnificent trees for 0.2 mile, and then abruptly descend switchbacks to Horseshoe Lake, the headwaters of East Lambert Creek, on a steep, oak- and fir-forested, west-facing slope.

Equestrians and **mountain bikers** continue on the graveled road, a relatively level, wide route that curves around the northeast side of the ridge that the hiker's route traverses, and meet **hikers** on the east side of Horseshoe Lake.

Hikers and **mountain bikers** proceed southwest around Horseshoe Lake to the dam; to reach the Horseshoe Lake trailhead and parking area from the dam, both groups take parallel routes on the west side of the lake, going north to the handicapped parking area. They then proceed uphill (northeast) on the same trail and cross a sloping meadow to the preserve's Horseshoe Lake north parking area.

Equestrians leave the hiker, bicyclist, and equestrian junction on the east side of the lake and proceed north through woods of oak and buckeye to the equestrian parking area.

Before you leave Horseshoe Lake, note that the lake does indeed resemble an equine shoe, with arms wrapped around the base of a high, tree-thatched knoll. Home to redwinged blackbirds and several species of ducks, Horseshoe Lake is known to attract a pair of black-shouldered kites. These large white birds with black-tipped wings are often seen here searching the lakeshore for the frogs and water snakes that make up their diet.

You too can enjoy this scene by circling the lake on the foot trails that reach the picnic tables at the tip of the knoll above the lake—a delightful spot to enjoy a knapsack lunch or snack and savor your experiences on this beautiful segment of the Bay Area Ridge Trail.

From the handicapped parking area, **wheelchair users** can take the gently graded Ridge Trail route along the lake's reed-lined west shore, cross the bridge over the dam on the south side, and then circle the wooded east side of the lake.

◆ ◆ ◆

The next leg of the Bay Area Ridge Trail continues northward from the Horseshoe Lake parking areas. Adding this 4.8-mile trip, with a car shuttle at Russian Ridge, makes it possible for the trail user to spend a full day and 12.6 miles in the finest of coastal, mixed-evergreen forests and on untrammeled grasslands with unsurpassed views. A round trip from Saratoga Gap to Horseshoe Lake and back makes for an almost 16-mile excursion.

Skyline Ridge and Russian Ridge Open Space Preserves

From Horseshoe Lake to Rapley Ranch Road

Length	4.8 miles
Accessibility	Hikers, equestrians, and mountain bikers; wheelchair users have access to two lakeside trails around Horseshoe and Alpine lakes
Agency	Midpeninsula Regional Open Space District
Regulations	Preserves are open from dawn to a half hour after sunset. Dogs are prohibited. Mountain bikers must wear helmets and observe 15 MPH speed limit.
Facilities	Drinking fountain at Skyline Boulevard/Highway 9 parking area; water and restrooms at Alpine Pond and Horseshoe Lake parking areas; restrooms at junction of Skyline Boulevard and Alpine Road

Enjoy the Peninsula's finest views and most spectacular spring wildflower displays on these ridgeline trails through Skyline Ridge and Russian Ridge Open Space Preserves. Climb through open grasslands to high knolls on trails that vary in surface from duff-covered to gravelly or rocky, and in width from narrow (hikers only) to wide, paved and unpaved ranch roads. Expect gradual ridgetop elevation gains and loses. These exposed ridgetops can be foggy and windy; trails on south- and west-facing slopes offer only intermittent shade.

Getting There

SOUTH TRAILHEAD, SKYLINE RIDGE OPEN SPACE PRESERVE, HORSESHOE LAKE: Take Page Mill Road to Skyline Boulevard (Highway 35), turn left (south), and go 0.75 mile to the preserve entrance on the west side of the road.

NORTH TRAILHEAD, RUSSIAN RIDGE OPEN SPACE PRESERVE, RAPLEY RANCH ROAD: Take Page Mill Road to Skyline Boulevard (Highway 35), turn right (north), and go 2.7 miles to roadside parking on the west side of the road at Rapley Ranch Road.

On the Trail

Wheelchair users can follow the gently graded trail around Horseshoe Lake's west shore to the bridge over the dam on the south side and then circle the wooded east side of the lake. The trail around Alpine Pond is also accessible to wheelchairs from the Alpine Road parking area.

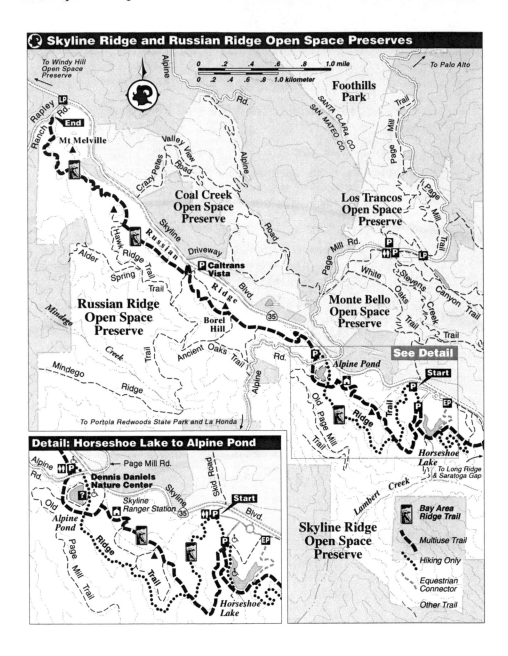

Skyline Ridge and Russian Ridge Open Space Preserves

To Windy Hill Open Space Preserve

To Palo Alto

Rapley Rd.

LP

End

Ranch Rd.

Mt Melville

Alpine

0   .2   .4   .6   .8   1.0 mile
0   .2   .4   .6   .8   1.0 kilometer

Foothills Park

SANTA CLARA CO.
SAN MATEO CO.

Page Mill Trail

Valley View Road

Crazy Pete's

Alpine Road

Coal Creek Open Space Preserve

Los Trancos Open Space Preserve

Page Mill Trail

Hawk Ridge Trail

Russian Ridge

Skyline

Alder Trail

Spring Trail

Driveway

Caltrans Vista

P

H P

LP

Page Mill Rd.

White Oaks Trail

Stevens Creek Canyon Trail

Russian Ridge Open Space Preserve

R i d g e

Borel Hill

Blvd.

35

Monte Bello Open Space Preserve

Trail

Mindego

Creek

Ancient Oaks Trail

Rd.

Alpine

P

Alpine Pond

See Detail

Start

P

EP

Mindego Ridge

Old Page Mill Trail

Ridge Trail

Horseshoe Lake

To Portola Redwoods State Park and La Honda

To Long Ridge & Saratoga Gap

Lambert Creek

Detail: Horseshoe Lake to Alpine Pond

Alpine Rd.

H P

Page Mill Rd.

Dennis Daniels Nature Center

?

Skyline Ranger Station

Skid Road

Skyline

35

Start

Blvd.

Old

Alpine Pond

Ridge

Page Mill Trail

Trail

H P

P

EP

Horseshoe Lake

Skyline Ridge Open Space Preserve

Bay Area Ridge Trail

━ ━ ━ Multiuse Trail

• • • • Hiking Only

Equestrian Connector

Other Trail

Hikers begin this Ridge Trail segment on a different route than equestrians and mountain bikers. From the northwest parking area at Horseshoe Lake, make a long, gradual ascent southwest on a steep, grassy hillside above East Lambert Creek. In late spring, a striking display of lemon-yellow mariposa lilies and blue brodiaea rise above drying oat grass.

After 0.9 mile, swing around to the west side of the preserve, and walk through pungent chaparral punctuated by occasional small oaks. From a dramatic parapet chipped out of a sheer sandstone butte, a 180-degree sweep of forests, stream canyons, ridges, and grasslands unfolds below you. On clear days, you can see the ocean, and in almost any weather, you can find Butano Ridge, which forms the western rampart above Portola Redwoods State Park and Pescadero and Memorial county parks. You can reach these parks from the Bay Area Ridge Trail via Ward Road in Long Ridge Open Space Preserve, and someday Old Page Mill Road in Portola Redwoods State Park will connect to the Bay Area Ridge Trail through Skyline Ridge Open Space Preserve.

The trail bends into folds of the mountain and traverses sloping grasslands for about a half mile and then enters a brief forested section, where great canyon live oaks flank the trail. A knoll above the Old Page Mill Road junction is the site of former Governor James Rolph's 1930s "Summer Capital," which was topped by a gold-painted, papier-mâché dome. "Sunny Jim" owned this land, as well as present-day Russian Ridge Open Space Preserve. Many years earlier, before the settlers arrived, the Ohlone came here to gather acorns, which they ground on nearby rocks. Continuing on the Bay Area Ridge Trail, round the east side of reed-lined Alpine Pond, cross Alpine Road to the Russian Ridge OSP parking area, and rejoin the mountain bikers and equestrians.

Mountain bikers and **equestrians** leave the Horseshoe Lake parking areas (mountain bikers use the northwest area, equestrians the northeast) and follow the marked routes down to the patrol road above the handicapped parking area at Horseshoe Lake. Here you go over a stile, veer right (south), and then bend northwest for a steep climb out of East Lambert Creek canyon. Cross the hikers' route and continue uphill (northwest) on an old, hard-surfaced, farm road through the preserve lands, now cleared of Christmas trees and replanted with native oaks by volunteers. At Alpine Pond, use the trail on the west side and cross Alpine Road to the Russian Ridge OSP parking area.

From the north side of the parking area, **hikers, equestrians,** and **mountain bikers** take the multiuse Ridge Trail route that zigzags up through grasslands toward 2572-foot Borel Hill. Although this hill was named for former owner Antoine Borel, a San Francisco banker and peninsula resident, the preserve's name commemorates a Russian emigrant who lived east of the ridge from 1920 until 1950.

In years of ample rain, this ridge in springtime is a wondrous wildflower sight. On both sides of the trail as far as you can see, extravagant palettes of color sweep over the hillsides and knolls. Often beginning in January you will find perky Johnny-jump-ups turning their yellow-orange faces to the sun. Then goldfields, cream cups, orange poppies, pink checkerblooms, red maids, and blue lupines follow. These beautiful flower fields may approximate what John Muir saw on his trips across California.

After 0.7 mile, just before you reach Borel Hill, a fork in the trail invites you to veer left (northwest) and follow the gently graded, multiuse Bay Area Ridge Trail route around the west side of the ridge. From this trail you can look past the preserve's boundary to Mindego Hill, an ancient, extinct volcano. Beyond lies a succession of rounded, grassy hills creased by almost a dozen streams that join San Gregorio Creek on its way to the San Mateo County coast. This west fork of the Ridge Trail descends to a cleft in the ridgeline from where the Mindego Ridge Trail goes right (east) to reach the Cal-trans Vista Point on Skyline Boulevard, a convenient parking area where you could put a shuttle car.

However, to continue toward the Russian Ridge north boundary, make a slight jog (less than 0.1 mile) to the left (west) on the Mindego Ridge Trail and then turn right (northwest) on the Bay Area Ridge Trail. A short, steep climb to a 2400-foot ridgetop will reward you with wonderful views of the Bay Area—north lie San Francisco and Mt. Tamalpais; across the bay is Mt. Diablo, and farther south of it are Mission and Monument peaks, where another Bay Area Ridge Trail segment traverses East Bay ridgetops; southeast beyond San Jose is Mt. Hamilton. If you look due south on very clear days, you can see the Santa Lucia Mountains rising beyond Monterey Bay. After 0.5 mile on this top-of-the-world trail, look right for a Ridge Trail turnoff marked Rapley Ranch Road, where **all trail users** bear right; the Hawk Ridge Trail angles sharply left.

A 1.6-mile segment proceeds to the junction of Skyline Boulevard and Rapley Ranch Road. Follow the old ranch fence line, curving around the south and east sides of another 2400-foot hill crowned by telephone-relay and electric-transmission-line towers. Abruptly you enter woods of tall oak trees that shade both you and the low-growing shrubs of elderberry, hazelnut, gooseberry, and thimbleberry. As the trail straightens out on the north side of the hill, you pass a wooden platform, a perfect picnic site for your backpack lunch or early evening supper.

Continue north on a long, downhill switchback, under a canopy of broad-branching oaks with lichen- and moss-covered trunks. Looking back, note the transmission towers outlined against the sky contrasting with an earlier, but still operative, form of energy—a windmill. When strong ocean winds blow across this ridge, you can hear the power lines singing.

A few more switchbacks carry you downhill, across a service road, and below a fascinating, glass-fronted, circular private home high above on the crest of the hill. In the wooded ravine far below the trail another windmill is set in a pretty garden. Follow the contour of the trail around a few curves midway between the woods and the ridgecrest; you pass great boulders splattered with lichen and bedecked with healthy patches of poison oak. In late summer the pearly everlasting's tufted, creamy flowers edge the trail cut into a steep hillside.

After passing through a little woods nourished by an intermittent stream, you skirt a small meadow, round a shoulder of the ridge with a close-to-vertical drop-off, and then enter another woods. At the preserve gate at Rapley Ranch Road, use the stile beside the brown pipe gate, and carry on to the right for just 0.1 mile to roadside parking on Skyline Boulevard.

◆ ◆ ◆

Someday the Bay Area Ridge Trail will bridge the short gap from here to Windy Hill Open Space Preserve. In the meantime, plan a car shuttle at Skyline Boulevard, or retrace your steps to the Alpine Road parking area. If you are making a round-trip, try an alternate and longer return route, using the Hawk Ridge, Alder Spring, and Mindego Ridge trails to reach the Bay Area Ridge Trail going south.

Windy Hill Open Space Preserve

From Upper Razorback Ridge to Spring Ridge

Length 3.2 miles

Accessibility Hikers, equestrians, and mountain bikers

Agency Midpeninsula Regional Open Space District

Regulations Preserve is open from dawn to a half hour after sunset. Dogs are prohibited on the Lost or Connector trails; dogs must be on leash on the Anniversary Trail and at the top of Spring Ridge.

Facilities Restrooms at picnic area

Follow the Windy Hill ridgeline through a sheltered forest and across rolling grasslands on a narrow footpath and broad wagon road. After initially descending 320 feet, you gradually gain 234 feet on a final short climb to the knobs of Windy Hill, a peninsula landmark. Expect sweeping views of the San Mateo Coast and the Santa Clara Valley. True to its name, strong winds are possible in this preserve, as is coastal fog.

Getting There

SOUTH TRAILHEAD, UPPER RAZORBACK RIDGE: Take Skyline Boulevard (Highway 35) south 4.3 miles from La Honda Road (Highway 84) at Skylonda or north 3 miles from Page Mill Road. There is off-road parking for 6 cars at the trail entrance.

NORTH TRAILHEAD, SPRING RIDGE, GATE 1 (WHO1): Take Skyline Boulevard (Highway 35) south 1.8 miles from La Honda Road or 5.5 miles north from Page Mill Road. There is ample off-road parking.

SPRING RIDGE PICNIC AREA, SKYLINE BOULEVARD: Take Skyline Boulevard 2.3 miles south from La Honda Road or 4.9 miles north from Page Mill Road.

On the Trail

Mountain bikers' access to Windy Hill Preserve begins at Spring Ridge Picnic Area. A Midpeninsula Regional Open Space District sign and Bay Area Ridge Trail logo at the Razorback Ridge Trail direct **hikers** and **equestrians** left and downhill. Leaving the whir of Skyline Boulevard traffic behind, hikers and equestrians take the wide trail, an old farm road, through a mixed woodland where feathery moss and clusters of lichen decorate the trees. After 0.4 mile and a couple of zigzags on the steep hillside you reach the Razorback Ridge Trail, which branches right (east), downhill. You bear left on the Lost Trail, and for the next 1.7 miles, traverse the upper reaches of the preserve.

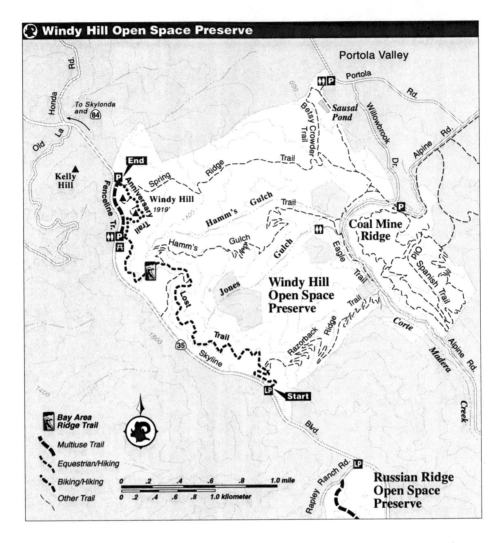

Windy Hill Open Space Preserve

Head northwest on the Lost Trail through a fir forest at approximately 1700 feet. You wind in and out of little ravines and cross headwaters of streams named for settlers who once farmed this mountainside. Water seeping from the hillside and onto the trail feeds the creeks that empty into perennial Corte Madera Creek on the lower east side of the preserve.

After 1.3 miles from the start, you emerge from the dense forest at the head of Jones Gulch. The former Lauriston estate, a forested private inholding, lies in Jones Gulch. In 1915, Herbert E. Law began to purchase land in the area and eventually accumulated 627 acres of meadows, mountains and valleys. His holdings, known as Willow Brook Farm, included the magnificent villa, Lauriston, and acres of lath houses for his agricultural enterprises. In 1937, John Francis Neylan, a San Francisco attorney, purchased the estate. Subsequent owners Ryland Kelley and partners gave part of the estate to the Peninsula Open Space Trust. Sold to MROSD in the early 1980s, this land became the original Windy Hill Open Space Preserve.

Primeval Redwood Forest

This mountainside was once part of a huge land grant known as Rancho El Corte de Madera, deeded to Maximo Martinez and Domingo Peralta in 1834 by Governor José Figueroa. Its name translates as "the wood-cutting ranch." As you travel through the forest, try to picture its former grandeur. Before the mid-19th century, redwood trees 8 to 10 feet in diameter covered the mountains above present-day Portola Valley and Woodside. These primeval redwood forests supplied the wood that built Mission Santa Clara and the Pueblo of San José. Severe logging to build Gold Rush San Francisco in the 1850s and a disastrous fire in the 1860s left hardly a tree standing here.

Today, a second-growth forest of Douglas firs and redwoods flourishes in the 1130-acre Windy Hill Open Space Preserve. Some trees have grown to considerable girth, aided by natural springs, heavy rainfall, and coastal fogs that often shroud this ridgetop.

For several years after this trail was completed, a rusty wheelbarrow chained to a tree reminded passers-by of former trail workdays. A few rotting fence posts once marked boundaries of old ranches. High sandstone cliffs draped with ferns and berry bushes may have been the site of Herbert Law's quarry.

Skirting a chaparral-clothed, south-facing flank of the mountain you cross a dirt access road from Skyline Boulevard. Then bending west toward Skyline, you tread an area that is fed by springs that empty into Hamm's Gulch. Where the trail that bears this settler's name turns right, you veer left along the edge of the gulch where several immense Douglas firs cling to the hillside. (The Hamm's Gulch Trail zigzags downhill for 2.4 miles to a stone bridge over Corte Madera Creek and the ornate iron gates of the former Lauriston estate.)

You continue north on the Bay Area Ridge Trail route in Windy Hill Open Space Preserve just off Skyline Boulevard. You pass Bob's Bench, named for the first executive director of POST, Bob Augsburger. A large wooden sign thanks contributors to the Windy Hill Loop Trail and the trail crews, under the direction of Jane Ames, who built the 8.4-mile loop trail up, down, and around this preserve.

Shortly you reach the picnic area next to Skyline Boulevard near the site of the pioneering Brown Ranch. Settlers Brown and his neighbor to the north, Orton, must have traversed the Lost Trail route you just followed. Until Skyline Boulevard was built in the 1920s, this old wagon road, known as the Ridge Road, stayed below the ridgecrest. From the picnic area, all users begin the northbound leg of this trip on the Anniversary Trail but soon split ways.

Hikers continue on the Anniversary Trail where the Fence Line Trail branches left. The 0.75-mile Anniversary Trail was constructed with funds from POST to mark the tenth anniversary of the establishment of the Windy Hill Preserve. Gradually ascend the east side of the Windy Hill knobs and climb to the summit on one of the small side trails you pass. These treeless protrusions above the long sweep of grasslands descending to Portola Valley are prominent landmarks on the Peninsula. On a clear day, they offer views of the entire Bay Area and the San Mateo coast. On a day true to its name, the 1917-foot summit can be a challenge to steady footing, yet a delight for kite flyers and

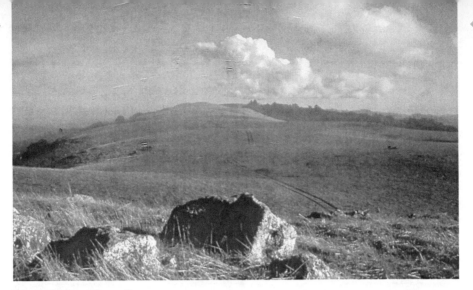

Windy Hill Open Space Preserve

model-glider enthusiasts. From the summit, it is a quick descent to the north parking area at the top of Spring Ridge, the end of this Bay Area Ridge Trail segment.

Equestrians and **mountain bikers** leave the Anniversary Trail at the first swale and veer left on the Fence Line Trail. The trail, which heads north above Skyline Boulevard, offers splendid ocean views when the day is clear. They join hikers at the top of Spring Ridge.

Since this is a relatively short trip, **hikers** and **equestrians** may want to do the 6.4-mile round-trip. If not, park a shuttle car at the picnic area or at the top of Spring Ridge and do the shorter trip.

◆ ◆ ◆

The next segment begins in Wunderlich County Park, about 5 miles north of Windy Hill.

Wunderlich County Park to Huddart County Park

The Skyline Trail from Wunderlich West Gate to Purisima Creek Trailhead

Length	5.8 miles
Accessibility	Hikers and equestrians
Agency	San Mateo County Parks Department
Regulations	Parks are open from 8 AM to sunset and prohibit dogs and bicycles.
Facilities	Restrooms on Redwood Trail in Purisima Creek Redwoods Open Space Preserve across Skyline Boulevard from the north trailhead

Follow the gently graded Skyline Trail through redwood and Douglas-fir forests just below the crest of the Santa Cruz Mountains. You'll discover unusual spring wildflowers along one of the few remaining segments of the old California Riding and Hiking Trail, a trail system established in 1954. Take this easy, shaded trail on a summer day when you need a retreat from the valley heat.

Getting There

SOUTH TRAILHEAD, WUNDERLICH PARK: Take Skyline Boulevard (Highway 35) 3 miles north from La Honda Road (Highway 84) junction or 10 miles south from Half Moon Bay Road (Highway 92) junction. Parking is limited on the west side of Skyline Boulevard. The trailhead is on the east side of Skyline.

NORTH TRAILHEAD, HUDDART PARK: Take Skyline Boulevard (Highway 35) 6.5 miles south from Half Moon Bay Road (Highway 92) or 6.5 miles north from La Honda Road (Highway 84) to parking at the Purisima Creek Trailhead on the west side of Skyline Boulevard. The trailhead is on the east side of Skyline.

On the Trail

Hikers and **equestrians** begin this trail from the northwest corner of Wunderlich Park and quickly lose 100 feet in elevation on switchbacks through a redwood forest. You cross private Bear Gulch Road and then head north below a subdivision in the shade of redwoods and firs, grown tall since most logging ended here in the mid-1860s.

For the next 4 miles, you are on the upper slopes of the California Water Service Company watershed (formerly the Bear Gulch Water Company). You wind in and out of small ravines, often close enough to Skyline Boulevard to hear the murmur of traffic, but not so close that you cannot hear the calls of Steller's jays, the crested blue-black cousins of the blue (scrub) jays of the foothill woodlands.

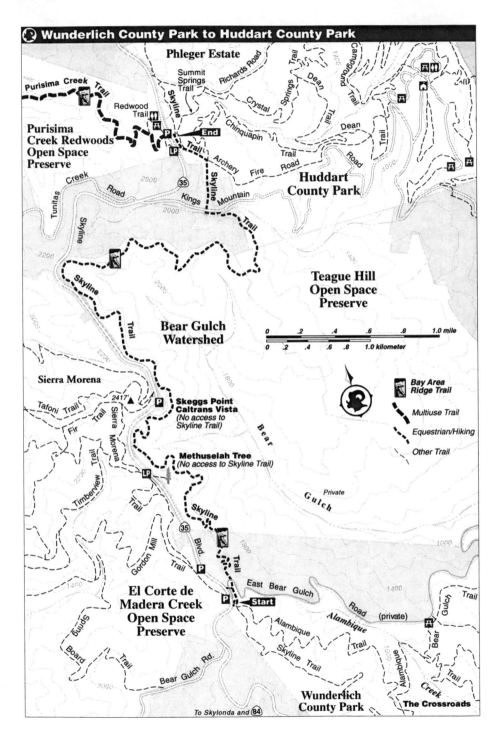

Wunderlich County Park to Huddart County Park

Phleger Estate

Purisima Creek Trail

Summit Springs Trail

Richards Road

Dean Springs Trail

Campground Trail

Redwood Trail

Crystal

Purisima Creek Redwoods Open Space Preserve

Skyline

End

Chinquapin

Dean Road

Trail

P

LP

Archery Fire Road

Trail

Huddart County Park

Tunitas Creek Road

Skyline

(35)

Kings Mountain Trail

Skyline Trail

Skyline Trail

Bear Gulch Watershed

Teague Hill Open Space Preserve

| 0 | .2 | .4 | .6 | .8 | 1.0 mile |
| 0 | .2 | .4 | .6 | .8 | 1.0 kilometer |

Sierra Morena

Tafoni Trail

Fir

2417'

Sierra Morena Trail

P

Skeggs Point Caltrans Vista
(No access to Skyline Trail)

Bear

Bay Area Ridge Trail

Multiuse Trail

Equestrian/Hiking

Other Trail

Timberview Trail

Methuselah Tree
(No access to Skyline Trail)

LP

Private Gulch

Skyline

(35)

Blvd.

Gordon Mill Trail

Trail

P

P

East Bear Gulch

El Corte de Madera Creek Open Space Preserve

P

Start

Alambique

Alambique Road *(private)*

Trail

Spring

Board Trail

Bear Gulch Rd.

Skyline Trail

Bear Gulch Trail

Wunderlich County Park

The Crossroads

To Skylonda and (84)

Camping

On the east side of Skyline Boulevard, the Skyline Trail continues north for almost 2 miles through Huddart Park and the Phleger Estate lands. From the Huddart Park northwest boundary, the Crystal Springs Trail descends 2 miles to a woodsy setting in the park where group campsites with picnic tables and restrooms are available for **equestrian** and **hiker groups** by reservation only—a pleasant place to camp before continuing on to the next leg of your Ridge Trail trek.

On clear days, you'll catch occasional glimpses through the trees of the valley below, though fog often shrouds the view. In all weather, the forest in all its variety delights at every turn. Tall Douglas firs are part of the new forest taking hold here after the logging of the 1800s. A contrast to the dark conifers is the light foliage of bigleaf maples growing in ravines where water is plentiful.

By the edge of the trail, blue hound's tongue blooms in early spring, followed by masses of Douglas iris in shades of lavender. In May you will find the bright, rose-red flower clusters of the uncommon Clintonia and the elegant, lacy-leafed, pink bleeding heart nestled in damp ravines.

After traveling 1.5 miles along the trail, you will see old moss-covered stumps of the largest redwood trees, some 10 feet or more in diameter. These immense trees, some of which were 2000 years old, flourished in the heavy rainfall—as much as 40 inches a year—along the ridge with frequent fogs adding to the precipitation.

After rounding a wide curve in the trail below Skeggs Point, you come to a wooden bench and memorial plaque, dedicated by the local Sierra Club chapter to Clara May Lazarus, an ardent trail advocate. Here is a peaceful place for enjoying the forest's solitude.

The Pulgas Redwoods

The size of the redwood stumps along this trail gives you an idea of the scale of the ancient forest. Known to the Spanish as the Pulgas Redwoods, the forest once covered the eastern slopes of the Santa Cruz Mountains above present-day Woodside and Portola Valley. Note the horizontal slots in the stumps, cut about 6 feet from the ground, which held boards on which loggers stood to fell the trees. This whole forest was cut to supply redwood to build Gold Rush San Francisco. Oxen dragged the logs down the steep hills to sawmills; the wood was then taken to the port of Redwood City and sent up the bay on barges. So great was the demand for wood that by 1870 hardly a redwood remained standing on this mountainside. Logging finally ceased here because the water of Bear Gulch Creek, formerly used in the sawmills, was needed for other uses—first to supply a grist mill and then for the growing communities in the valley.

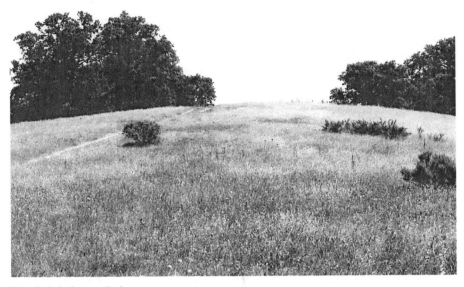

Wunderlich County Park

You continue through forest and beside occasional meadows, flower-filled in spring, and skirt a few mountaintop homes. After a short climb, about 2.5 miles from Wunderlich Park, the trail veers east, bringing spectacular views south as far as Black Mountain in Santa Clara County. You follow a south-facing ridge through oak woodland and chaparral to Teague Hill Open Space Preserve and then begin a gentle descent northwest through a redwood forest to Kings Mountain Road. Follow the footpath beside the road to a marked pedestrian crossing leading to Huddart County Park.

The trail passes a large, private home on a hill and enters redwood forest again at a Huddart Park crossroads. The Bay Area Ridge Trail route, also the Skyline Trail, turns west on a graveled service road through open woodland and continues 0.3 mile to Skyline Boulevard, where this segment of the Bay Area Ridge Trail ends.

◆ ◆ ◆

The next segment of the Ridge Trail in Purisima Creek Redwoods Open Space Preserve begins across the road on the west side of Skyline Boulevard.

Purisima Creek Redwoods Open Space Preserve

From Purisima Creek Trailhead to Preserve's North Entrance

Length 5.7 miles for hikers; 7.7 miles for equestrians and mountain bikers

Accessibility Hikers, equestrians, mountain bikers, and wheelchair users

Agency Midpeninsula Regional Open Space District

Regulations Preserve is open from dawn to a half hour after sunset. Dogs are prohibited. Mountain bikers must obey the 15 MPH speed limit and wear helmets.

Facilities Restrooms at south and north ends of trail

Five trails in Purisima Creek Redwoods Open Space Preserve link together for a challenging loop through forested canyons and over high ridges. You'll lose 1000 feet in elevation in the first 2 miles and regain it on a steady climb out of the canyon. Summer fog sometimes bathes the forested areas, while the open, south-facing ridges may be hot.

Getting There

SOUTH TRAILHEAD, PURISIMA CREEK TRAILHEAD: Take Skyline Boulevard (Highway 35) 6.5 miles south from Half Moon Bay Road (Highway 92) or 6.5 miles north from La Honda Road (Highway 84) to parking at Purisima Creek Trailhead on the west side of Skyline Boulevard. Parking for wheelchair users is 0.1 mile farther south at the head of the Redwood Trail on west side of Skyline Boulevard.

NORTH TRAILHEAD, PURISIMA CREEK TRAILHEAD: Take Skyline Boulevard (Highway 35) 4.5 miles south from Half Moon Bay Road (Highway 92) or 8.5 miles north from La Honda Road (Highway 84) to a large parking area on the west side of the road; parking is available for equestrian trailers here as well.

On the Trail

Wheelchair users start at the head of the Redwood Trail and follow the well-graded path northwest through a beautiful redwood grove, where shade-loving wildflowers and shiny-leaved huckleberry shrubs thrive at trailside. Your path crosses the Purisima Creek Trail and continues 0.2 mile to a flat where a picnic table affords a place to have a snack and enjoy the forest view.

Hikers, equestrians, and **mountain bikers** descend into a deep canyon on the Purisima Creek Trail under tall, second-growth redwoods and tanoaks. The trees in this 2511-acre preserve were heavily logged in the late 19th century. The forest scene here was very different from what you see now—loggers felled redwoods by hand, several streamside mills cut the wood into shingles, and oxen teams pulled wagons loaded with logs up the steep mountainside.

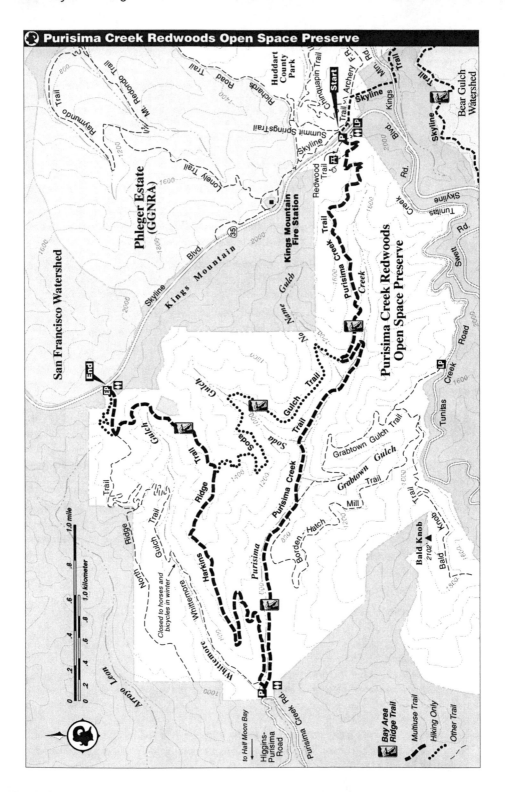

Purisima Creek Redwoods Open Space Preserve

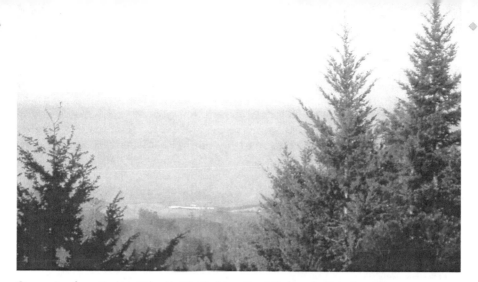

Ocean view from Harkins Ridge Trail in Purisima Creek Redwoods Open Space Preserve

Logging continued sporadically into the 20th century, until Midpeninsula Regional Open Space District completed its purchase of this land in 1984. Today, historic logging roads, linked by newly built footpaths, make fine trails. The wide openings in the forest were once used as landings for the logs and are now springtime gardens of blue ceanothus, scarlet columbine, and the yellow blossoms of invasive Scotch broom. In fall, the brilliant yellow of bigleaf maples accents the forest greens.

After 1.8 miles of steady downhill (an elevation loss of 1000 feet) on the Purisima Creek Trail, **hikers** split ways from **mountain bikers** and **equestrians. Equestrians** and **mountain bikers** continue downhill to the western terminus of the Purisima Creek Trail, losing 1630 feet in elevation. Then turn right, uphill, on the Harkins Ridge Trail.

Hikers turn right on the 2.5-mile, hiker-only Soda Gulch Trail, its secluded entrance marked by a Bay Area Ridge Trail sign on the right side of a hairpin turn. The trail follows the forested east side of No Name Gulch, where delicate springtime flowers abound. You cross a bridge over a tributary and another over the main creek and then switch to the drier, south-facing slope. Tanoaks, cream bush, and even an evergreen oak or two flourish in this sunny zone.

You reach Soda Gulch and return to deep forest, where circles of second-growth trees surround redwood stumps 5 to 6 feet in diameter. One of the largest trees on the steep-sided trail is a towering, double-trunked redwood, whose scarred bark may indicate it was used to anchor cables for hauling logs uphill.

A handsome wooden bridge crosses the upper reaches of Soda Gulch Creek, full in spring, though sometimes dry by fall. Now more than halfway along the Soda Gulch Trail, you again leave the moist redwood forest and begin to ascend open chaparral slopes. At a bend in the trail, you will find welcome shade under a lone, wide-spreading tanoak tree.

Turn right (east) when you reach the Harkins Ridge Trail junction and meet the equestrian/bicyclist route, 1.4 miles from the north parking area. **Hikers, equestrians,** and **mountain bikers** climb steeply on the wide Harkins Ridge Trail, formerly known as the Harkins Fire Road. Low chaparral and a scattering of trees line the trail, which veers left and levels off to cross over the headwall of Whittemore Gulch. Look west to the ocean to see breakers crashing on the beach near Half Moon Bay. Past sizable redwoods, clusters of Douglas fir, and abundant seasonal flowers, you come to the North Ridge Trail junction.

Hikers cross the wide North Ridge Trail to a well-graded footpath that zigzags up through a fir and tanoak forest. At one of the bends in the footpath, you can see other high points of the Santa Cruz Mountains to the northwest—Montara Mountain, Scarper Peak, and the long central Cahill Ridge in the San Francisco Watershed. Soon you reach the parking area at the crest of the Skyline ridge, having regained the 1000 feet in elevation you lost in Purisima Creek Canyon. **Equestrians** and **mountain bikers** veer right (east) and follow the North Ridge Trail to the parking area.

On a beautiful day in May 1989, this 5.7-mile segment and the one just south, Wunderlich County Park to Huddart County Park, were dedicated as the first Ridge Trail segments in San Mateo County. The occasion was marked by speeches congratulating all trail advocates and volunteers. There were hikes and rides on both legs of the Bay Area Ridge Trail, followed by refreshments for all.

◆ ◆ ◆

From the northern terminus of this trail to the San Francisco Watershed on Highway 92, there is a 6-mile gap in the Bay Area Ridge Trail route.

San Francisco Watershed Trail

Quarry Road to Sneath Lane

Length	9.5 miles one-way
Accessibility	Hikers, equestrians, and mountain bikers on guided trips only (shuttle return is arranged)
Agency	San Francisco Public Utility Commission
Regulations	The trail is only open for twice-monthly, docent-led group trips on Wednesday, Saturday, and Sunday during daylight hours for a fee (register at www.sfwater.org on "Natural Resources" page). Dogs are prohibited.
Facilities	Restrooms at Quarry Road and Sweeney Ridge entrances and at Five Points. The hikers' trip north to Sneath Lane requires a car shuttle. Equestrians can enter the trail from stables in Pacifica.

In this remote open space dedicated volunteers will lead you through dense forests and over hilly grasslands to extensive views of the entire Bay Area.

Getting There

SOUTH TRAILHEAD, OLD WATERSHED QUARRY ROAD: Going west on Highway 92; shortly after crossing causeway over lakes, look for Quarry Road entrance sign on the north side of the road. Going east on Highway 92, pass the entrance sign, continue to the junction of Skyline Boulevard and Highway 92, make a **U**-turn and proceed west on Highway 92. Follow directions above.

NORTH TRAILHEAD, SNEATH LANE: From Skyline Boulevard (Highway 35) in San Bruno go west on Sneath Lane to off-street parking at gate.

On the Trail

Beginning at the quarry you follow an old road up a steep hill for about 1.5 miles to reach the Cahill Ridge Road. From there this service road meanders along the middle ridge of the Watershed lands, at first through a mature forest of tall Douglas firs interspersed with occasional redwood trees. Also growing along the route are occasional, escaped plants from urban gardens, such as English holly and cotoneaster plants.

From a few openings in the forest you catch glimpses of San Francisco, Mt. Diablo, and the hills of the East Bay. Below you lies San Andreas Lake, though it will appear later on the trip. A few patches of open grassland offer views west of the canyon of Pilarcitos Creek up to the heights of Starker Peak. After about 4 miles on Cahill Ridge Road you reach Five Points, where the shorter Watershed trip returns to the quarry road entrance.

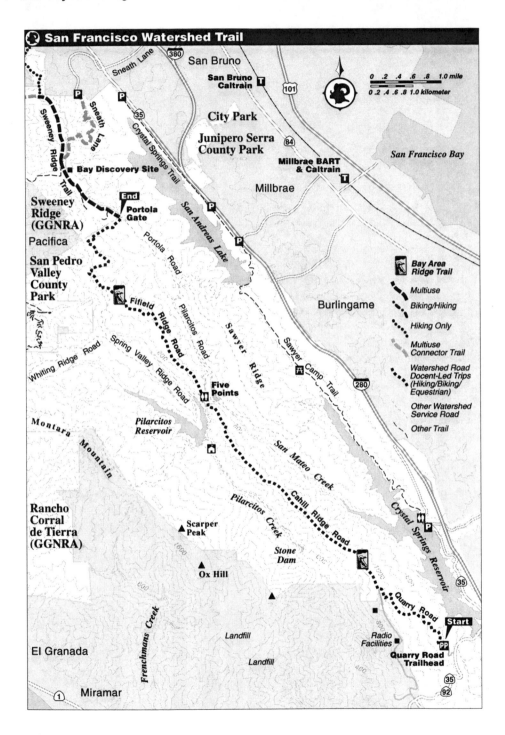

San Francisco Watershed Trail

Sneath Lane

San Bruno

380

San Bruno Caltrain

101

City Park

35

Junipero Serra County Park

84

Millbrae BART & Caltrain

San Francisco Bay

Crystal Springs Trail

Bay Discovery Site

Millbrae

Sweeney Ridge Trail

Sweeney Ridge Road

Sneath Lane

P

P

End

Portola Gate

San Andreas Lake

P

Sweeney Ridge (GGNRA)

Pacifica

San Pedro Valley County Park

Portola Road

P

Fifield

Burlingame

Bay Area Ridge Trail

Multiuse

Biking/Hiking

Hiking Only

Multiuse Connector Trail

Watershed Road Docent-Led Trips (Hiking/Biking/ Equestrian)

Other Watershed Service Road

Other Trail

Ridge Road

Pilarcitos Road

Sawyer Ridge

Sawyer Camp Trail

280

Whiting Ridge Road

Spring Valley Ridge Road

Five Points

Montara Mountain

Pilarcitos Reservoir

San Mateo Creek

Cahill Ridge Road

Crystal Springs Reservoir

P

Rancho Corral de Tierra (GGNRA)

Scarper Peak

Pilarcitos Creek

Stone Dam

Ox Hill

Quarry Road

35

El Granada

Frenchmans Creek

Landfill

Radio Facilities

Start

PP

Landfill

Quarry Road Trailhead

35

92

Miramar

1

0 .2 .4 .6 .8 1.0 mile

0 .2 .4 .6 .8 1.0 kilometer

If you take the entire Ridge Trail trip, you will follow your guide north for another 5-plus miles. Now on the Fifield Ridge Trail you can look back west to Pilarcitos Reservoir nestled in a deep canyon surrounded by wooded hillsides. As you proceed up and down over low hills with very little shade, low-growing shrubs permit very fine views of the Bay and the mountains surrounding it. To the north lies Mt. Tamalpais, east is Mt. Diablo and south lies Mt. Hamilton. Some other Ridge Trail trips reach the slopes of these Bay Area landmarks.

The near view takes in the full length of San Andreas Lake and Crystal Springs Reservoir and the curve of San Francisco Bay shoreline beyond. At your feet in the spring are fields of glorious wildflowers covering the rolling grasslands. As you near the junction of the Sneath Lane Trail with this segment of the Ridge Trail, look for the San Francisco Bay Discovery Site on the east side of the trail. Marble monuments here commemorate Don Gaspar de Portolá's sighting of San Francisco Bay while he was searching for a land route to Monterey Bay.

At the Portola Gate in Sweeney Ridge or at the Sneath Lane entrance 3.5 miles farther north there is a shuttle for **hikers**. Ridge Trail guides will arrange for **bikers** and **equestrians** who may want to return to the quarry gate or for shuttles at Sneath Lane. Check the website listed above for reservations for this trip, one of the longest on the Ridge Trail route around the Bay.

◆ ◆ ◆

The next leg of the Bay Area Ridge Trail, Sweeney Ridge to Milagra Ridge, begins in the San Francisco Watershed just past the Discovery Site before the Sneath Lane Trail heads downhill to the locked gate at the parking area.

Crystal Springs Reservoir in the San Francisco Watershed

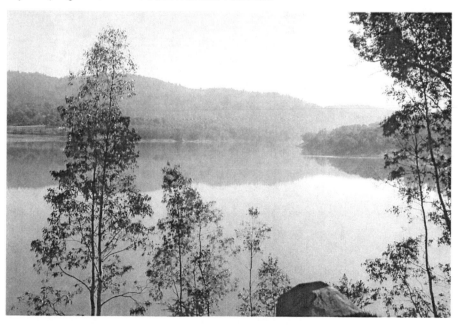

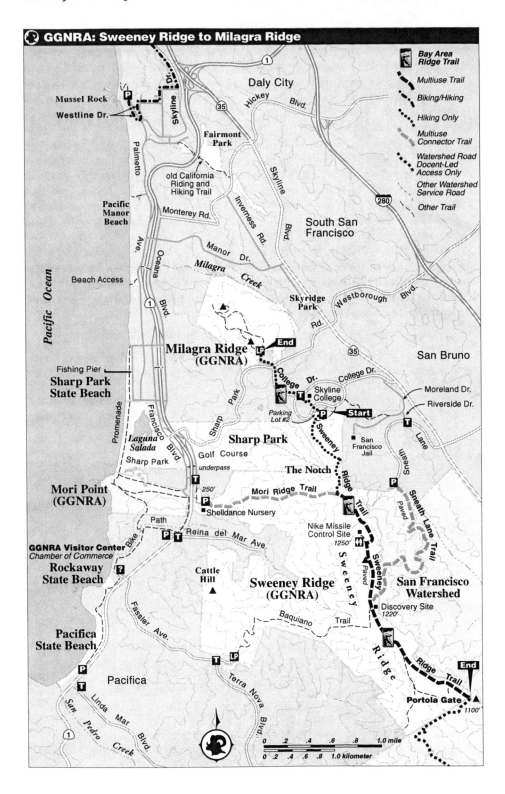

GGNRA: Sweeney Ridge to Milagra Ridge

Bay Area
Ridge Trail

Multiuse Trail

Biking/Hiking

Hiking Only

Multiuse
Connector Trail

Watershed Road
Docent-Led
Access Only

Other Watershed
Service Road

Other Trail

Daly City

Mussel Rock
Westline Dr.
Skyline Dr.

Fairmont
Park

Pacific
Manor
Beach

old California
Riding and
Hiking Trail

Monterey Rd.

Palmetto

Hickey Blvd.

Skyline Blvd.

Inverness Rd.

South San
Francisco

280

Beach Access

Pacific Ocean

Milagra Creek

Manor Dr.

Oceana Ave.

Skyridge
Park

Westborough Blvd.

Milagra Ridge
(GGNRA)

End

35

San Bruno

Fishing Pier

Sharp Park
State Beach

Sharp Park

College Dr.

College Dr.

Skyline
College

Moreland Dr.

Riverside Dr.

Francisco Blvd.

Sharp Park

Parking
Lot #2

Start

Sneath Lane

Promenade

Laguna
Salada

Golf Course

Sharp Park

underpass

250'

The Notch

Sweeney

San
Francisco
Jail

Ridge Trail

Mori Point
(GGNRA)

Mori Ridge Trail

Shelldance Nursery

Nike Missile
Control Site
1250'

Sweeney Paved

Sneath Lane Trail

Paved

GGNRA Visitor Center
Chamber of Commerce

Rockaway
State Beach

Path

Bike

Reina del Mar Ave.

Cattle
Hill

Sweeney Ridge
(GGNRA)

Sweeney

Sweeney Paved

San Francisco
Watershed

Discovery Site
1220'

Pacifica
State Beach

Fassler Ave.

Baquiano Trail

Ridge

Ridge Trail

End

Pacifica

Terra Nova Blvd.

Portola Gate
1100'

Linda Mar Blvd.

San Pedro Creek

1

0   .2   .4   .6   .8   1.0 mile
0   .2   .4   .6   .8   1.0 kilometer

Golden Gate National Recreation Area: Sweeney Ridge to Milagra Ridge

From Portola Gate to Milagra Ridge Gate

Length 7.0 miles from Sneath Lane trailhead, 7.6 miles from Mori Ridge Trailhead (includes round-trip to Portola Gate from Discovery Site and then north to Milagra Ridge Gate)

Accessibility Hikers, equestrians, and mountain bikers

Agency Golden Gate National Recreation Area

Regulations Sweeney Ridge is open from 8 AM to a half hour after sunset. Dogs must be on leash. Skyline College is open during school hours, prohibits dogs, and requires mountain bikers to use campus roads.

Facilities Restroom at Nike site on Sweeney Ridge; water, restroom, and telephone at vista point on west side of Skyline College campus

A trek along this 1000-acre ridgetop visits the San Francisco Bay Discovery Site, unique coastal plant communities, and the Skyline College campus and offers sweeping views of the coast and mountains. The long, rounded Sweeney Ridge, separating north Peninsula bayside and coastal communities, was slated to become Interstate 380—the route from Highway 101 to Highway 1—until the Golden Gate National Recreation Area purchased it in 1982. The exposed ridge can be windy, foggy, or hot and is subject to sudden changes in weather. Choose from two trailheads, on the east and west sides of the ridge: You'll gain 550 feet from the Sneath Lane trailhead and 850 feet from the Mori Ridge trailhead. The trail from Sneath Lane to the Nike site is a paved road; all other trails are wide and unpaved.

Getting There

By Car

SOUTH TRAILHEAD, PORTOLA GATE: This trailhead is only accessible by car on some guided Golden Gate National Recreation Area hikes.

SNEATH LANE TRAILHEAD: From Skyline Boulevard (Highway 35) in San Bruno, go west on Sneath Lane to off-street parking at gate.

MORI RIDGE TRAILHEAD: Going north on Highway 1 in Pacifica, pass Reina del Mar Avenue, and turn abruptly right into the Shelldance Nursery. Continue past nursery buildings to parking at the end of the dirt road. Going south on Highway 1 in Pacifica, make a **U**-turn at Reina del Mar Avenue and go north, following directions above.

SKYLINE COLLEGE: From Skyline Boulevard (Highway 35) in San Bruno, go west on College Drive, turn left at the college entrance, and proceed to Parking Lot 2. Several spaces are reserved for Golden Gate National Recreation Area trail use.

NORTH TRAILHEAD, MILAGRA RIDGE: From Highway 1 or from Skyline Boulevard (Highway 35), take Sharp Park Road, turn north on College Drive Extension North, and continue to roadside parking at the Milagra Ridge gate.

By Bus

SamTrans buses run to Skyline College on weekdays and on Saturdays. SamTrans stops at the intersection of Sneath Lane and Monterey Drive on weekdays and runs on Highway 1 to Westport Drive or Reina del Mar Avenue near the Mori Ridge Trailhead in Pacifica.

On the Trail

This segment of the Bay Area Ridge Trail can now be reached by traversing the San Francisco Watershed lands starting at the southern Watershed gate at the intersection of Skyline Boulevard and Highway 92 on guided trips. However, by starting at the north end of this 10-plus-mile trail, you can take a shorter round-trip that reaches the Discovery Site and returns to Sweeney Ridge. Therefore, your trip begins with an ascent from Sneath Lane in San Bruno or from Mori Ridge in Pacifica to the Discovery Site; you then go south and/or north on the Sweeney Ridge Trail. Equestrians begin from the private Park Pacific Stables to reach the Sweeney Ridge Trail.

To start from the bayside, **hikers** and **mountain bikers** go around the locked gate at the end of Sneath Lane and pick up the paved road that climbs through a dense growth of chaparral and coastal scrub. The trail curves into ravines and rounds shoulders of the ridge. A rich variety of native shrubs—red-berried toyon, cream-colored Queen Anne's lace, coyote bush, arroyo willows, elderberry bushes, and blue-blossomed California lilac—border the route. In springtime, scarlet and yellow columbines, orange poppies, and lavender yerba santa brighten your way.

At the crest of the ridge, the paved trail veers right (north), but you turn left to reach the San Francisco Bay Discovery Site. Almost immediately, you pass the right-branching Baquiano Trail, named for Portolá's scout, Sergeant José Francisco Ortega, who was the first European to see San Francisco Bay. This trail crosses private property at its western end and is open only for occasional ranger-led walks.

Continue a short distance beyond the Baquiano Trail to the San Francisco Bay Discovery Site on a 1200-foot knoll on your left, on the east side of the trail. Two monuments commemorate the sighting of San Francisco Bay on November 4, 1769, by Don Gaspar de Portolá's men. A bronze plaque on a weathered serpentine boulder on the left states that the men first saw the bay while searching for a land route to Monterey Bay. On the right (south) side of the knoll, a monument shows the outlines and names of the Bay Area's major peaks etched on a black granite cylinder. Among the peaks shown are Mt. Tamalpais, Mt. Hamilton, Mt. Diablo, San Bruno Mountain, and Montara Mountain.

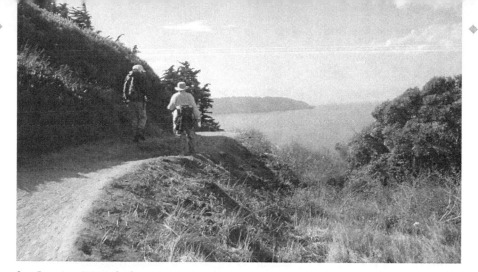

San Francisco Watershed

Portolá's men would have seen these same Bay Area peaks and ridges from this knoll. Portolá's commission was traveling north to establish a colony in Monterey to thwart British and Russian settlements in Alta California. Not until after Portolá's journey, when other expeditions recorded the vastness of the bay's waters, did the Spaniards realize the importance of their find. They then charted the extensive harbor and, in 1776, established their northern colony in present-day San Francisco on the shores of that bay.

Discovery Site South to Portola Gate

To reach the boundary between Sweeney Ridge and the San Francisco Watershed lands at the Portola Gate, you can make a 2.4-mile round-trip south from the Discovery Site on the Sweeney Ridge Trail. It takes you past luxurious clumps of Douglas irises, beautiful blue or creamy-white blossomed in May, and beside a few springs seeping from winter to early summer. You can locate the springs in summer by the patches of sedges and tall grasses that prosper in the damp soil of the seep. Along this trail in late summer, you may be lucky enough to see, half-concealed under the shrubs, tall, slim flower stalks clustered with whitish-green blossoms—one of California's native orchids.

En route to the Portola Gate, you pass the horse trail that leads to private stables in Pacifica outside the Sweeney Ridge property. Equestrians use this route to reach the Sweeney Ridge Trail and then go north to the Discovery Site or south to the Portola Gate. Toward the south end of the Sweeney Ridge Trail, crinkly-leaved ceanothus (California lilac) and orange-flowered twinberry have grown tall enough to provide a hedge and a modest but welcome windbreak. The vegetation soon opens up in a clearing at the watershed boundary, and a high fence and restrictive signs bar travel beyond the Portola Gate. However, the GGNRA rangers and Bay Area Ridge Trail docents frequently offer public nature hikes and discovery walks in the watershed. Management requires advance reservations and a fee for these events; contact the Bay Area Ridge Trail office in San Francisco. Retrace your steps to the Discovery Site.

North to Skyline College

From the Discovery Site, **hikers, equestrians,** and **mountain bikers** follow the paved service road with a yellow fog line past defunct buildings of a former Nike missile site—the highest point on the ridge at 1250 feet. As the trail swings west around the buildings, views of Mt. Tamalpais, Wolf Ridge in the GGNRA Marin Headlands, San Bruno Mountain, and the beautiful bay open up. Even when fog lies in the valleys, the peaks might be visible, giving you the feeling of overlooking a vast, misty sea, pierced by isolated islands.

Soon the Sweeney Ridge Trail meets the Mori Ridge Trail, the coastside connector from Pacifica. The Mori Ridge Trail gains 850 feet in elevation in 1.3 miles, in a series of steep pitches that alternate with more gentle climbs. It offers magnificent views of the coast, from San Pedro Point in the south to the tip of Point Reyes Peninsula in the north. In the southwest, Montara Mountain's long sweep to the sea stands dark against the sky, its many antennae piercing the blue.

Diverse species of coastal scrub cover the hillside along the Mori Ridge Trail, from pungent sage to aromatic coyote mint. The moist ocean air enhances and intensifies the color of the plants' blossoms, particularly the blue-flowered lupine and the bushy yellow lizardtail. Crimson stalks of Indian paintbrush glow among the wind-sculpted coyote bush and California coffeeberry.

From the junction of Mori Ridge and Sweeney Ridge trails, **mountain bikers** and **equestrians** return to their starting points. **Hikers** veer right (northeast) at the junction, to follow the Sweeney Ridge Trail to Skyline Community College and on to Milagra Ridge. Dedicated on October 12, 1996, the Ridge Trail route from here descends a very steep ravine known as "The Notch." Broad steps defined by rope handrails strung through pressure-treated posts offer a safer grade and protect native plants that host the endangered Mission Blue butterfly.

Rift Zone Lakes

On clear days, you can see long lakes that fill the linear valley at the east base of the ridge, San Andreas Lake and the Crystal Springs Reservoir, from north to south. The linear valleys continue farther south, though they aren't dammed for water storage. On a visit to California in the 1890s, Andrew Lawson, a pioneering geologist, recognized these linear valleys as typical of a rift zone and after the 1906 San Francisco earthquake, named the great California earthquake fault, the San Andreas Fault, for the valley containing the northernmost lake.

Water from the Hetch Hetchy Reservoir in the Sierra Nevada is transported through huge pipes to be stored in these lakes and is then purveyed to more than 1 million users in San Francisco and on the peninsula. Local water runoff from the east side of Sweeney Ridge and those ridges to the south, Fifield and Cahill, also stored in these lakes, amounts to less than 5 percent of the drinking water supplied by the San Francisco Water Department to its patrons.

On the other side of the steep ravine, you traverse a high ridge with views of the coastline. On clear days, you'll see waves crashing against the rocky cliffs and lapping at the sandy beaches. At your feet is evidence of the geologic beginnings of this land. A trained eye will distinguish Franciscan Formation rocks such as greenstone (a rounded basalt), some sandstone, and a red chert. White patches you may see on some rocks are remnants of the Calera limestone, which is found in abundance in the Rockaway Quarry just west of here. These Franciscan rocks formed underwater, then were stressed and modified through the ages by action deep within the earth's crust and along the San Andreas Fault.

The Bay Area Ridge Trail descends from the ridge to Parking Lot 2 at Skyline College. Cross the lot and go down 78 broad steps through a tall conifer forest. Then cross the road to a pretty plaza, its left side sheltered by mature cypress trees in huge planters. On a large campus map, you can note the route through the inner campus.

Proceed through the plaza to the bookstore, turn left (west), mount a series of steps, and pass the north side of Buildings 1 and 2. Between these buildings is another tree-filled plaza where the dedication of the Skyline College Ridge Trail Connection took place. Skyline College marked its 25th anniversary by celebrating the completion of this important link between Sweeney and Milagra ridges and the opening of the first Bay Area Ridge Trail segment to pass through a college campus. Continue past this plaza, pausing at the north corner of Building 1 to read a bronze plaque commemorating Skyline College's dedication on May 17, 1970. Then turn right (north), pass Building 7, and cross the street to a bus stop, which is often crowded with children, college students, and Bay Area Ridge Trail travelers.

North to Milagra Ridge Gate

Bay Area Ridge Trail directional arrows placed high on lampposts and street signs mark the route from here. Go around the corner and veer right (north) on sidewalks beside College Drive. Shortly the Ridge Trail route shifts a few feet east onto parallel Ysabel Drive and continues north to Sharp Park Road. Crosswalks at stoplights take you to the opposite side of the street, where you use the road past a residential complex to continue north to the Milagra Ridge gate. You could park a shuttle car here or leave one at Parking Lot 2 on the college campus. A few places on the south side of this lot are reserved for those using the trail.

Negotiations are underway to complete a short gap between the northwest end of Milagra Ridge Preserve and city streets in Pacifica. For now, you can take a brisk round-trip along the trail that traverses the ridgetop to the end of the preserve. Thanks to revegetation efforts by the National Park Service, once-rampant pampas grass is gone, the lupine plant that is host to the Mission Blue butterfly is being protected, and new plants native to this region are being set out. On crisp, clear days, the fabulous views of ocean and coastline are well worth a trip on this ridge. Retrace your route along College Drive North to Parking Lot 2 at Skyline College, or have a shuttle car waiting to take you to the Sneath Lane or Mori Ridge parking areas.

◆ ◆ ◆

The next segment of the Bay Area Ridge Trail begins at Mussel Rock in Daly City, about 5 miles north of Milagra Ridge.

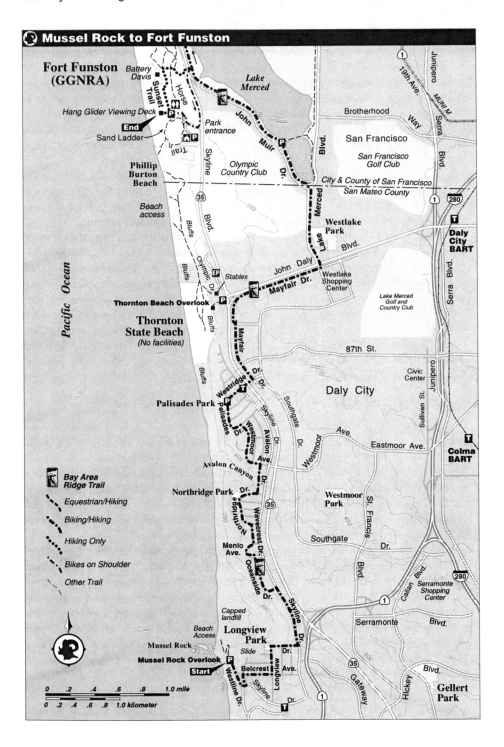

Mussel Rock to Fort Funston

Fort Funston
(GGNRA)

Battery Davis

Lake Merced

Hang Glider Viewing Deck

End

Sand Ladder

Park entrance

Brotherhood

San Francisco

San Francisco Golf Club

Phillip Burton Beach

Olympic Country Club

City & County of San Francisco
San Mateo County

Beach access

Westlake Park

Daly City BART

Stables

Westlake Shopping Center

Thornton Beach Overlook

Lake Merced Golf and Country Club

Thornton State Beach
(No facilities)

87th St.

Daly City

Civic Center

Palisades Park

Eastmoor Ave.

Colma BART

Avalon Canyon

Northridge Park

Westmoor Park

Bay Area Ridge Trail

Equestrian/Hiking

Biking/Hiking

Hiking Only

Bikes on Shoulder

Other Trail

Menlo Ave.

Southgate

Serramonte Shopping Center

Capped landfill

Serramonte

Beach Access

Longview Park

Mussel Rock

Slide

Mussel Rock Overlook

Start

Belcrest Ave.

Gateway

Gellert Park

Pacific Ocean

0   .2   .4   .6   .8   1.0 mile
0   .2   .4   .6   .8   1.0 kilometer

Mussel Rock to Fort Funston

From Mussel Rock Overlook Through Daly City Neighborhoods to Fort Funston

Length 2.9 miles through Daly City neighborhoods; 2.4 miles round-trip through Fort Funston

Accessibility Hikers, equestrians, mountain bikers

Agencies Golden Gate National Recreation Area and Daly City

Regulations The city portion is open during daylight hours and permits dogs on leashes. Fort Funston is open from sunrise to sunset and permits dogs on leashes (but owners must pick up after them).

Facilities Water, restrooms, and telephone at Fort Funston

On the southern segment, take in impressive coastal views from parking above Mussel Rock and then travel north on Daly City streets to Fort Funston. These exposed bluff-tops offer no shade and can be breezy and foggy. You'll gain 550 feet in elevation in the first 0.75 mile from Mussel Rock.

Getting There

By Car

SOUTH TRAILHEAD, MUSSEL ROCK PARKING AREA: Going south, take Skyline Boulevard (Highway 35) to Westmoor Avenue in Daly City and turn right (west). Immediately turn left (south) on Skyline Drive, continue 1.75 miles to Belcrest Avenue and turn right. Go 4 blocks to Westline Drive, turn left, and then go right to continue north to entrance road of Mussel Rock parking area.

Going north, take Highway 1 to Manor Drive exit in Pacifica, turn left at the first stop sign, go two blocks, turn left on Manor Drive, and cross the highway. Immediately turn right onto Palmetto Avenue and continue for almost 1 mile to Westline Drive in Daly City. Turn left on Westline Drive and then veer left on entrance road to Mussel Rock parking area.

NORTH TRAILHEAD, FORT FUNSTON: Going south on Skyline Boulevard (Highway 35) towards Lake Merced, go 0.1 mile past John Muir Drive, and turn right (west) into Fort Funston. At a fork in the road, bear right and continue to an extensive parking area. The entrance for Sunset Trail is on the north side of the parking area near the hang glider viewing deck (on a bluff above the beach).

Going north on Skyline Boulevard (Highway 35), make a U-turn at John Muir Drive, go south on Skyline Boulevard 0.1 mile, turn right (west) into Fort Funston, and follow directions above.

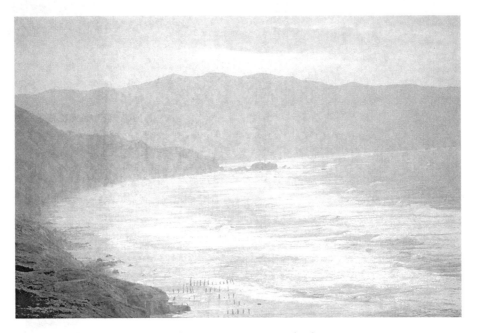

Mussel Rock from Fort Funston, with Montara Mountain in the distance

When leaving Fort Funston, drivers and bicyclists must turn right (south). To go north, continue south on Skyline Boulevard to John Daly Boulevard and make a **U**-turn.

EQUESTRIAN TRAILHEAD: Going south, take Skyline Boulevard (Highway 35), turn right (west) on Olympic Way, and proceed south to stables and equestrian parking. Going north, take Skyline Boulevard (Highway 35) to John Muir Drive, make a **U**-turn, and follow directions going south as above.

By Bus

SamTrans serves the intersection of Palmetto and Westline daily from the Daly City BART Station and serves Daly City and Pacifica daily (except Sundays) from Serramonte Shopping Center.

On the Trail

North Through Daly City

Before setting off from the vista point above Mussel Rock, take in the view of several jagged, rocky islets just offshore. The largest of these, topped by a navigational marker, is Mussel Rock. These small, offshore islands are inhabited by black-coated, long-necked cormorants and a variety of other shorebirds. However, these islets also present a formidable boating hazard and a tempting, but risky destination for fishermen and adventurers. It is exceedingly dangerous to attempt to reach them due to erratic wave patterns off this coast.

The San Andreas Fault enters the Pacific Ocean at Mussel Rock and reappears on the Point Reyes Peninsula. Look south from the vista point along the gentle curve of beaches and rocky shoreline beyond the Pacifica pier to see Point San Pedro jutting into the sea. Just east of Pacifica lies the rounded flank of Sweeney Ridge in the 74,000-acre Golden Gate National Recreation Area, where another segment of the Bay Area Ridge Trail traverses the 3-mile-long ridgeline.

Fort Funston lies to the north, and beyond, San Francisco's Ocean Beach stretches all the way to the Golden Gate. On a very clear day, the Marin Headlands and Point Reyes are visible farther north. Twenty-five miles offshore, the Farallon Islands appear from this perspective to stand guard over the narrow entrance to San Francisco Bay.

Landward and immediately north of the vista point in a deep canyon, a former dumpsite has been replaced by the refuse transfer station housed in the large concrete building above the parking area. This canyon developed when heavy winter storms washed out great chunks of coastal bluffs.

Almost hidden, north of the canyon on a shelf midway between the cliffs and the ocean, lies more testimony to the relentless force of Pacific Ocean storms. The northern leg of the Ocean Shore Railroad ran along this coast from 1907 until its demise in 1920. Although planned to connect San Francisco and Santa Cruz, the tracks never bridged the gap south of Half Moon Bay between Tunitas Creek and Davenport Landing. However, passengers were transported by Stanley Steamer on a scenic ride across the unfinished section. Your Bay Area Ridge Trail trip approximates the old railroad route north on a safer alignment.

After orienting yourself at the vista point above Mussel Rock, **hikers** and **mountain bikers** go back along the entry road to the first corner, where Westline Drive curves north. Turn left (east) on Westline Drive. **Hikers** use the sidewalks on the left side of the street; **mountain bikers** ride on the street. After just one block, turn right on Belcrest Avenue. Then go left (north) on Longview Drive. In three blocks you come to Longview City Park, where you'll find attractive benches. Follow Longview Drive as it curves right (east), around the corner.

At each intersection on this trip, a Bay Area Ridge Trail marker on a signpost tells you which way to turn. For most of the trip north through Daly City, houses sit between you and the bluffs. However, occasional openings between the houses and three cliff-top city parks offer ocean views. In this Daly City neighborhood each home has its plot of lawn, often graced with small, rock-bordered flower beds of ferns and roses and accented by a palm tree.

At Skyline Drive, turn left and follow it north. When you pass a water tower on the right at Fog Cap 3, you've reached the summit of your invigorating climb—it's downhill from here to the end of the first leg of this Ridge Trail segment.

There are a few benches and remnants of playing fields at Daly City's Northridge Park, but storm damage has destroyed much of this park. On balmy days, neighborhood residents still relax in protected, sunny areas. Each of the city parks you pass has fencing and hedges atop the bluff, and breaks in the hedges afford sea views. Even when it's foggy, the sound of the surf reminds the visitor of the ocean's incessant action below the cliffs.

Disastrous winter storms eroded cliffs and rendered cliffside houses unsafe just beyond Northridge on Avalon Drive. Gone are those houses, but you can walk on Skyline Drive or the east side of the street and look out to sea.

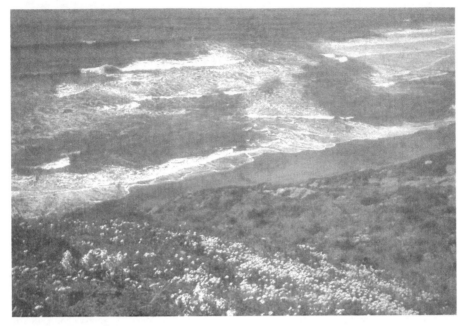

San Mateo County Coast

This first section ends at Palisades Park at the corner of Palisades Drive and Westridge Drive. You can return to Mussel Rock on foot or bike or have a shuttle car waiting on Palisades Drive by the park.

North to Fort Funston

Hikers and **mountain bikers** begin the second part of this Bay Area Ridge Trail segment at the corner of Palisades and Westridge Drives in Daly City. Follow Westridge Drive across Skyline Drive and cross Highway 35 (Skyline Boulevard) with the signal. Turn left (north) on Mayfair Drive where **hikers** continue north on sidewalks and **mountain bikers** proceed along the street. Follow Mayfair as it curves east paralleling John Daly Boulevard.

At the corner of Lake Merced Boulevard and John Daly Boulevard (the west corner of the Westlake Shopping Center), **hikers** and **mountain bikers** turn left and follow Lake Merced Boulevard north. In less than a half mile you reach John Muir Drive, where you turn left and proceed along its off-road path to the junction with Highway 35. **Hikers** cross the street at the signal and turn south at this intersection. Look here for a rather steep trail up to Fort Funston and its road out to the viewing deck.

Mountain bikers follow the edge of Highway 35 south to the Fort Funston entrance and take the park road out to join **hikers** on the hang glider viewing deck. If you arrived by car, be sure to join **all users** on the viewing deck. Here behind the protection of wind-sculpted trees by the viewing deck, the parked hang gliders look like a swarm of butterflies with outspread, brilliantly colored wings. You may see some other aerial adventurers—paragliders—rise above the beach, floating, suspended by ropes from a longitudinal sliver of double-layered, multicolored parachute cloth.

When the fog hangs over the shore, there is a sense of solitude here, broken only by the shrieks of gulls. When coastal breezes sweep in and the surf crashes on the beach, the closeness to nature's power makes this almost a wilderness experience. And on clear, sunny days with the glint of sunshine on the breaking waves and flocks of shorebirds searching for clams, this is truly a glorious place to be.

Watching the stream of ship traffic move in and out of the Golden Gate can test your knowledge of seagoing vessels. Especially on weekends, the brightly colored hang gliders' silent take off and flight above the strand can provide hours of vicarious aerial thrills. If the day is clear, you may want to stroll north along the Sunset Trail or linger longer on the viewing deck for a picnic and more views of this dramatic coast.

Although the Ridge Trail route no longer goes along the beach from Fort Funston, it is possible to walk south along this strand for a few miles.

◆ ◆ ◆

The next leg of the Bay Area Ridge Trail starts in Fort Funston and goes to Stern Grove.

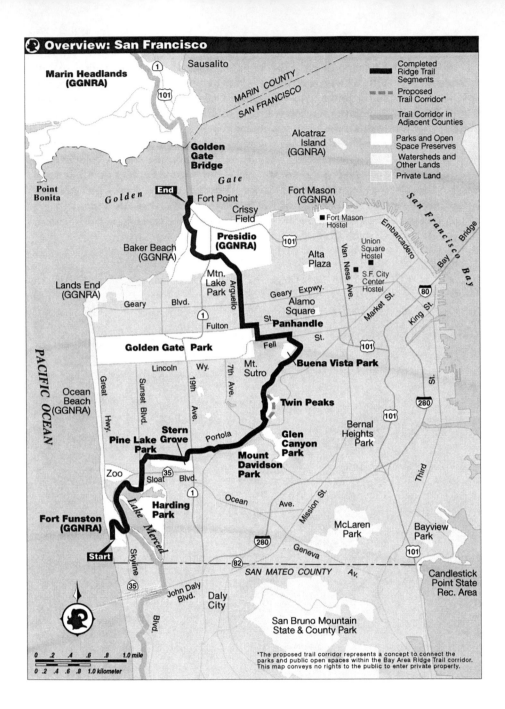

Marin Headlands (GGNRA)

Sausalito

MARIN COUNTY
SAN FRANCISCO

Completed Ridge Trail Segments

Proposed Trail Corridor*

Trail Corridor in Adjacent Counties

Parks and Open Space Preserves

Watersheds and Other Lands

Private Land

Golden Gate Bridge

Alcatraz Island (GGNRA)

Gate

Point Bonita

Golden

End

Fort Point

Crissy Field

Fort Mason (GGNRA)

■ Fort Mason Hostel

Presidio (GGNRA)

Baker Beach (GGNRA)

Embarcadero

Union Square Hostel

■ S.F. City Center Hostel

Lands End (GGNRA)

Mtn. Lake Park

Alta Plaza

Geary

Blvd.

Alamo Square

Market St.

Fulton

Panhandle

Golden Gate Park

Fell St.

Buena Vista Park

Lincoln Wy.

Mt. Sutro

Ocean Beach (GGNRA)

Twin Peaks

Portola

Stern Grove
Pine Lake Park

Glen Canyon Park

Bernal Heights Park

Zoo

Mount Davidson Park

Sloat Blvd.

Ocean Ave.

Harding Park

Fort Funston (GGNRA)

McLaren Park

Bayview Park

Start

Geneva

Lake Merced

Skyline

SAN MATEO COUNTY

Av.

Candlestick Point State Rec. Area

John Daly Blvd.

Daly City

San Bruno Mountain State & County Park

PACIFIC OCEAN

0 .2 .4 .6 .8 1.0 mile

0 .2 .4 .6 .8 1.0 kilometer

*The proposed trail corridor represents a concept to connect the parks and public open spaces within the Bay Area Ridge Trail corridor. This map conveys no rights to the public to enter private property.

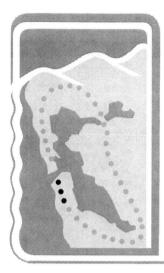

SAN FRANCISCO

Fort Funston to Stern Grove 257

Stern Grove to the Presidio 261

San Francisco Presidio 267

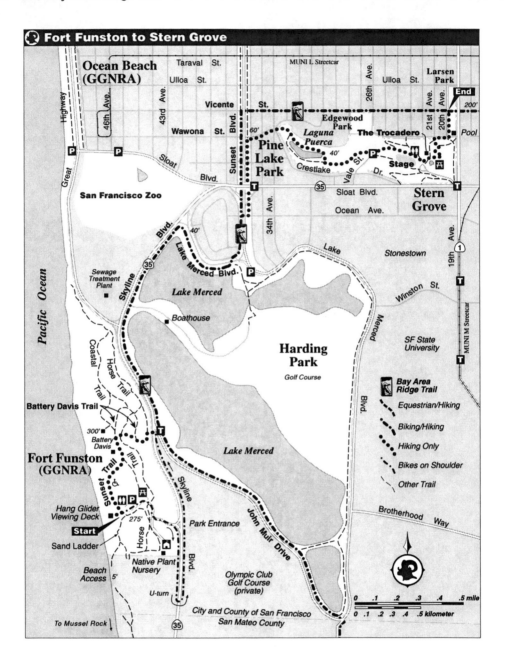

Fort Funston to Stern Grove

Ocean Beach (GGNRA)

Taraval St.

Ulloa St.

MUNI L Streetcar

26th Ave.

Ulloa St.

Larsen Park

End

200'

Vicente St.

Edgewood Park

The Trocadero

21st Ave.

20th Ave.

Pool

Wawona St.

Laguna Puerca

60'

Pine Lake Park

Sunset Blvd.

40'

Stage

San Francisco Zoo

43rd Ave.

46th Ave.

Highway

Great Highway

P

P

P

Sloat Blvd.

Crestlake

Vale St.

Dr.

Stern Grove

35

Sloat Blvd.

Ocean Ave.

34th Ave.

T

P

Lake Merced Blvd.

Lake

Stonestown

Skyline Blvd.

35

Sewage Treatment Plant

40'

Lake Merced

Boathouse

Merced Blvd.

Winston St.

19th Ave.

1

T

MUNI M Streetcar

T

Pacific Ocean

Harding Park

Golf Course

SF State University

Bay Area Ridge Trail

Equestrian/Hiking

Biking/Hiking

Hiking Only

Bikes on Shoulder

Other Trail

Coastal Trail

Horse Trail

Battery Davis Trail

300'

Battery Davis

T

Lake Merced

Fort Funston (GGNRA)

Sunset Trail

Skyline Blvd.

Hang Glider Viewing Deck

Start

275'

Horse Trail

Park Entrance

John Muir Drive

Brotherhood Way

Sand Ladder

Native Plant Nursery

Beach Access

5'

U-turn

35

Olympic Club Golf Course (private)

City and County of San Francisco
San Mateo County

To Mussel Rock

0   .1   .2   .3   .4   .5 mile
0 .1 .2 .3 .4 .5 kilometer

Fort Funston to Stern Grove

From Hang Glider Viewing Deck to Trocadero Inn

Length	3.2 miles
Accessibility	Hikers, bicyclists, and wheelchair users
Agencies	Golden Gate National Recreation Area and San Francisco Recreation and Park Department
Regulations	Fort Funston is open from sunrise to sunset and permits dogs that are on a 6-foot or shorter leash. Pine Lake Park and Stern Grove are open from 7 AM to 10 PM; dogs must be on a leash on park trails and city streets.
Facilities	Water, restrooms, and telephone at Fort Funston; water, restrooms, and telephones at Stern Grove

Watch hang gliders soar on ocean breezes at the launching site in Fort Funston and take in sweeping vistas from a former military observation point. Begin this diverse San Francisco stroll on foggy, bluff-top dunes at a defunct military site, now part of Golden Gate National Recreation Area. On your way to historic Stern Grove you'll pass two freshwater lakes, dip into sunny and protected glens, and cross residential neighborhoods on mostly paved trails. A steep 115-foot climb in the last 0.1 mile gives you a sense of accomplishment.

Getting There

By Car

SOUTH TRAILHEAD, FORT FUNSTON: Going south on Skyline Boulevard (Highway 35) toward Lake Merced, go 0.1 mile past John Muir Drive and turn right (west) into Fort Funston. At a fork in the road, bear right and continue to an extensive parking area. The Sunset Trail entrance is on the north side of the parking area near the hang glider viewing deck on a bluff above the beach.

Going north on Skyline Boulevard (Highway 35), make a U-turn at John Muir Drive and go south on Skyline Boulevard 0.1 mile, turn right (west) into Fort Funston, and follow directions above.

When leaving Fort Funston, drivers and bicyclists must turn right. Thus, to go north, continue south on Skyline Boulevard to John Daly Boulevard and make a U-turn.

NORTH TRAILHEAD, STERN GROVE: This trailhead is between Sloat Boulevard and Wawona Street, just west of 19th Avenue. Traveling north on 19th Avenue, no left turns are allowed. Therefore, pass Stern Grove and turn right on Ulloa Street. Turn right on the next street, 18th Avenue, and then right again on Vicente Street. Cross 19th Avenue, turn left on 20th Avenue, and go one block to Wawona Street, where there is on-street parking. To park in the grove, go left (east) on Wawona Street and then turn right on 19th Avenue. Continue to the corner of Sloat Boulevard and 19th Avenue and then turn right to parking at Stern Grove.

Traveling south on 19th Avenue, turn right into the Stern Grove parking area from the corner of Sloat Boulevard and 19th Avenue. For on-street parking, turn right on Wawona Street from 19th Avenue, or turn right on Sloat Boulevard from 19th Avenue and right again on Vale Avenue to park in Pine Lake Park.

By Bus

San Francisco MUNI runs daily from Market Street to Skyline Boulevard at John Muir Drive and from Market Street to Stern Grove.

On the Trail

As you leave Skyline Boulevard for Fort Funston, consider how "beating swords into ploughshares" benefits the Bay Area and the Ridge Trail. This former military site, as well as several others used in World Wars I and II for coastal defense, is now open for public enjoyment as part of the vast Golden Gate National Recreation Area. Today Fort Funston's paved parking area covers the site of former Nike silos, and the elevated hang glider viewing deck and the adjacent hang glider launching site encompass an earlier military observation point.

Be sure to walk out to the viewing deck for sweeping vistas of the Pacific Ocean from Point San Pedro in the south to Point Reyes in the north. On a clear day, the view extends 25 miles offshore to the Farallon Islands. You may see an aerial display by hang gliders soaring on the ocean breezes.

To start the trip from the parking area, **hikers** and **wheelchair users** take the wide, paved Sunset Trail north along the bluffs. At a junction after about 200 yards, go left on the Sunset Trail to continue on the Ridge Trail route. Soon the trail veers east and passes through the concrete arch of Battery Davis, the site of a World War II gun emplacement.

Wheelchair users turn right (south) at a junction on the other side of the battery tunnel and return to the trailhead on a paved trail that rejoins the first segment of the Sunset Trail. From this junction they then return to the parking area.

Hikers continue east, cross an equestrian trail, and after 100 yards take a footpath to the top of a sandy hill. From here, you descend on a flexible ladder made of wooden crossbars secured on each side to heavy ropes. The ropes are attached to sturdy posts at the top and bottom of the sand dune. When they're wet, the wooden crossbars can be slippery. At the foot of the dunes, you make a short jog north to the intersection of Skyline Boulevard and John Muir Drive. Cross with the signal and go left (north) on the paved path beside fenced Lake Merced.

To access the Bay Area Ridge Trail from the hang glider viewing deck, **mountain bikers** must take the paved road in Fort Funston to Skyline Boulevard (Highway 35) and go right (south) to John Daly Boulevard. Make a **U**-turn and ride north on Skyline Boulevard to John Muir Drive. Across John Muir Drive, join the paved path around Lake Merced.

Hikers and **bicyclists** share the path with runners and parents pushing strollers around Lake Merced. This now-freshwater lake occupies an ancient valley that was flooded at the end of the last ice age. As the sea coast rose, dunes built up, thus isolating

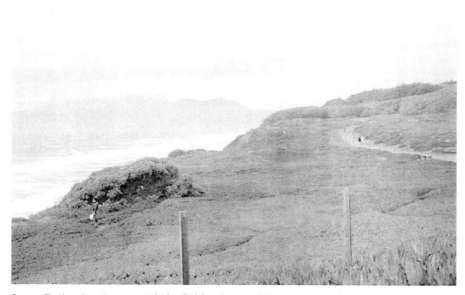

Sunset Trail at Fort Funston with the Golden Gate and Marin Headlands in the distance

this lake and Pine Lake in Stern Grove. Gradually, springs and groundwater changed the new lakes into a freshwater environment.

As you round the northwest corner of Lake Merced, you may hear the roar of a lion or the piercing scream of a peacock emanating from the forested west side of the street, which bounds one side of the San Francisco Zoo. The Bay Area Ridge Trail route now turns southeast following the path between Lake Merced and the boulevard of the same name. After passing parcourse stations set in a broad lakeside band, you cross Lake Merced Boulevard to the west side of Sunset Boulevard. This wide avenue, laid out in the tradition of the grand boulevards of Paris and Washington, D.C., has landscaped borders and a parklike center strip and runs from Lake Merced to Golden Gate Park.

Bicyclists cross Ocean Avenue at Sunset Boulevard and follow the westside path to Vicente Street. Here you cross Sunset Boulevard and travel east on Vicente Street to 20th Avenue, the end of this Ridge Trail trip for bicyclists. Follow the next segment of the Ridge Trail another 7 miles to the Presidio for a longer ride.

At Ocean Avenue, **hikers** cross Sunset Boulevard and take the graveled path on its east side. Follow this path for four blocks, then turn right (east) on Wawona Street, continuing for three blocks to Pine Lake Park at Crestlake Drive and 34th Avenue.

Now you leave city streets to enter a steep-sided, tree-lined canyon. The paved path, often strewn with fragrant eucalyptus and cypress seedpods, descends rather steeply to marshy Laguna Puerca and then levels off on a dirt footpath hugging the north edge of the lake. (Although early Spanish settlers used this name, which translates as "Sow Lake," no pigs are in sight today. However, you will still see the pine trees that give this park its name.) Blackberry bushes and tall reeds crowd the path, which soon emerges at the first of four narrow meadows filling the rest of the canyon.

Take the asphalt path that heads east up the meadow to a parking area. Beside two large eucalyptus trees at the north edge of the lot, you will find a trail, constructed by volunteers, which joins paths above Stern Grove's West Meadow and Stage Meadow. The paths are edged with handsome, low stone walls that also serve as additional seats for the crowds that come on summer Sundays to enjoy the free concerts held here. The long-standing tradition of fine public performances was started by Mrs. Sigmund Stern in 1931, when she gave the grove to San Francisco in honor of her husband.

Beyond Stage Meadow on the north hillside sits the charming Trocadero Inn, built in 1892 as a public hotel by George M. Greene, who owned the land for 40 years. The Trocadero Inn, with its deer park, restaurant, dancing pavilion, rowing lake, and trout farm, flourished until the Prohibition Amendment to the Constitution took effect in 1920. Refurbished in 1986, the Trocadero today appears much as it did at the turn of the century.

You'll find picnic tables beside a small lily pond in a dense redwood grove near the Trocadero. When the day is warm, this is a shady place for a backpack lunch after your hike. If your shuttle car is parked in Stern Grove or at Pine Lake, you have a short walk to reach it. If your shuttle car is parked on Wawona Street, however, you will need to climb the steep hillside on a zigzag asphalt path just east of the Trocadero to its end at 21st Avenue and Wawona Street. For those returning to Fort Funston, another 3.2 miles of views from a new perspective await. Sunsets over the ocean are particularly dramatic from the hang glider viewing deck.

◆ ◆ ◆

If you are continuing north to the Presidio on the Bay Area Ridge Trail, see the next segment for descriptions of attractive parks to visit along the route.

Stern Grove to the Presidio

From Wawona Street at 21st Avenue to Arguello Gate

Length 7.0 miles

Accessibility Hikers and bicyclists

Agencies San Francisco Recreation and Park Department and Golden Gate National Recreation Area

Regulations Dogs must be on leash.

Facilities Water, restrooms, and telephone at Stern Grove

San Francisco's spectacular bay and ocean views reward you on gradual climbs along city streets and park paths. Visit unique and lively neighborhoods, parks, and playgrounds. You'll gain significant elevation on detours to the city's high peaks—a steep stairway to Mt. Olympus and a 685-foot ascent to Twin Peaks, plus three other climbs to viewpoints. Be prepared for San Francisco's foggy and breezy weather.

Getting There

By Car

NORTH TRAILHEAD, STERN GROVE: The north trailhead is between Sloat Boulevard and Wawona Street, just west of 19th Avenue. Traveling north on 19th Avenue, left turns are prohibited. Therefore, pass Stern Grove and turn right on Ulloa Street. Turn right on the next street, 18th Avenue, and then right again on Vicente Street. Cross 19th Avenue, turn left on 20th Avenue, and go one block to Wawona Street, where there is on-street parking. To park in the grove, go left (east) on Wawona Street and then turn right on 19th Avenue. Continue to the corner of Sloat Boulevard and 19th Avenue and then turn right to parking at Stern Grove.

Traveling south on 19th Avenue, turn right into the Stern Grove parking area from the corner of Sloat Boulevard and 19th Avenue. For on-street parking, turn right on Wawona Street from 19th Avenue, or turn right on Sloat Boulevard from 19th Avenue and right again on Vale Avenue to park in Pine Lake Park.

NORTH TRAILHEAD, SAN FRANCISCO PRESIDIO, ARGUELLO GATE: Take Arguello Boulevard to the Presidio. Limited parking is available on the west side of Arguello Boulevard 100 yards inside the Presidio or at Inspiration Point less than 0.1 mile farther north on Arguello Boulevard.

By Bus

Public transportation is the best way to reach this Ridge Trail segment. Some MUNI lines serve Stern Grove, and several others stop on Arguello Boulevard several blocks south of the Presidio.

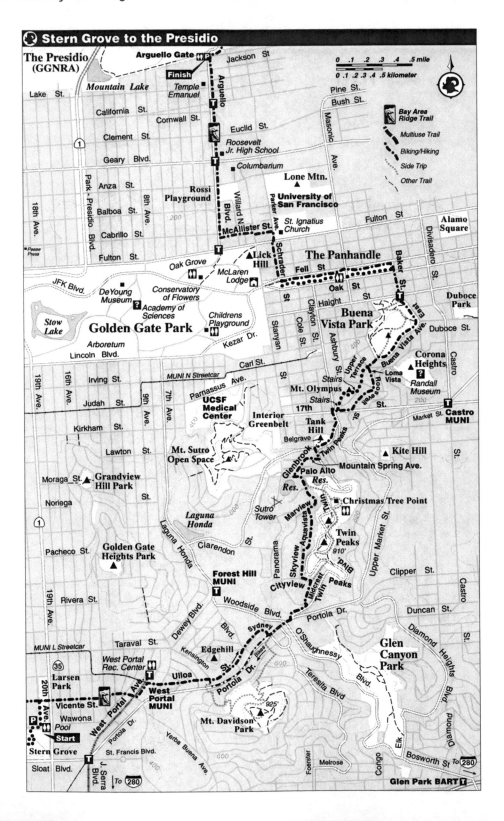

Stern Grove to the Presidio

The Presidio (GGNRA)

Arguello Gate

Finish

Jackson St.

Lake St.

Mountain Lake

Temple Emanuel

California St.

Cornwall St.

Pine St.

Bush St.

Clement St.

Euclid St.

Roosevelt Jr. High School

Masonic

Geary Blvd.

Columbarium

Anza St.

Rossi Playground

Lone Mtn.

Balboa St.

University of San Francisco

Cabrillo St.

St. Ignatius Church

Fulton St.

Fulton St.

Alamo Square

McAllister St.

Oak Grove

Lick Hill

The Panhandle

Fell St.

McLaren Lodge

Oak St.

Duboce Park

JFK Blvd.

DeYoung Museum

Conservatory of Flowers

Haight St.

Buena Vista Park

Duboce St.

Academy of Sciences

Childrens Playground

Corona Heights

Stow Lake

Golden Gate Park

Kezar Dr.

Loma Vista

Randall Museum

Castro

Arboretum

Lincoln Blvd.

Carl St.

Upper Terrace

MUNI N Streetcar

Stairs

Mt. Olympus

Irving St.

Parnassus Ave.

UCSF Medical Center

Stairs

17th

Market St.

Castro MUNI

Judah St.

Interior Greenbelt

Tank Hill

Belgrave

Kirkham St.

Kite Hill

Lawton St.

Mt. Sutro Open Space

Mountain Spring Ave.

Moraga St.

Grandview Hill Park

Palo Alto Res.

Noriega St.

Christmas Tree Point

Laguna Honda

Sutro Tower

Twin Peaks 910'

Pacheco St.

Golden Gate Heights Park

Clarendon

Clipper St.

Rivera St.

Forest Hill MUNI

Cityview

Glen Canyon Park

MUNI L Streetcar

Woodside Blvd.

Portola Dr.

Duncan St.

Taraval St.

West Portal Rec. Center

Edgehill

Larsen Park

Ulloa

West Portal MUNI

Vicente St.

Wawona Pool

Start

Stern Grove

Mt. Davidson Park

Sloat Blvd.

St. Francis Blvd.

Bosworth St.

Glen Park BART

To 280

On the Trail

Hikers and **bicyclists** start this trip where the paved trail emerges from Stern Grove at 21st Avenue and Wawona Street. Following the Bay Area Ridge Trail signs, you go east one block on Wawona Street, turn left on 20th Avenue and skirt the Larsen Park greensward. At the turn of the century, Carl Larsen had a chicken ranch here, which supplied eggs for his Tivoli restaurant downtown. Today, a swimming pool, tennis courts, and children's play equipment serve neighborhood families.

From the corner of Vicente Street and 20th Avenue, proceed east, cross 19th Avenue and continue uphill on Vicente Street. Saint Cecelia's, with a façade graced by handsome bronze doors, is the first of several churches you'll see on this trip.

Soon eucalyptus-covered Mt. Davidson in Mt. Davidson Park and its 103-foot concrete cross looms on your right; the soaring, spare, rusty-orange frame of Sutro Tower rises on your left. These will be landmarks for the first half of your trip. Mt. Davidson, the city's highest peak at 927 feet, commemorates surveyor George Davidson for exposing a false ownership claim to vast acreage in the southwest quarter of the city.

You leave Vicente Street's flowery front gardens and curve left (northeast) onto West Portal Avenue. Here is a one-block opportunity to stop at a neighborhood restaurant or buy a deli lunch for a picnic later in Buena Vista Park. Turn right, uphill, on Ulloa Street, just before the streetcar line disappears into its tunnel. As you progress along Ulloa Street, look on your left above the houses for a steep cliff with wavy lines of red chert. This rock is composed of layers of silica and clay, uplifted from the ocean floor and deposited on the edge of California by movement of the earth's tectonic plates.

Continue to the heights of Rockridge Terrace, crowned by the colorful mosaic bell tower of St. Brendan's Church. At the intersection of Ulloa and Laguna Honda streets, you'll have a sweeping view across the Bay to the Marin Headlands and Mt. Tamalpais.

Now you descend gradually and curve right (east) onto Sydney Way, before turning left (northeast) on Portola Drive. Across Portola Drive there are more neighborhood

San Francisco's Past

This trip begins at Stern Grove in San Francisco's Sunset District in the area of the former San Miguel Rancho. The rancho was originally granted to José Noé in 1839 and passed to Adolph Sutro. Sutro was the entrepreneur of the former Sutro Baths, now part of the Golden Gate National Recreation Area, as well as a philanthropist and former mayor of San Francisco. Rancho San Miguel was mostly composed of shifting sand dunes beyond city limits at the time and remained undeveloped for nearly 40 years—used only for horse racing and some farming and cattle grazing.

When the Twin Peaks Tunnel opened in 1918, and rapid transportation by trolley to downtown became possible, an era of residential building away from the city center began. It culminated in San Francisco's feverish expansion in post–World War II years. Row upon row of houses of varied façades and trims filled the former sand dunes. The wooded glen now known as Stern Grove escaped development because it was occupied by the George M. Greene family from 1847 until 1931, when Mrs. Sigmund Stern gave it to the City of San Francisco.

shops and restaurants. In a few blocks you bear left onto Twin Peaks Boulevard. Pause at the Portola Drive/Twin Peaks Boulevard junction and glance southeast across tree-filled Glen Canyon Park to see Mt. Diablo rising above the East Bay Hills across the bay.

Onward and upward, make a quick left turn on Panoramic Drive and in 50 yards a sharp right onto Midcrest Way. After turning left on Cityview Way, make a right turn (north) on Skyview Way. The street names attest to the remarkable vistas this Bay Area Ridge Trail route offers. In a quick succession of right turns on Aquavista and Marview ways, you skirt the steep sides of Twin Peaks. On windy days you may see people flying kites from the top.

Hiker Side Trips

Twin Peaks Summit

To get the kite-flyer's view from Twin Peaks, **hikers** turn right onto a foot trail at the junction of Marview and Farview ways. You'll pass a reservoir the city set aside for fighting fires, remembering the conflagration after the 1906 earthquake. **Bicyclists** can lock their bikes to the chain-link fence surrounding the reservoir and make the trek to the summit. From the foot trail, you emerge beside Twin Peaks Boulevard and walk south to the summit path that is flanked by boulders of weathered red chert. The windswept, rocky soil beside the path supports one of San Francisco's last remaining habitats of native plants that harbor the endangered Mission Blue butterfly. In spring, indigenous pink checkerblooms, blue and white lupines, and orange poppies brighten the landscape.

You have a 360-degree view from your vantage point at 910 feet above sea level: the Pacific Ocean, the Golden Gate, and the Coast Range mountains that encircle San Francisco Bay. Other segments of the Bay Area Ridge Trail lie along the ridges of these mountains: Mt. Tamalpais and Sonoma Mountain to the north; Vollmer, Mission, and Monument peaks to the east; and Mt. Madonna and Kings Mountain to the south. Spread out before you is the magical city of San Francisco. With a good map you can identify its famous hills, its historic buildings, its new skyscrapers, its bracelets of bridges across the bay, and its many parks. When you've had your fill of vistas near and far (on very clear days you can see north to Mt. St. Helena), retrace your steps.

Buena Vista Park

Hikers can take a short side trip into Buena Vista Park, a 36-acre hilltop preserved in 1894 for its trees and views. Take the wide, paved path from the end of Upper Terrace and follow it to a grassy summit knoll with lacy, tree-framed views—a fine lunch stop. It's said that the ornate marble gutters edging the path that circles the knoll are recycled tombstones from relocated cemeteries. Rejoin the signed Bay Area Ridge Trail route on Buena Vista Avenue East by retracing your steps or by taking one of many paths descending the park's east side.

If you don't make the trek to Twin Peaks' summit, go past San Francisco's Central Radio Station to the lee of Christmas Tree Point for a more intimate view east, north, and south of city neighborhoods, hilltop parks, and landmark public structures, such as the bronze-domed City Hall.

Bear northwest on Marview Way. At the intersection with Palo Alto Avenue, a path to the left through the trees circumnavigates yet another reservoir.

You pass houses with intricate brickwork facing, charming garden gates, and handsome redwood siding and jog right (northeast) on Glenbrook Avenue for a quick, steady descent. Bear right on Mountain Spring Avenue and then arc sharply left (north) on Twin Peaks Boulevard. In the late 1860s, the popular roadhouse, Mountain Spring House, was situated near here on Corbett Road, a predecessor of present-day Twin Peaks Boulevard. Corbett Road continued past the Trocadero Inn, still standing in Stern Grove, to the now-defunct San Miguel Ocean House and its nearby racetrack at the beach.

Watch for the Bay Area Ridge Trail signs and stay on Twin Peaks Boulevard as it turns right (east), past a former water tank site, Tank Hill Open Space, pausing to note its exposed, convoluted, layered chert and greenstone rocks. Sighting northwest from here, beyond the Golden Gate you see the Point Bonita Lighthouse, and on a clear day, farther still to the tip of Point Reyes. Twin Peaks Boulevard becomes Clayton Street, where another reservoir sits encased in a solid steel tank.

Hikers and **bicyclists** diverge here and rejoin at Buena Vista Park. **Hikers** turn right (east) on 17th Street, walk a few yards on its north side, and then mount a steep stairway to Upper Terrace. Head left (northeast) at the top, continuing to Mt. Olympus Park, a tiny, circular green space in the geographical center of the city, which surrounds a raised pedestal.

You then descend the stairway on the circle's north side to the lower leg of Upper Terrace and pass well-kept gardens and attractive homes, following a fairly level route to Buena Vista Park. If the day is sunny, you can see the ocean sparkling at the end of intersecting side streets, named for surveyors and developers of this area. At the entrance to Buena Vista Park your view northwest points to the forested Presidio, where you are headed.

Bicyclists turn right (east) as well on 17th Street and go left (northeast) on Roosevelt Way, which then becomes Loma Vista. Turn right (northeast) on Upper Terrace before rejoining **hikers** at Buena Vista Park.

Along Buena Vista Avenue East, **hikers** and **bicyclists** pass several refurbished Victorian mansions and a former hospital converted to residences. Continue downhill on this avenue to cross Haight Street. On the other side of Haight Street, Buena Vista Avenue East becomes Baker Street; follow Baker Street for two blocks north to the Panhandle, a long, tree-canopied, grassy strip that leads to Golden Gate Park.

Hikers bear left (west) on a park path in the Panhandle that parallels Oak Street. **Bicyclists** continue one block on Baker Street and then turn left on the Panhandle's Fell Street path. Rambling under some of the city's oldest trees, these paths replace a boulevard that once cut through the middle of the park, a space now filled with basketball courts, hopscotch games, and children's play equipment.

Just before Golden Gate Park, **hikers** and **bicyclists** turn right (north) onto Schrader Street and pass St. Mary's Hospital. Schrader Street ends at Fulton Street; the Ridge Trail route makes a slight jog right on Fulton Street and continues north on Parker Avenue. You go one block on Parker Avenue past twin-towered St. Ignatius Church on the University of San Francisco campus to McAllister Street, where you turn left (west).

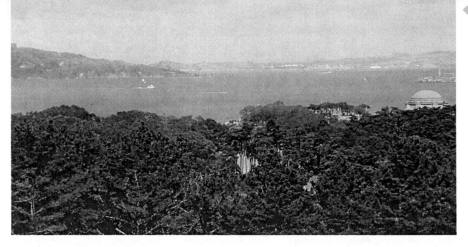

View from Inspiration Point

Admire the tight row of venerable, tiny, stick-style homes, each trimmed in different, but harmonious, dark colors.

Turn right onto Stanyan Street, jog north slightly, and cross Stanyan to pick up McAllister again. At the corner of Willard North and McAllister, note two small houses on the right, vestiges of pre-1906 San Francisco, tucked in among taller homes and apartments. Growing next to a white picket fence surrounding the corner house is a patriarch among buckeye trees with gnarled, twisted limbs.

The last leg of this trip brings more San Franciscana to those who travel it slowly. Turn right (north) onto Arguello Boulevard from McAllister Street. In a few blocks, you'll come to a playground donated by former mayor Angelo J. Rossi. Mount the concrete steps graced by circular flower-filled planters to see the playing fields, tennis courts, and swimming pool. To continue your trip, descend the second set of steps 50 yards to the north. In the last mile of your trip along this busy boulevard, look on its west side for Roosevelt Junior High School, an imposing, brick-faced public school, designed by distinguished architect Timothy Pflueger.

Two houses of worship stand on opposite corners of the intersection of Lake Street and Arguello Boulevard. The brown-shingled St. John's Presbyterian Church, dating from 1905, contains stained glass windows from two churches built in the late 1800s. The monumental, neobyzantine style Temple Emanu-El, has a fine courtyard and stained-glass windows designed by Mark Adams. (It's possible to enter these churches at posted times to see their windows and to sample the architectural and cultural variety of this City of Saint Francis.)

After climbing a little in the last two blocks, you reach the Arguello Gate of the Presidio of San Francisco. The Spaniards established the Presidio here in 1776 to guard their colony at the edge of the Pacific Ocean.

◆ ◆ ◆

On the next segment of the Bay Area Ridge Trail, **hikers** and **bicyclists** leave from Arguello Gate to explore the Presidio's northwest-trending ridges, between the military station and the mission settlement. The trip ends at the Golden Gate Bridge.

San Francisco Presidio

From Arguello Gate to the Golden Gate

Length	2.7 miles
Accessibility	Hikers, bicyclists, and wheelchair users
Agency	Golden Gate National Recreation Area
Regulations	Presidio trails are open during daylight hours. Dogs must be on leash. Horses are prohibited.
Facilities	Water, restrooms, and telephone at clubhouse and at Rob Hill Campground and Picnic Area; water, restrooms, and telephone at Golden Gate Bridge Plaza and Vista Point

Explore the charm, seclusion, natural wonders, and historic and cultural variety of the Presidio. Stunning views await you on this short trip through forests and grasslands and along coastal bluffs, from the Presidio's south-central entrance to its northwest tip. You'll travel sidewalks along the Fort Scott segment and gently sloping unpaved paths elsewhere. Handsome Presidio signs identify the Bay Area Ridge Trail, the Anza Trail, and the American Discovery Trail on this interesting, informative route. Dress for possible coastal fog that often lingers until afternoon.

Getting There

By Car

SOUTH TRAILHEAD, ARGUELLO GATE: Take Arguello Boulevard to the Presidio. Limited parking is available on the west side of Arguello Boulevard, 100 yards inside the Presidio adjacent to the golf course, or at Inspiration Point less than 0.1 mile farther north on Arguello Boulevard. (There is a time limit for parking at Inspiration Point.) Cross Arguello Boulevard in a crosswalk from the southern Presidio Golf Course parking lot to join the trail there.

NORTH TRAILHEAD, GOLDEN GATE BRIDGE TOLL PLAZA: Going north on Highway 1, turn right into the parking plaza immediately before the toll booths. Going south on Highway 1, turn right immediately after the toll booth, turn right again, and turn right yet again. Then go under the bridge approach and into toll plaza and metered parking area.

To continue to Lincoln Boulevard for free parking area east of the toll plaza, leave the plaza on the road going downhill (south), and turn left (east) on Lincoln Boulevard. An unpaved parking area is on your left. Look for the battery east sign. To reach alternative north parking, from Lincoln Boulevard just west of Fort Winfield Scott, turn west on Langdon Court to an unpaved parking area near Battery Godfrey beside the Coastal Trail.

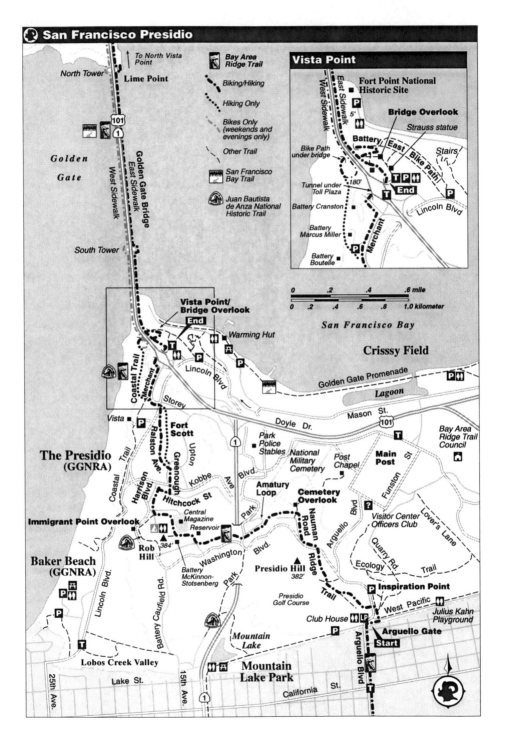

San Francisco Presidio

To North Vista Point

North Tower
Lime Point

Golden Gate Bridge
West Sidewalk
East Sidewalk

Golden
Gate

South Tower

Bay Area Ridge Trail

Biking/Hiking

Hiking Only

Bikes Only
(weekends and
evenings only)

Other Trail

San Francisco
Bay Trail

Juan Bautista
de Anza National
Historic Trail

Vista Point

West Sidewalk
East Sidewalk

Fort Point National
Historic Site

5'

Bridge Overlook

Strauss statue

Battery

Bike Path
under bridge

East Bike Path

Stairs

Tunnel under
Toll Plaza

180'

End

Battery Cranston

Lincoln Blvd

Merchant

Battery
Marcus Miller

Battery
Boutelle

0   .2   .4   .6 mile
0   .2   .4   .6   .8   1.0 kilometer

San Francisco Bay

**Vista Point/
Bridge Overlook**

End

Warming Hut

Coastal Trail
Merchant

Lincoln Blvd

Storey

Crisssy Field

Golden Gate Promenade

Lagoon

Vista

Fort
Scott

Mason St.
Doyle Dr.

101

Park
Police
Stables

National
Military
Cemetery

Post
Chapel

**Main
Post**

Bay Area
Ridge Trail
Council

**The Presidio
(GGNRA)**

Coastal Trail

Harrison Blvd.
Ralston Ave.
Upton Ave.
Greenough
Kobbe

Hitchcock St

Central
Magazine
Reservoir

**Amatury
Loop**

**Cemetery
Overlook**

Park Blvd.

Nauman
Road

Funston St.

Visitor Center
Officers Club

Lover's Lane

Immigrant Point Overlook

Rob
Hill
384'

Washington

Blvd.

Presidio
Ridge
382'

Arguello Blvd.

Quarry Rd.

Ecology

Trail

**Baker Beach
(GGNRA)**

Lincoln Blvd.

Battery Caufield Rd.

Battery
McKinnon-
Stotsenberg

Park

Presidio
Golf Course

Trail

P Inspiration Point

West Pacific

Julius Kahn
Playground

Club House

**Arguello Gate
Start**

Mountain
Lake

Arguello Blvd

25th Ave.
15th Ave.

Lobos Creek Valley

Lake St.

1

**Mountain
Lake Park**

California St.

By Bus

SOUTH TRAILHEAD, ARGUELLO GATE: Several MUNI lines stop on Arguello Boulevard a few blocks south of the Presidio.

NORTH TRAILHEAD, GOLDEN GATE BRIDGE TOLL PLAZA: Any Golden Gate Transit bus southbound to San Francisco from Marin and Sonoma counties will stop at the plaza on request. Some MUNI lines run daily to the toll plaza, and others stop there on Sundays and holidays.

On the Trail

As you enter the Presidio through the Arguello Gate, take note of the gate's flanking stone columns. A prominent stars-and-stripes emblem proclaims the founding of the Presidio in 1776, and the insignia of the Infantry, Cavalry, and Artillery decorate the columns. In the more than 200 years since the founding of the Presidio, these gates have been closed only once—at the beginning of World War II.

Beyond the gate, **hikers** and **bicyclists** veer right, cross West Pacific Street, and bear right on the paved trail. In less than 50 yards the trail swings left and proceeds north beside Arguello Boulevard. After 100 yards, take the crosswalk that leads to the Presidio Golf Course clubhouse. The signed entrance to the Bay Area Ridge Trail is just north of the clubhouse driveway and leads up Presidio Hill into the forest. (If you have parked at Inspiration Point, go south on Arguello to this crosswalk.)

Side Trip to Inspiration Point

Before or after your trip, visit Inspiration Point, less than 0.1 mile north from Arguello Gate on Arguello Boulevard. From this vantage point, Spanish soldiers scanned the Golden Gate for incoming ships carrying supplies from the Old World. They scouted the waters for unfriendly ships—British, French, and Russian—that might threaten this tiny toehold at the entrance to San Francisco Bay; in its early days, the Presidio was Spain's northernmost outpost.

Steps lead downhill from Inspiration Point to a new, unpaved trail that joins the Ecology Trail as it meanders around the southern quarter of the Presidio. A large area of serpentinite, California's state rock, is exposed along this trail. Several placards tell about plant species that thrive on soils composed of this rock, bringing luxurious spring wildflower displays to California's grasslands.

On the hillside north of Inspiration Point, you can also glimpse a remnant of the native serpentine grassland that once stretched across San Francisco. Here the National Park Service has protected small colonies of two endangered species—the Presidio clarkia and the Marin dwarf flax. If you would like to learn more about the native flora here, you can join a wildflower walk led by a park naturalist. Inquire at the Visitor Center, Building 102, at the Main Post Parade Ground.

Side Trip to San Francisco National Military Cemetery

On a short side trip, follow Naumann Road along a unique urban wildlife habitat. The huge blackberry bramble is perfect cover for quail and rabbits; in early morning or at dusk, you may see quail at the bramble's edge or even on the road. At almost any time of day, you can hear the quail's distinctive call, "Be careful, be careful." Halfway around curving Naumann Road, look into the eucalyptus forest on your right for a trail surfaced with decomposed granite that leads downhill to a corner of the San Francisco National Military Cemetery. Built in the 1850s, this was the Presidio's first post cemetery; in 1884, it was converted to a National Military Cemetery. Robert Todd Lincoln, son of Abe, is buried here. General Funston, who commanded the rebuilding of the Presidio after the 1906 quake and for whom the southernmost coastal fort of the Golden Gate National Recreation Area is named, also rests here.

Among the many famous people also interred here are the relatively un-known Native American scout "2 Bits" and Pauline Cushman Fryer, a Union spy in the Civil War. Phillip and Sala Burton, heroes today for preserving the Marin Headlands and the San Francisco beaches and bay fronts in the GGNRA, are also buried here. Here too, lie the remains of 400 "Buffalo Sol-diers," outstanding African-American soldiers, many of them Medal of Honor winners. You can walk to a locked gate in the fence that surrounds the cem-etery to see a few historic grave markers.

From this vantage point, you can look beyond the cemetery's white mark-ers, arranged in symmetrical rows on a gentle slope, to the opposite side of the Golden Gate. There, you'll see the World War II bunkers of Fort Barry and the Coast Guard installations at East Fort Baker, more recent military installations.

On the hill you thread through mature forests of Monterey pine and cypress and a scattering of redwoods. In 1883, Major W. A. Jones had trees planted on three ridgetops and around the parade ground. He intended to beautify the windswept sand dunes and the coastal scrub landscape, as well as to provide much-needed wind protection and to camouflage the military fort.

Today, angled sunlight glancing through these trees creates an ethereal, peaceful effect as you traverse this trail. Major Jones would be amazed to see the height and pro-liferation of the forest. The ridgetop trees grew so well that they spread into the valleys, where abundant moisture encouraged vigorous growth. Today's forest is composed of tall, spindly trees, so closely spaced that most of their branches are clustered at the top reach-ing for sunlight. The National Park Service is selectively removing some nearly dead trees to afford better bay views and to introduce sunshine into the forest, grasslands, val-leys, and riparian corridors.

As you continue up a gentle rise, you see the fence that surrounds the post reservoir in a eucalyptus grove uphill on your left. Through the trees on your right you can glimpse San Francisco's famous skyline.

The trail splits and you bear right, descending gradually to Washington Boulevard. After crossing the street, turn left and stay on the roadside trail for a short distance to Naumann Road, where a spur trail skirts the back side of former Army officers' housing and another spur trail leads to the San Francisco National Military Cemetery surrounded by a metal picket fence.

You bear right and descend to Armatury Loop following it past more housing and a children's playground with gaily painted slides, swings, and other imaginative play equipment. At busy Park Boulevard, which has no crosswalk, a sign gently reminds visitors that quail still inhabit these forests and to please be careful when crossing the street. It also says: 1.7 MILES TO THE GOLDEN GATE BRIDGE. On the other side you dip into woods of Monterey pine and cypress (as well as some thriving acacia and Cape Ivy destined for removal as part of an effort to clothe the park with California native plants). Here too are some fine specimens of native lavender-flowered bush lupine.

Curving west, the trail follows an unpaved road between Battery McKinnon-Stotsenberg (unseen to the left) and the old armory bunkers to the right dating from 1892. (Today, an enterprising company uses the ideal temperature conditions of these bunkers for wine storage.) Go about 100 yards on this minor road (no path) bordered by blackberry brambles, native grasses, and clumps of native iris that bloom in purple springtime splendor. Then turn right (uphill) onto a wide path covered with soft duff. On your left is a raised area topped by yellow bush lupine—the former Battery McKinnon-Stotsenberg. Then on your right is a sunken concrete structure, the fenced-off 1938 Central Magazine. Though in disuse, the mossy complex is still surveyed by a raised wooden guard tower.

Past the bunkers is an intersection—straight ahead is the Rob Hill Group Camp, but the main Ridge Trail turns right along the fence around the Central Magazine. If you

Former officers' quarters at the Presidio

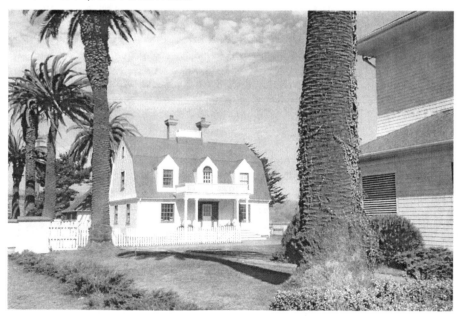

have reservations for the campground, go straight to the picnic grounds and campsites. If they are not occupied, **hikers** and **bicyclists** may use the picnic tables for a quite civilized lunch stop.

Taking the main trail you turn right, following the west side of the fenced-off Central Magazine and shortly curve left downhill. You meet the entry road to Rob Hill Group Camp, the highest point in the Presidio. Here the Juan Bautista de Anza Trail comes in from Immigrant Point. A nearby signpost bears its symbol and that of another long-distance trail, the American Discovery Trail, as well as the Ridge Trail emblem.

Passing between lichen-covered posts, you continue on a quiet stretch of trail under a tall forest canopy. Follow the trail parallel to Harrison Boulevard for one block. Then turn right (east) on Hitchcock Street, a little-used road, walk on the right side in the bike lane for about 150 yards, and watch for a low board-and-batten building (a warehouse) on your left, #1340. Just beyond it, turn left (north) downhill on a short path lined with stone pavers to Kobbe Avenue, cross it, pass a low brick building (#1339), and then follow Greenough Street due north to the Fort Winfield Scott Parade Ground. On this route you pass a brick wall surrounding the spacious garden of a 1915 officer's residence, its Georgian style façade contrasting with the presently unused wood barracks on your left.

Shortly you reach Ralston Avenue, where the hiker and mountain biker routes briefly diverge: **Bicyclists** go left on the marked Ridge Trail route. **Hikers** go a few feet farther to walk through the arched entrance to Fort Winfield Scott and veer left (west) on the broad Fort Scott promenade in front of the buildings, which are awaiting rehabilitation. (This promenade is suitable for wheelchair use.)

Named for a commanding general of the U.S. Army during the Mexican-American War, Fort Winfield Scott became the headquarters for the coastal defenses of San Francisco in 1912. The Post Parade Ground, an elongated, open greensward, is partially surrounded by former U.S. Army buildings.

When the fort was built, this extensive open space commanded an uninterrupted view of the Marin Headlands, the Golden Gate, and Richardson Bay. Now trees block some of the near view, but you can still see these landmarks and the Golden Gate Bridge's dramatic, rust-colored towers, which clearly define the entrance to the bay. Even on foggy days, the towers' tops might be visible, swept clear of fog by fresh ocean winds.

As you walk along around the parade ground on a clear day, look out at the blue bay waters filled with sailboats heeling in the wind, windsurfers skimming across the waves, and great ships, mostly ocean-going freighters, cruising to or from distant ports. Alcatraz Island sits in a swirl of swift bay currents, first a fortress, then a federal prison, and is now a national park and part of Golden Gate National Recreation Area. You can reach it by ferry from San Francisco.

To the east lie Coit Tower, the Transamerica Pyramid, other downtown skyscrapers, and the Bay Bridge leading to the populous East Bay cities. The Campanile's tall shaft rises on the University of California–Berkeley campus, and forested public parklands crown the surrounding hills. Topping the distant view are two East Bay landmarks— triangular-shaped Mt. Diablo and half-spherical Round Top, both within public parklands.

Continuing north along the west side of the Fort Winfield Scott Parade Ground, you pass buildings constructed in Mission Revival style, popular in the early 20th century. The square, two-story building on the far northern side is the former Fort Scott stockade, now devoid of inmates.

Side Trip to Fort Point

Before you cross the Golden Gate Bridge to Marin County, take a short, 0.4-mile walk from the toll plaza to Fort Point. Return to the Coastal Trail from the Toll Plaza and descend north toward the bay on a series of wide steps. Fort Point stands directly beneath the bridge, reminding us of over 200 years of Golden Gate defenses. The Spaniards first established Castillo de San Joaquin here at White Cliff Point, with a small bastion of 13 guns. It fell into disrepair during the Spanish and Mexican periods, and was claimed by Army Lieutenant John C. Fremont in 1846.

In the late 1850s, the U.S. Army planned to build three forts to defend the bay and the Golden Gate from attack. A fortification of about 109 cannon batteries and 2 mortars was established on Alcatraz Island; a fort planned for rocky Lime Point in Marin County, directly across the Golden Gate on the east side of the bridge, was never completed. Fort Point, a massive three-story brick fortress, was first occupied in 1861 and used intermittently through World War II. Now a national historic site, it is open for guided day tours and special evening programs by the National Park Service.

When **hikers** arrive at a passageway between Buildings 1207 and 1208, they go left and then swing right on Lincoln Boulevard sidewalks joining bicyclists as all proceed to the corner of Storey Avenue and Merchant Road.

At this writing, the Landfill Remediation Project is working on the coastal bluffs northwest of this intersection. Thus **hikers** use the Merchant Road sidewalks to go north to the Golden Gate Bridge and the end of this trip, and **bicyclists** continue right (north) on Merchant Road to reach the bridge.

When the reconstruction work is complete sometime in 2008, the Ridge and Coastal trails will again pass the coastal defense batteries, and a short description of these fortifications built from 1891 to 1900 is given here: Plaques on the batteries tell their story, the earliest of which had a one-mile range. Later, Nike missiles had a 75-mile range. Just seaward from Fort Scott is Battery Godfrey. On its landward side you see a ramp used to transport ammunition stored below ground to guns behind low walls on upper concrete platforms. Its rifles were mounted on disappearing carriages and retracted below the battery's walls after firing so the soldiers could safely load the guns.

Beyond the next battery, Battery Boutelle, you reach an opening with a fabulous view of Land's End, the Point Bonita Lighthouse, and the Marin Headlands. The Golden Gate's high cliffs are indented by small, crescent-shaped beaches. In good weather, these picturesque cliffs and rugged shores seem quite benign. But when it's foggy, the many-voiced warning horns, now computer-driven, announce the imminent danger of rocky points, small islets, and treacherous tides to ship traffic navigating the hazardous waters at the entrance to San Francisco Bay. On a clear day, you'll see west to the Farallons—small, rocky islands 25 miles offshore.

After Battery Boutelle, **bicyclists** go straight on Merchant Road. Turn left just before the freeway entrance, then turn right and go through the narrow tunnel beneath the Golden Gate Bridge Toll Plaza.

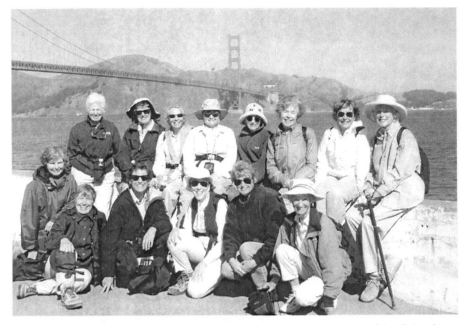

The Walkie-Talkies, a group of about 60 women, mostly from the Peninsula and South Bay, have taken monthly hikes together since the 1970s. They explore local trails and take longer yearly trips to places farther afield.

Hikers continue to the next battery, Marcus Miller. It retains a small, square, concrete lookout, known as a base-end station, which in conjunction with another such station could triangulate the position of its targets or the site of its shell landing.

To continue toward the Golden Gate Bridge, stay on the cliff-top path, the Coastal Trail and the Bay Area Ridge Trail route. You'll hear the crashing surf and screeching seagulls and get a slight approximation of a ship's view as it enters the Golden Gate. After traversing the wild and scenic bluffs west of Battery Marcus Miller and Battery Cranston, the Coastal Trail dips under the bridge and reaches a paved trail. Go uphill (south) to the Golden Gate Bridge Plaza, where tourists and locals alike flock on clear days to enjoy the world-class views of the Golden Gate, the bridge, San Francisco, the bay, and its enclosing hills.

If the weather is too windy and foggy to appreciate the bluffs, **hikers** can take the bicycle route on the east side of Battery Marcus Miller. Follow it through the bridge-maintenance yard, cross to the sidewalk under the bridge's south portal, and emerge at the Golden Gate Bridge Plaza. From the plaza you can take a bus back to the Presidio.

To reach the Lincoln Boulevard parking area on the east side of the bridge plaza, return to the Coastal Trail and follow it east through a short tunnel, part of the original Battery East (1876). Beyond the tunnel, you can climb to an observation deck to look down at the top of the fortifications, the Bay, and Fort Point.

As you continue east on the Coastal Trail, look for a path that bears right (south) to the alternate parking area on Lincoln Boulevard, where you could have a shuttle car waiting. From this parking area, you drive along Lincoln Boulevard southeast under Highway 101, pass the National Military Cemetery, and reach the Presidio's Main Post

Parade Ground and Visitor Information Center and the parking area from which you started this trip.

This trip only samples the remarkable story of the Presidio at San Francisco—from establishment of the first Spanish military outpost in 1776 through Spanish and Mexican settlements, the Gold Rush, and the early California statehood period to its present national park status. Although the military presence is diminished, its influence will stay on with an outstanding military museum, the 19th- and 20th-century coastal defenses, and the intact, historic Civil War building, Fort Point. Many interesting tours led by experienced volunteers and National Park Service staff offer more detailed information about this historic site. Inquire at the Visitor Information Center, at the former officer's club, 50 Moraga Avenue, facing the Main Post Parade Ground.

◆ ◆ ◆

The next leg of the Bay Area Ridge Trail begins at the South Vista Point on the Golden Gate Bridge; see the first trip in this guidebook, which crosses the Golden Gate Bridge. If you had begun your journey along the Bay Area Ridge Trail here at the south end of the Golden Gate Bridge and followed all the trips in this guidebook described clockwise around San Francisco Bay, you would have traveled more than 300 miles along the ridges above the bay. Each trip offers outstanding views and different perspectives on some very special features of the San Francisco Bay Area.

Appendix 1

Summary of Trail Features

	Dogs Allowed	Water	Toilet	Parking Fee	Phone
The North Bay					
The Golden Gate Bridge	On leash only	Yes	Yes	Yes	Yes
Marin Headlands from the Golden Gate Bridge to Tennessee Valley		Yes	Yes	Yes	Yes
Marin Headlands from Tennessee Valley to Shoreline Highway	Yes (on Ridge Trail only)		Yes	Yes	Yes
Mount Tamalpais State Park		Yes (at Pantoll)	Yes (at Pantoll)	Yes	Yes
Mount Tamalpais State Park and Golden Gate National Recreation Area	On leash in GGNRA; prohibited in state park	Yes (at Pantoll)		Yes (at Pantoll)	Yes (at Pantoll)
Golden Gate National Recreation Area and Samuel P. Taylor State Park		Yes	Yes	Yes	Yes
Samuel P. Taylor State Park to Loma Alta Open Space Preserve	On leash			Yes (roadside)	
Loma Alta Open Space Preserve to Lucas Valley Open Space Preserve	On leash			Yes (roadside)	
Lucas Valley Open Space Preserve	on leash			Yes (roadside)	
Indian Tree Open Space Preserve to O'Hair Park	Yes			Yes (roadside)	
Mount Burdell Open Space Preserve	Yes (except on Dwarf Oaks Trail)		Yes	Yes	
Helen Putnam Regional Park and McNear Park to Petaluma Adobe State Historic Park	On leash	Yes	Yes	Yes	
Jack London State Historic Park		Yes	Yes	Yes	Yes
Annadel State Park		Yes	Yes	Yes	Yes (near ranger station)

Picnic Tables	Visitor Center	Camping	Ranger Station	Horses Allowed	Wheelchair Accessible	Other
	Yes				Yes	
	Yes					Headlands Institute and Golden Gate Hostel
Yes		Yes		Yes	Yes	
Yes						Bus runs on weekends to Pantoll and Stinson Beach
Yes						Parking fee at Pantoll
Yes		Yes		Yes	Yes	
				Yes		Tunnel under Lucas Valley Road to facilitate safe crossing from south to north
						Tunnel under Lucas Valley Road to facilitate safe crossing from south to north
	Yes (Indian artifacts)	Yes		Yes		Hitch racks and rails and youth camping
	Yes	Yes (at Petaluma Adobe)				Historic buildings in Petaluma; bus stops at Petaluma Adobe SHP and Helen Putnam RP; fee at Petaluma Adobe SHP
Yes	Yes (London's cottage)	Yes	Yes	Yes		Beauty ranch buildings, winery, distillery, and rock wall remains of Wolf House
Yes			Yes	Yes		Parking fee; hitch rack at Marsh-Burma trails junction

	Dogs Allowed	Water	Toilet	Parking Fee	Phone
Hood Mountain Regional Park and Open Space Preserve		Yes		Yes	
Sugarloaf Ridge State Park		Yes	Yes	Yes	Yes
Yountville Cross Road		Yes	Yes		Yes
River-to-Ridge Trail		Yes	Yes	Yes	
Skyline Wilderness Park and Napa Solano Ridge Trail		Yes	Yes	Yes	
Rockville Hills Regional Park				Yes	
Lynch Canyon Open Space			Yes		
Hiddenbrooke Trail					
Vallejo-Benicia Buffer		Yes	Yes	Yes	Yes
Vallejo-Benicia Waterfront		Yes	Yes		Yes
The East Bay					
Al Zampa Memorial Bridge	Yes	Yes	Yes	Yes	Yes
Martinez City Streets to Carquinez Strait Regional Shoreline	On leash	Yes	Yes	Yes	
Carquinez Strait Regional Shoreline to John Muir National Historic Site on the Hulet Hornbeck Trail	On leash	Yes	Yes	Yes	

Picnic Tables	Visitor Center	Camping	Ranger Station	Horses Allowed	Wheelchair Accessible	Other
			Yes	Yes		Parking fee; historic Hood Mansion; horse trailer parking
Yes	Yes	Yes		Yes		Parking fee and guided horse rides only (horse rentals)
Yes	Yes			On unpaved sections		Napa Wine Train stops here; several parking lots and a visitor center in Yountville
Yes	Yes (tent and RV)					Boat launch and marina in Kennedy Park
Yes	Yes	Yes		Yes		All amenities in Skyline only; parking fee; archery range, disc golf, native habitat garden, horse arena, and RV park
Yes						No parking at north end of trail or on Green Valley Road; nature programs
				Yes		Portable toilet at entrance
						Views west to the Golden Gate and peaks in the Sierra Nevada
Yes						Parking fee, phone, and water flume at Blue Rock Springs Park
Yes (at Benecia State Recreation Area)				Yes (only in Benicia State Recreation Area)	Yes	Hikers only on Carquinez Overlook Trail; no bikes on unpaved trails
Yes					Yes	Water, restrooms, parking, and picnic tables in Carquinez Park but not on bridge
Yes				Yes	Yes	Public fishing pier, restaurants, city park, history museum, historic buildings, boat launching ramp, sand beaches, bocce ball, baseball, soccer, and horse arena
Yes	Yes			Yes	At Muir house	Dogs on leash in staging area and under voice control in open space

	Dogs Allowed	Water	Toilet	Parking Fee	Phone
Mount Wanda Trail				Yes (at Muir House)	
Crockett Hills Regional Park		Yes	Yes		
Sobrante Ridge Regional Preserve	Yes	Yes (at Coast Drive)	Yes		Yes
Kennedy Grove to Tilden Park	On leash in parking and picnic areas and under voice control on Nimitz Way	Yes	Yes	Yes (at Tilden)	Yes
Tilden Regional Park to Redwood Regional Park	Yes	Yes	Yes	Yes	Yes
Redwood and Anthony Chabot Regional Parks	Yes		Yes	Yes	
Anthony Chabot Regional Park	Yes	Yes (at picnic sites)	Yes	Yes	Yes
East Bay Municipal Utility District Lands to Independent School	On leash and under voice control in open spaces (not in EBMUD)	Yes	Yes	Yes	
Independent School to Five Canyons	On leash	Yes	Yes		Yes
Mission Peak Regional Preserve and Ed R. Levin County Park	On leash in parking areas and under voice control in open spaces	Yes (Ohlone College)	Yes (Ohlone College)	Yes (on weekends)	Yes
The South Bay					
Alum Rock Park and the Boccardo Trail Corridor		Yes	Yes	Yes	Yes

Picnic Tables	Visitor Center	Camping	Ranger Station	Horses Allowed	Wheelchair Accessible	Other
				Yes		Contra Costa Connection bus stops at the park
Yes (staging area)				Yes		
Yes				Yes		Trail begins in Pinole Valley Park, which has water, restrooms, and parking
Yes					Yes (Nature Trail on Nimitz Way)	AC Transit bus stops at Tilden; bikes allowed from Fish Ranch Road to Huckleberry Botanic Preserve; parking fee; picnic tables in Tilden can be reserved; playground, volleyball, horseshoes, playing field, and senior citizen's center
Yes		Yes (group)				Group camping by reservation
Yes		Yes (family camp at Lake Chabot)		Yes (on Golden Spike in rainy weather)	Yes	Lake Chabot Marina, Anthony Chabot Family Camp; golf course in northwest corner
				Yes		EBMUD prohibits dog and bikes and requires a permit for hiking; sign in on register at staging area
				Yes (in Don Castro Recreation Area)		Bikes allowed from Don Castro Recreation Area to Five Canyons
Yes		Yes (group)		Yes		Bikes allowed on Hidden Valley and Eagle Trails; cattle grazing on some trails; Ed Levin has hang glider facilities and an equestrian staging area at Stanford Avenue entrance
Yes	Yes			Yes	Yes (Creek Trail)	Parking fee; barbecues, playground, Youth Science Institute, and nature programs

	Dogs Allowed	Water	Toilet	Parking Fee	Phone
Joseph D. Grant County Park	Limited areas, not on trails; must be on leash	Yes	Yes	Yes	Yes
Coyote Lake-Harvey Bear Ranch Trail	Limited areas, not on trails; must be on leash	Yes	Yes	Yes	Yes
Mount Madonna County Park	On leash (prohibited from trails)	Yes	Yes		Yes
Sierra Azul Open Space Preserve	Yes (except on Wood Trail)	Yes	Yes	Yes	
Coyote Creek Parkway North	On leash	Yes	Yes	Yes	Yes
Coyote Creek Parkway South	On leash	Yes	Yes		Yes
Santa Teresa County Park	On leash	Yes	Yes	Yes	
Almaden Quicksilver County Park	On leash	Yes	Yes	Yes	
Sanborn County Park	Yes (except on Sunnyvale Mountain)	Yes	Yes	Yes	Yes
Castle Rock State Park		Yes	Yes	Yes	Yes
The Peninsula					
Saratoga Gap Open Space Preserve	On leash				
Skyline Ridge Open Space Preserve	On leash		Yes	Yes	Yes
Russian Ridge Open Space Preserve	On leash		Yes	Yes	Yes
Windy Hill Open Space Preserve	On Anniversary Trail only	Yes	Yes	Yes	Yes
Wunderlich County Park		Yes	Yes	Yes	Yes

Picnic Tables	Visitor Center	Camping	Ranger Station	Horses Allowed	Wheelchair Accessible	Other
Yes	Yes	Yes	Yes	Yes		Parking fee; equestrian staging area and fishing
Yes (at both entrances)		Yes	Yes	Yes		Parking fee; camping at lakeside in Harvey Bear and at Coyote Lake entrance
		Yes		Yes		Bikes are prohibited
Yes				Yes		Hitch rail at Hicks Road
					Yes	Parking fee; tiny tots playground and skateboard park at Metcalf
			Yes	Yes	Yes	
Yes				Yes	Yes	
	Yes		Yes	Yes		Visitor center, ranger station, and horse amenities are all at Mockingbird Hill entrance only
Yes	Yes	Yes				Welch Hurst Sanborn Hostel; Bikes and dogs are prohibited on Sunnyvale Mountain
		Yes				Parking fee
			Yes	Yes	Yes	
Yes			Yes		Yes	Telephone and water at Saratoga Summit Fire Station; nature center with observation deck and displays
Yes				On Fence Line Trail only		Dogs on Anniversary Trail and top of Spring Ridge
Yes		Yes (use Huddart park)		Yes		Bikes are prohibited

	Dogs Allowed	Water	Toilet	Parking Fee	Phone
Huddart County Park		Yes	Yes	Yes	Yes
Purisima Creek Redwoods Open Space Preserve			Yes	Yes	Yes
San Francisco Watershed Trail			Yes	Yes	
Golden Gate National Recreation Area: Sweeney Ridge to Milagra Ridge	On leash			Yes (at Sneath Lane)	
Mussel Rock to Fort Funston	On leash	Yes	Yes	Yes	Yes
San Francisco					
Fort Funston to Stern Grove	On leash	Yes	Yes	Yes	Yes
Stern Grove to the Presidio	On leash	Yes	Yes	Yes	Yes
San Francisco Presidio	On leash	Yes	Yes	Yes	Yes

Picnic Tables	Visitor Center	Camping	Ranger Station	Horses Allowed	Wheelchair Accessible	Other
Yes		Yes		Yes		Barbecue pits, nature trail, play structures, play fields, archery range, youth and adult camps by reservation
Yes				Yes	Yes	0.2-mile segment for wheelchair users
				Yes		Access on guided tours through Watershed by advance reservation for a fee
					At Fort Funston	Musssel Rock to Funston beach route closed; follows city streets and bike paths
Yes	Yes	Yes	Yes	Yes	Yes	Native plant nursery, hang glider viewing deck
Yes						Summer Sunday concerts at Stern Grove
Yes (only 1)	Yes	Yes (youth groups)			Yes	Wheelchair users can access this trail segment at Arguello entrance, the south entrance of the Golden Gate Bridge, and at Rob Hill Campground

Appendix 2

Trail Sampler: Trips for Many Reasons

THE NORTH BAY

Mount Tamalpais State Park: Mt. Tamalpais's East Peak, 2571 feet
Lucas Valley Open Space Preserve: Big Rock Ridge, 1895 feet
Mt. Burdell Open Space Preserve: Mt. Burdell, 1480 feet
Jack London State Historic Park: Trail reaches upper flanks of Sonoma Mountain, approximately 2000 feet
Hood Mountain: 2730 feet, "sister mountain" to Sugarloaf Ridge
Sugarloaf Ridge State Park: Bald Mountain, 2720 feet

THE EAST BAY

Tilden Regional Park to Redwood Regional Park: Vollmer Peak, 1905 feet
Mount Wanda Trail, John Muir National Historic Site: Mt. Wanda, 660 feet
Redwood Regional Park to Anthony Chabot Regional Park: Redwood Peak, 1619 feet, and Round Top Mountain, 1763 feet
East Bay Municipal Utility District Lands to Cull Canyon Regional Recreation Area: Dinosaur Ridge, 1000 feet
Mission Peak Regional Preserve and Ed R. Levin County Park: Mission Peak, 2517 feet, and Monument Peak, 2594 feet

THE SOUTH BAY

Boccardo Trail Corridor: Unnamed hill on side trip, 1896 feet
Alum Rock Park: Eagle Rock, 796 feet
Santa Teresa County Park and Los Alamitos/Calero Creek Trail: Coyote Peak, 1155 feet
Mt. Madonna County Park: Mt. Madonna, 1897 feet

THE PENINSULA

Skyline Ridge and Russian Ridge Open Space Preserves: Borel Hill, 2572 feet, and Mt. Melville, 2190 feet
Windy Hill Open Space Preserve: Windy Hill summit, 1919 feet

SAN FRANCISCO

Stern Grove to the Presidio: Twin Peaks, 910 feet

NORTH BAY

The Golden Gate Bridge: Views west to the Farallons and east throughout the Bay Area
Marin Headlands from the Golden Gate Bridge to Tennessee Valley

Marin Headlands from Tennessee Valley to Shoreline Highway
Mount Tamalpais State Park
Mount Tamalpais State Park and Golden Gate National Recreation Area
Golden Gate National Recreation Area and Samuel P. Taylor State Park

THE EAST BAY

Kennedy Grove to Tilden Regional Park: From Inspiration Point
Tilden Regional Park to Redwood Regional Park: From Sea View Trail

THE SOUTH BAY

Sanborn County Park and Castle Rock State Park: Views of Monterey Bay

THE PENINSULA

Saratoga Gap Open Space Preserve to Skyline Ridge Open Space
   Preserve: From Long Ridge Open Space Preserve
Skyline Ridge and Russian Ridge Open Space Preserves: From Borel Hill
Windy Hill Open Space Preserve: From Windy Hill summit
Purisima Creek Redwoods Open Space Preserve: From Harkins Ridge Trail
Golden Gate National Recreation Area: Sweeney Ridge and Milagra Ridge: From Mori
   Ridge and the Discovery Site
Mussel Rock to Fort Funston: From both ends of the trail

SAN FRANCISCO

Fort Funston to Stern Grove: See the Farallons from the hang glider viewing deck
Stern Grove to the Presidio: From Twin Peaks and adjoining streets

For San Francisco Bay Area Views: Sparkling Blue or Fog-Shrouded, It's Always Impressive

THE NORTH BAY

Golden Gate Bridge: West to Farallons and east to Mt. Diablo
Marin Headlands from the Golden Gate Bridge to Tennessee Valley
Marin Headlands from Tennessee Valley to Shoreline Highway: Richardson Bay and Angel
   Island
Mount Tamalpais State Park: From Shoreline Highway to Pantoll
Indian Tree Open Space Preserve: From Indian Tree summit
Mt. Burdell Open Space Preserve: From the summit of Mt. Burdell
Jack London State Historic Park: From Sonoma Mountain summit
Hood Mountain Regional Park: From the summit of Hood Mountain
Sugarloaf Ridge State Park: From Bald Mountain
Skyline Wilderness Park: Napa Marshlands on San Pablo Bay
Hiddenbrooke Trail: Views of the Golden Gate, the bridge, and the Napa Marshlands
Vallejo-Benicia Buffer: On the upper trail
Vallejo-Benicia Waterfront: On the west trail

THE EAST BAY

Carquinez Strait Regional Shoreline to John Muir National Historic Site:
   San Pablo Bay

Mount Wanda Trail: Carquinez Strait

Sobrante Ridge Regional Preserve: Views especially of San Pablo Bay

Kennedy Grove to Tilden Regional Park: From Nimitz Way

Tilden Regional Park to Redwood Regional Park: From Sea View Trail

Mission Peak Regional Preserve and Ed R. Levin County Park: South Bay and its wetlands

THE SOUTH BAY

Boccardo Trail Corridor: South Bay and its wetlands

Mt. Madonna County Park: Views south to the Santa Lucia Mountains and east to the Diablo Range

Sanborn County Park: To the Diablo Range from Indian Rock

THE PENINSULA

Skyline Ridge and Russian Ridge Open Space Preserves

Windy Hill Open Space Preserve: Views up and down the bay from the summit

Sweeney Ridge to Milagra Ridge: This is where Don Gaspar de Portolá first saw San Francisco Bay.

SAN FRANCISCO

Stern Grove to the Presidio: From Twin Peaks

San Francisco Presidio: Especially Golden Gate Bridge, Richardson Bay, and Alcatraz

For a Child's Birthday Party (Picnic Tables and Restrooms Nearby)

THE NORTH BAY

Mount Tamalpais State Park: Rock Spring or Bootjack Picnic Areas

Golden Gate National Recreation Area and Samuel P. Taylor State Park: Walk or ride on the Cross Marin Trail and picnic in the park.

Helen Putnam Regional Park and McNear Park to Petaluma Adobe State Historic Park: Picnic and play areas at the west end; picnic areas at parks along the way and at Petaluma Adobe State Historic Park

Jack London State Historic Park: Sample a bit of history and picnic afterward.

Annadel State Park: Picnic at Spring Lake Park and walk or ride the Connector Trail to Annadel.

Sugarloaf Ridge State Park: Enjoy a round-trip on Stern Trail and picnic by Sonoma Creek.

Skyline Wilderness Park: Play areas and picnic sites

Blue Rock Springs Park, Vallejo-Benicia Buffer: Picnic tables and play area

Vallejo-Benicia Waterfront: Walk, bike, or roller-blade on level, paved trail and picnic at one of several park sites along the way.

THE EAST BAY

Martinez Regional Shoreline: Picnic and play areas, large playing fields, and fishing pier

Sobrante Ridge Regional Preserve: At Pinole Valley Park, many picnic tables on the ridge (after an uphill climb)

Kennedy Grove to Tilden Regional Park: Picnic sites and level trail at both ends

Tilden Regional Park to Redwood Regional Park: Many sites at several entry points; Steam Trains and Merry-Go-Round at Tilden

Redwood and Anthony Chabot Regional Parks: Picnic at Redwood Bowl beside the Ridge Trail or after a trip to Chabot Science Center, or walk from the Redwood Regional Park's Moon Gate to the Redwood Bowl (less than 1 mile); other sites available at Redwood Gate and at Bort Meadow

East Bay Municipal Utility District Lands to Independent School: Cull Canyon Recreation Area especially suited to birthday parties, with swimming available

Independent School to Five Canyons: Picnic and play areas, swimming, and playing fields at Don Castro Regional Park

Mission Peak Regional Preserve and Ed R. Levin County Park: Sandy Wool Lake picnic sites and children's play area

THE SOUTH BAY

Alum Rock Park: Play area in middle of park and picnic tables throughout park

Joseph D. Grant County Park: Picnic tables and group camping

Mount Madonna County Park: Picnic tables near visitor center and at amphitheater; white deer and more picnic tables near Ridge Trail

Coyote Creek Parkway North: Walk or ride bikes on the trail and return to birthday treats at several parks along the trail.

Coyote Creek Parkway South: Walk or ride bikes or horses; picnic facilities at trail's south end

Santa Teresa County Park and Los Alamitos/Calero Creek Trail: Work off extra energy before the party on a short Ridge Trail trip from Santa Teresa Pueblo Group Area

THE PENINSULA

Skyline Ridge and Russian Ridge Open Space Preserves: Hike the trail before picnicking at Horseshoe Lake or Alpine Pond; Nature Center at Alpine Pond open on spring and summer weekends

Windy Hill Open Space Preserve: Picnic area adjacent to Skyline Boulevard entrance and at Spring Ridge entrance

Mussel Rock to Fort Funston: Neighborhood parks along the trail in Daly City; watch the hang gliders and picnic on the viewing deck at Fort Funston

SAN FRANCISCO

Stern Grove to the Presidio: Many parks along the Ridge Trail route with picnic facilities; restrooms at Stern Grove and Golden Gate Park only

San Francsico Presidio: See the World War II gun emplacements and picnic at Rob Hill; visitors center at Main Post Parade Ground

For Spring Wildflowers' Beautiful Blossoms, Especially in the Grasslands

THE NORTH BAY

Marin Headlands from the Golden Gate Bridge to Tennessee Valley: Swaths of mule ears and bush lupines

Marin Headlands from Tennessee Valley to Shoreline Highway: Irises in many hues

Mount Tamalpais State Park: Lavender bush lupine

Mount Burdell Open Space Preserve: Milkmaids herald spring

Annadel State Park: White fritillary

Sugarloaf Ridge State Park: Lewisia

Rockville Hills Regional Park: Blue iris, orange sticky monkeyflower

Lynch Canyon Open Space: Dazzling array of spring wildflowers

Vallejo-Benicia Buffer: Tall blue brodiaea

THE EAST BAY

Carquinez Strait Regional Shoreline Park to John Muir National Historic Site: Poppies and blue-eyed grass

Mount Wanda Trail: Woodland stars

Anthony Chabot Regional Park: Trillium garden

Mission Peak Regional Preserve and Ed R. Levin County Park: Poppies and white phacelia on high grasslands between peaks

THE SOUTH BAY

Joseph D. Grant County Park: Some of earliest and largest displays in the Bay Area

Sierra Azul Open Space Preserve: Unusual species on Barlow Trail side trip

Santa Teresa County Park and Los Alamitos/Calero Creek Trail: Jewel flower and magenta Clarkia on Stile Ranch Trail

THE PENINSULA

Saratoga Gap Open Space Preserve to Skyline Ridge Open Space Preserve: Masses of blue- and cream-colored irises

Skyline Ridge and Russian Ridge Open Space Preserves: Acres of wildflowers, especially on Russian Ridge; yellow Johnny-jump-ups early in spring

Windy Hill Open Space Preserve: Columbine in particular but many flowers late into summer

Wunderlich County Park to Huddart County Park: Especially Clintonia and bleeding heart

Purisima Creek Redwoods Open Space Preserve: Shade-loving plants: columbine and Clintonia

Golden Gate National Recreation Area: Sweeney Ridge and Milagra Ridge: Native orchids and host plants for Mission Blue butterfly

Mussel Rock to Fort Funston: Seaside flowers, yellow lizard tail

SAN FRANCISCO

San Francisco Presidio: Rare native flower in garden near Inspiration Point

To Historic Sites
(Ranches, Homes, Forts, and Inns)

THE NORTH BAY

The Golden Gate Bridge: Most visited site in San Francisco, a San Francisco icon

Marin Headlands: Military site, historic lighthouse at Point Bonita

McNear Park to Petaluma Adobe State Historic Park: Victorian homes and General Vallejo's ranch house

Jack London State Historic Park: Ranch buildings and cottage of literary figure

Annadel State Park: Former Rancho Los Guilicos

Hood Mountain Regional Park and Open Space Preserve: Historic Hood Mansion

Vallejo-Benicia Buffer and Vallejo-Benicia Waterfront: Former General Vallejo rancho; former state capital

THE EAST BAY

Mount Wanda, John Muir National Historic Site: John Muir's home and favorite walking site

Mission Peak Regional Preserve and Ed R. Levin County Park: Former Mission San José lands

THE SOUTH BAY

Alum Rock Park: California's first and oldest park; remnants of former steam railroad

Joseph D. Grant County Park: Historic home and ranch of former Stanford University trustee on former Mexican land grant

Mount Madonna County Park: Summer home of land and cattle baron Henry Miller

Santa Teresa County Park and Los Alamitos/Calero Creek Trail: Joaquin Bernal's former Rancho Santa Teresa

Sanborn County Park: Homesites of early pioneers and vestiges of Capt. Seagraves homesite

THE PENINSULA

Skyline Ridge and Russian Ridge Open Space Preserves: Former "summer capital" of California Governor James Rolph; historic logging road from west side forests to Bay

Windy Hill Open Space Preserve: Former Rancho El Corte de Madera

Golden Gate National Recreation Area: Sweeney Ridge to Milagra Ridge: First sighting of San Francisco Bay by Don Gaspar de Portolá's scout; World War II military sites

SAN FRANCISCO

Fort Funston to Stern Grove: Military site and Trocadero Inn

San Francisco Presidio: Historic Spanish military site and U.S. military base

Almost Level and Mostly Paved Trails

THE NORTH BAY

The Golden Gate Bridge
Helen Putnam Regional Park and McNear Park to Petaluma Adobe State
   Historic Park
Yountville Cross Road
River-to-Ridge Trail
Vallejo-Benicia Waterfront

THE EAST BAY

Al Zampa Memorial Bridge
Martinez City Streets to Carquinez Strait Regional Shoreline
Kennedy Grove to Tilden Regional Park: Nimitz Way segment from Wildcat Canyon
   Regional Park gate to Inspiration Point

THE SOUTH BAY

Alum Rock Park: Creek Trail
Joseph D. Grant County Park: Trails around Grant Lake and near park office
Mount Madonna County Park: Short trail to Henry Miller homesite
Coyote Creek Parkway North
Coyote Creek Parkway South
Santa Teresa County Park and Los Alamitos/Calero Creek Trail: Segment on Los
   Alamitos/Calero Creek Trail
Sanborn County Park: Peterson Grove and Trail

THE PENINSULA

Skyline Ridge Open Space Preserve: Trails around Alpine Pond and
   Horseshoe Lake
Mussel Rock to Fort Funston: Trail on city streets

SAN FRANCISCO

Fort Funston to Stern Grove: Entire trail
San Francisco Presidio: All trails

Short Trips: Less than 5 Miles Round-Trip or One-Way with a Shuttle

THE NORTH BAY

The Golden Gate Bridge: Round-trip
Marin Headlands from the Golden Gate Bridge to Tennessee Valley
Marin Headlands from Tennessee Valley to Shoreline Highway
Loma Alta Open Space Preserve to Lucas Valley Open Space Preserve
Vallejo-Benicia Buffer
Vallejo-Benicia Waterfront

THE EAST BAY

Al Zampa Memorial Bridge
Martinez City Streets to Carquinez Strait Regional Shoreline
Carquinez Strait Regional Shoreline to John Muir National Historic Site
Mount Wanda Trail, John Muir National Historic Site: From Muir's home to ridgetop
Kennedy Grove to Tilden Regional Park

THE SOUTH BAY

Mount Madonna County Park
Sanborn County Park and Castle Rock State Park

THE PENINSULA

Windy Hill Open Space Preserve

SAN FRANCISCO

Fort Funston to Stern Grove
San Francisco Presidio

Trips 5 to 10 Miles One-Way with a Shuttle

THE NORTH BAY

Mount Tamalpais State Park
Indian Tree Open Space Preserve to O'Hair Park and on to Mount Burdell Open
   Space Preserve
Helen Putnam Regional Park and McNear Park to Petaluma Adobe State Historic
   Park
Annadel State Park
Yountville Cross Road

THE EAST BAY

Tilden Regional Park to Redwood Regional Park
Redwood and Anthony Chabot Regional Parks
Anthony Chabot Regional Park
East Bay Municipal Utility District Lands to Independent School
Independent School to Five Canyons
Mission Peak Regional Preserve and Ed R. Levin County Park

THE SOUTH BAY

Coyote Creek Parkway North
Coyote Creek Parkway South
Santa Teresa County Park and Los Alamitos/Calero Creek Trail
Sanborn County Park and Castle Rock State Park

THE PENINSULA

Saratoga Gap Open Space Preserve to Skyline Ridge Open
   Space Preserve
Wunderlich County Park to Huddart County Park

Purisima Creek Redwoods Open Space Preserve
Golden Gate National Recreation Area: Sweeney Ridge to Milagra Ridge

SAN FRANCISCO

Stern Grove to the Presidio

Trips 5 to 10 Miles Round-Trip on the Ridge Trail

THE NORTH BAY

Loma Alta Open Space Preserve to Lucas Valley Open Space Preserve
Mt. Burdell Open Space Preserve
Sugarloaf Ridge State Park
Yountville Cross Road: From Van de Leur Park north to Napa River Ecological Reserve
Skyline Wilderness Park
Rockville Hills Regional Park
Lynch Canyon Open Space

THE SOUTH BAY

Alum Rock Park and Boccardo Trail Corridor

THE PENINSULA

Skyline Ridge and Russian Ridge Open Space Preserves
Windy Hill Open Space Preserve
Golden Gate National Recreation Area: Sweeney Ridge to Milagra Ridge

SAN FRANCISCO

Fort Funston to Stern Grove
Stern Grove to the Presidio
San Francisco Presidio

Long Trips: More than 10 Miles One-Way with a Shuttle or a Round-Trip on the Same Trail

THE NORTH BAY

Mount Tamalpais State Park: Round-trip
Mount Tamalpais State Park and Golden Gate National Recreation Area:
    Round-trip
Golden Gate National Recreation Area and Samuel P. Taylor State Park:
    One-way
Samuel P. Taylor State Park to Loma Alta Open Space Preserve: One-way

THE EAST BAY

Tilden Regional Park to Redwood Regional Park: Round-trip

THE SOUTH BAY

Coyote Creek Parkway North: One-way
Sanborn County Park to Horseshoe Lake in Skyline Ridge Open Space
    Preserve: One-way with shuttle

THE PENINSULA

San Francisco Watershed Trail: South entrance to Milagra Ridge summit, one-way with shuttle

SAN FRANCISCO

Stern Grove to the Presidio: Round-trip

Linger by a Lake

THE NORTH BAY

Mount Burdell Open Space Preserve: Seasonal
Jack London State Historic Park
Annadel State Park: Spring Lake Park and Lake Ilsanjo
Skyline Wilderness Park: Lake Marie
Rockville Hills Regional Park
Vallejo-Benicia Buffer

THE EAST BAY

Kennedy Grove to Tilden Regional Park
Anthony Chabot Regional Park: Short distance off the trail
East Bay Municipal Utility District Lands to Independent School, Cull Canyon Regional Recreation Area: Swimming in season, too
Mission Peak Regional Preserve and Ed R. Levin County Park

THE SOUTH BAY

Joseph D. Grant County Park
Coyote Lake-Harvey Bear Ranch Trail
Coyote Creek Parkway North

THE PENINSULA

Saratoga Gap Open Space Preserve to Skyline Ridge Open Space Preserve
Skyline Ridge and Russian Ridge Open Space Preserves: Horseshoe Lake and Alpine Pond
San Francisco Watershed Trail: San Andreas Trail at north end of watershed

SAN FRANCISCO

Fort Funston to Stern Grove: Lake Merced and Pine Lake

Trips Accessible by Bus

THE NORTH BAY

Marin Headlands: Golden Gate Transit at north end of Golden Gate Bridge
Mount Tamalpais State Park: Golden Gate Transit to Pantoll Ranger Station
Golden Gate National Recreation Area and Samuel P. Taylor State Park: Golden Gate Transit to State Park on Cross Marin Trail
Indian Tree Open Space Preserve: Golden Gate Transit to Novato at San Marin/ Novato Boulevard
Mount Burdell Open Space Preserve: Golden Gate Transit as in Indian Tree and at San Marin/San Andreas intersection in Novato

McNear Park to Petaluma Adobe State Historic Park: Golden Gate Transit
and Petaluma Transit
Annadel State Park: Santa Rosa city bus and Sonoma Transit
Vallejo-Benicia Buffer: Vallejo Transit
Vallejo-Benicia Waterfront: Benicia Transit

THE EAST BAY

Martinez Regional Shoreline: Contra Costa County Connection from BART
Carquinez Strait Regional Shoreline Park to John Muir National Historic Site:
Contra Costa County Connection and BART to historic site
Kennedy Grove to Tilden Regional Park: AC Transit
Tilden Regional Park to Redwood Regional Park: AC Transit
Redwood and Anthony Chabot Regional Parks: AC Transit to Chabot Space
and Science Center
Anthony Chabot Regional Park to Independent School: AC Transit from
Castro Valley BART to Cull Canyon Regional Recreation Area
Independent School to Five Canyons: AC Transit to Don Castro Regional
Recreation Area
Mission Peak Regional Preserve and Ed R. Levin County Park: AC Transit to
Ohlone College and Mission/Stanford Ave. intersection; climb the peak from
Ohlone College and return or continue on Hidden Valley Trail to intersection of
Mission Boulevard and Stanford Avenue

THE SOUTH BAY

Alum Rock Park: Valley Transit Authority
Coyote Creek Parkway: Valley Transit Authority to Yerba Buena Avenue
(northeast of Coyote Hellyer Park)
Santa Teresa County Park and Los Alamitos/Calero Creek Trail:
Valley Transit Authority Connections near both ends of trail

THE PENINSULA

Golden Gate National Recreation Area: Sweeney Ridge to Milagra Ridge: SamTrans
to Skyline College and Sneath
Lane; to Lundy Lane near Mori Ridge trailhead
Mussel Rock to Fort Funston: By BART and SamTrans to Palmetto/Westline from
Colma BART and Muni to intersection of John Muir Drive and Skyline Boulevard
and several locations in Daly City

SAN FRANCISCO

Stern Grove to the Presidio: San Francisco Muni at each end

"Fault-y" Trips

ALONG THE SAN ANDREAS FAULT

Mount Madonna County Park: This park lies between the Sargent and San Andreas
faults and the 1989 quake further destroyed remnants of Henry Miller's homesite.
Saratoga Gap Open Space Preserve north through Huddart County Park: These
trips lie close to the west side of the fault on the Pacific Plate.
Sweeney Ridge to Milagra Ridge: On Pacific Plate

At Mussel Rock: The fault drops into the Pacific Ocean and then reappears in Marin County.

San Francisco Watershed Trail: Fault lies just east of the trail.

Marin County: Trips from the Golden Gate Bridge north to Samuel P. Taylor State Park lie on the east side of the fault on the North American Plate.

ALONG THE HAYWARD FAULT

East Bay ridgetop parks: These trips parallel the Hayward Fault, which lies to the west.

ALONG THE CALAVERAS FAULT

Alum Rock Park and Boccardo Trail Corridor
Joseph D. Grant County Park: Halls Valley
Coyote Lake-Harvey Bear Ranch Trail

MORE FAULTS

Sugarloaf Ridge State Park: St. John's Mountain Fault
Annadel State Park: To the west lies Rodgers Creek Fault
Rockville Hills Regional Park: Concord-Green Valley Fault
Hiddenbrooke Trail: St. John's Mine Fault

Serpentine Strolls

Santa Teresa County Park: Two areas of serpentine outcrops
Sugarloaf Ridge State Park: Serpentine on trip to Bald Mountain
Loma Alta Open Space Preserve: Serpentine outcrops along Ridge Trail route
Mount Madonna County Park: Tanoak Trail passes ruins of Henry Miller's home, damaged by quakes of yesteryear
Santa Teresa County Park: Two areas of serpentine outcrops
Sweeney Ridge: A weathered serpentine column marks the Don Gaspar de Portolá Discovery Site
San Francisco Presidio: Large area of serpentine outcrops on Ecology Trail side trip

Three or More Continuous Ridge Trail Segments

38.4 miles: South entrance of the Golden Gate Bridge through the Marin Headlands, Golden Gate National Recreation Area, Samuel P. Taylor State Park, and Loma Alta Open Space Preserve to Buck's Bypass

41.9 miles: Kennedy Grove to Tilden Regional Park; Tilden Regional Park to Redwood Regional Park; Redwood and Anthony Chabot Regional Parks; East Bay Municipal Utility District Lands to Independent School and through Don Castro Regional Recreation Area to Five Canyons

18.6 miles: Sanborn County Park and Castle Rock State Park; Saratoga Gap Open Space Preserve to Skyline Ridge Open Space Preserve; Skyline Ridge and Russian Ridge Open Space Preserves

18.5 miles: San Francisco Watershed Trail to Sneath Lane Trailhead in Sweeney Ridge and round-trip to Milagra Ridge Trail from Sneath Lane Trailhead

12.7 miles: Fort Funston to Stern Grove and Stern Grove to the Presidio

Appendix 3

Information Sources and Contacts for Parks

National Park Service

Golden Gate National Recreation Area
Golden Gate National Parks
Fort Mason, Building 201
San Francisco, California 94123
415-561-4700
www.nps.gov/goga

  Fort Funston
  415-239-2366
  www.parksconservancy.org/visit/park
  asp?park=42

  Marin Headlands
  415-331-1540
  www.nps.gov/goga/marin-headlands.htm

  Milagra Ridge
  415-556-8642
  www.nps.gov/goga/miri.htm

  Muir Woods National Monument
  Mill Valley, California 94941
  415-388-2596
  www.nps.gov/muwo/

  Olema Valley
  415-464-5137
  www.nps.gov/goga/planyourvisit/
  olema-valley.htm

  San Francisco Presidio
  Presidio Interpretation
  Building 201, Fort Mason
  San Francisco, CA 94123
  415-556-4323
  www.nps.gov/prsf/

  Sweeney Ridge
  http://parksconservancy.org/visit/park
  asp?park=91

John Muir National Historic Site
4202 Alhambra Ave.
Martinez, CA 94553
925-228-8860
www.nps.gov/jomu/

Point Reyes National Seashore
415-464-5100
www.nps.gov/pore

California State Parks

Box 942896
Sacramento, CA 94296-0001
916-653-6995
www.parks.ca.gov/

  Annadel State Park
  707-539-3911

  Benicia State Recreation Area
  707-648-1911

  Castle Rock State Park
  15000 Skyline Blvd.
  Los Gatos, CA 95033-8291
  408-867-2952

  Jack London State Historic Park
  707-938-5216

  Mount Tamalpais State Park
  801 Panoramic Highway
  Mill Valley, CA 94941
  415-388-2070

  Petaluma Adobe State Historic Park
  3325 Adobe Road
  Petaluma, CA 94954
  707-762-4871

  Samuel P. Taylor State Park
  P.O. Box 251
  Lagunitas, CA 94938
  415-488-9897

  Sugarloaf Ridge State Park
  2605 Adobe Canyon Road
  Kenwood, CA 95452
  707-833-5712

Regional and County Agencies and Cities

City of Benicia Recreation Department
707-746-4285
www.ci.benicia.ca.us

City of Fairfield
1000 Webster Street
Fairfield, CA 94533
707-428-7428, ext. 100
www.ci.fairfield.ca.us

City of Petaluma Parks and Recreation
320 N. McDowell
Petaluma, CA 94954
707-778-4380
www.ci.petaluma.ca.us

East Bay Regional Park District
2950 Peralta Oaks Court
P.O. Box 5381
Oakland, CA 94605-0381
888-327-2757
www.ebparks.org

East Bay Municipal Utility District
500 San Pablo Dam Rd.
Orinda, CA 94563
510-254-3778
www.ebmud.com

Greater Vallejo Recreation District
395 Amador St.
Vallejo, CA 94590
707-648-4600
www.gvrd.org

Marin County Open Space District
Marin County Civic Center
San Rafael, CA 94903
415-499-6387
www.marinopenspace.org

Midpeninsula Regional Open Space District
330 Distel Circle
Los Altos, CA 94022
650-691-1200
www.openspace.org

San Francisco Recreation and Park Department
McLaren Lodge, Golden Gate Park
501 Stanyan St.
San Francisco, CA 9411
415-831-2700
www.parks.sfgov.org

San Jose Department of Parks, Recreation, and Neighborhood Services
4 North 2nd Street, Suite 600
San Jose CA 95113
408-277-4000
www.sanjoseca.gov/prns

San Mateo County Parks and Recreation Department
County Government Center
590 Hamilton St.
Redwood City, CA 94063
415-363-4020
www.sanmateocountyparks.org

Santa Clara County Open Space Authority
6830 Via del Oro, Ste. 200
San Jose, CA 95119
408-224-7476
www.openspaceauthority.org

Santa Clara County Parks and Recreation Department
298 Garden Hill Dr.
Los Gatos, CA 95030
408-358-3741
www.parkhere.org/portal/site/parks/

Solano County Parks
675 Texas St.
Fairfield, CA 94533
www.co.solano.ca.us

Sonoma County Regional Parks Department
2300 County Center Dr.
Santa Rosa, CA
707-527-2041
www.parks.sonoma.net/

Appendix 4

Transportation Agencies that Serve the Bay Area Ridge Trail Route

For all transit agencies, dial your Area Code and 511
or visit www.transit.511.org.trip planner.

AC Transit
www.actransit.org
510-891-4777

Bay Area Rapid Transit (BART)
www.bart.gov/stations
415-992-2278 or 510-465-2278

Caltrain
www.caltrain.org
800.660.4287

Contra Costa Transportation Authority
www.ccta.net/ and www.bart.org

Golden Gate Transit
www.goldengate.org/
415-332-6600 (from San Francisco and Southern Marin County)
415-453-2100 (from Central and Northern Marin County)
707-544-1323 or www.sctransit.com (from Sonoma County)

MUNI (San Francisco Municipal Railway)
www.sfmuni.com
415-673-6864

SamTrans (San Mateo County)
www.samtrans.com
800-660-4287

Solano County
www.baylink (Benicia to San Francisco)
www.solano.express (local routes)
707-648-1911

Valley Transit Authority (Santa Clara County)
www.vta.org
408-321-2300 or 800-894-9908

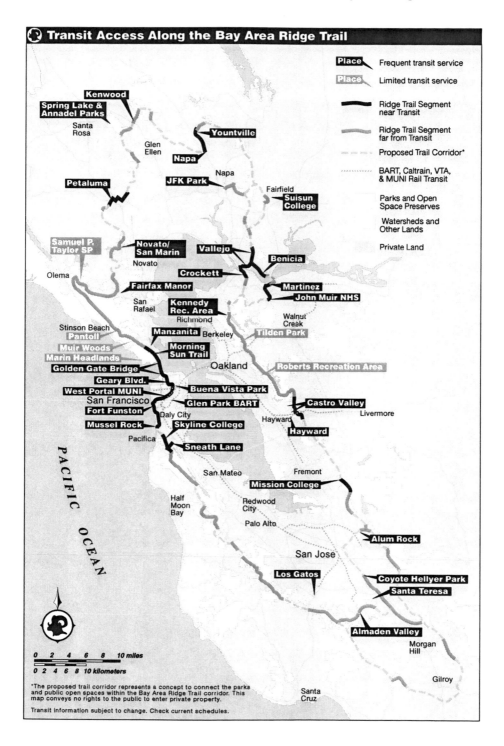

Transit Access Along the Bay Area Ridge Trail

Legend:

Place — Frequent transit service

Place — Limited transit service

▬▬ Ridge Trail Segment near Transit

▬▬ Ridge Trail Segment far from Transit

– – – Proposed Trail Corridor*

·········· BART, Caltrain, VTA, & MUNI Rail Transit

Parks and Open Space Preserves

Watersheds and Other Lands

Private Land

Kenwood
Spring Lake & Annadel Parks
Santa Rosa
Glen Ellen
Yountville
Napa
Napa
Petaluma
JFK Park
Fairfield
Suisun College
Samuel P. Taylor SP
Novato/San Marin
Novato
Vallejo
Benicia
Olema
Crockett
Fairfax Manor
Martinez
John Muir NHS
San Rafael
Kennedy Rec. Area
Richmond
Walnut Creek
Stinson Beach
Pantoll
Manzanita
Berkeley
Tilden Park
Muir Woods
Morning Sun Trail
Marin Headlands
Golden Gate Bridge
Oakland
Roberts Recreation Area
Geary Blvd.
West Portal MUNI
Buena Vista Park
San Francisco
Glen Park BART
Castro Valley
Fort Funston
Daly City
Livermore
Mussel Rock
Skyline College
Hayward
Pacifica
Hayward
Sneath Lane
San Mateo
Fremont
Mission College
Half Moon Bay
Redwood City
Palo Alto
Alum Rock
San Jose
Los Gatos
Coyote Hellyer Park
Santa Teresa
Almaden Valley
Morgan Hill
Santa Cruz
Gilroy

PACIFIC OCEAN

0 2 4 6 8 10 miles
0 2 4 6 8 10 kilometers

*The proposed trail corridor represents a concept to connect the parks and public open spaces within the Bay Area Ridge Trail corridor. This map conveys no rights to the public to enter private property.

Transit information subject to change. Check current schedules.

Index

A

Achistaga Trail 221
Agua Caliente Creek 171
Agua Caliente Trail 173
Alcatraz Island 273
Alhambra Valley 128
Almaden Lake 205
Almaden Quicksilver County Park 193, 204, 206–10
Alum Rock Park 176, 177–80
Alum Rock Steam Railroad 178
Al Zampa Memorial Bridge 117, 120–22
American Discovery Trail 272
Annadel State Park 78–82
Anniversary Trail 229–30
Anthony Chabot Regional Park 150, 151–59
Archery Center 153
Arguello Boulevard 261
Arguello Gate (Presidio) 266
Arroyo Aguague 180
Arroyo Trail 147
Ascot Parkway 110

B

Bald Knob 236
Bald Mountain 82, 86, 87, 89
Bald Mountain Trail 87, 88
Baquiano Trail 244
Basham, Gregory 110
Battery Godfrey 273
Battery Marcus Miller 274
Bay Area Ridge Trail. See also San Francisco Bay Area; specific locations in Bay Areas
  beginnings of the 7–8
  continued development of the 8–9
  guides available on 11
Bay Area Ridge Trail Council
  guides produced by 11
  mission and accomplishments of 8–9
  website of 12
Bear Gulch Watershed 232, 236
Bear Valley Trail 47
Beauty Ranch 76
Beauty Ranch Trail 77

Benicia
  Fisher-Hanlon House in 116
  touring Benicia Marina and historic 113, 114, 115–16
Benicia Marina 113, 115
Benicia State Recreation Area 112
Berkeley Hiking Club 143
Big Bear Trail 153
Big Rock Ridge Trail 56–57
Big Springs Trail 147
Big Trees Trail 60, 61
Big Valley Trail 133
biking. See also specific trails
  hazards to watch for when 14–15
  information on access for 11–12
  trail etiquette and rules for 14
  varying rules on 11
Bitakomtara tribe 81
Blackhawk Trail 189, 191
Blue Heron Pond 84–85
Blue Rock Springs Park 108, 109, 110, 112
Bobcat Trail 30
Bob's Bench 229
Boccardo Trail Corridor 176, 177–80
Bolinas-Fairfax Road
  from Pantoll Ranger Station to 39–42
  to Samuel P. Taylor State Park from 43–48
Bolinas Ridge logging 47
Bolinas Ridge Trail 50
Bonjetti Creek Canyon 213
boots 16
Borel, Antoine 225
Borel Hill 225
Bort Meadow Staging Area 154
  to Chabot Staging Area from 155–59
  from Skyline Gate to 151–54
Brandon Trail 157, 158, 159
Brewer, William H. 1
Broken Oak Trail 137
Brown Bridge 49, 51
Brush Trail 184
Buck's Bypass 56–57
Buena Vista Park 264, 265
Buffer Trail 110–12
Bunker Road Trailhead 25

Burdell Mountain Ridge Road 67
Burnett Ranger Station 199–200

C

Calera Creek Trail (East Bay) 173
Calero Creek Trail (San Jose) 204
Calero Reservoir Park 204
California Coastal Commission 4
California and Hawaiian Sugar Refinery
    Company 134
California Maritime Academy 117
California and Nevada Railroad 142,
    144
California Water Service Company
    (formerly Bear Gulch Water
    Company) 231
Call of the Wild (London) 76
Caltrans Vista Point 226
Campground Trail 187
camping sites 16–17, 233
Camp Tamarancho 51
Canyon Trail 80
Capehorn Pass 210
Carquinez Bridge Overlook 116–17
Carquinez Lighthouse and Life Saving
    Station 117
Carquinez Overlook Trail 116
Carquinez Park 121–22
Carquinez Regional Shoreline 133
Carquinez Strait 112, 133
Carquinez Strait waterfront 116
Casa Grande Road 71–72
Castle Rock State Park 211, 213–15
Chabot Regional Park 150, 151–59
Chabot Space and Science Center 153
Chabot Staging Area 155–59, 163
Chabot-to-Garin Regional Trail 163
Challenger maple trees commemoration
    153
Chaparral Trail 97
cinnabar (quicksilver) mining 206
clothing recommendations 15–16
Coastal Conservancy 3
Coastal Fire Road 37
Cobblestone Fire Road 67
Cobblestone Trail 66
coho salmon 50
Coit Tower 272

Columbus Parkway 110
Conestoga Way 135, 138
Conlon Trail 142, 143
Contour Trail 191
Corral Trail 184
Corte Madera Creek 228
County Historic Zoning District (New
    Almaden) 209
Cowan Meadow Trail 76–77
Cowell, Bob 9
Coyote Creek 197
Coyote Creek Parkway North 195–98
Coyote Creek Parkway South 199–200
Coyote Creek Trail 197–98
Coyote Hellyer County Park 195–97
Coyote Lake-Harvey Bear Ranch Trail
    185–87
Coyote Peak 203
Coyote Ridge Trail 33, 187
Creek Trail 180
Crissy Field 274
Crockett Hills Regional Park 132–34
Crockett Ranch 134
Cross Marin Trail 48, 50
Crowder, Betsy 14
Crystal Springs Lake 246
Crystal Springs Trail 233
Cull Canyon 163, 164
Cummings Skyway 133
Curran Trail 147

D

Dairy Trail 183
Daly City 250–52
Dead Fish restaurant 121, 122
Deer Camp Fire Road 66, 67
Deer Camp Trail 60
Deer Park Fire Road 35, 36
Del Valle Regional Park 171
Desai, Dinesh 9
Dias Ridge Trail 36
Dinosaur Ridge 158, 163
Dipsea Trail 36, 37
disabled individuals. *See* wheelchair
    access
Discovery Site 243, 244, 245
Doe Hill Fire Road 62

Don Castro Regional Recreation Area 165–67

Don Edwards San Francisco Bay National Wildlife Refuge 3–4

Douglas, David 100

Dutch Flat Trail 183–84

Dwarf Oaks Trail 62, 65

E

Eagle's Nest Trail 142

Eagle Trail 171

early Skyline setters (late 1800s) 213

East Bay
Al Zampa Memorial Bridge 120–22
Anthony Chabot Regional Park 150, 151–54
Crockett Hills Regional Park 132–34
Don Castro Regional Recreation Area 165–67
EBMUD (East Bay Municipal Utility District) lands 160, 161–64
Ed R. Levin County Park 168, 169–73
John Muir National Historic Site 124, 127–31
Martinez 123–26, 130
Mission Peak Regional Preserve 168, 169–73
overview of 118
Redwood Regional Park 146, 150, 151–54
Sobrante Ridge Regional Preserve 135–38
Tilden Regional Park 139–49

East Bay Trails (Weintraub) 14

East Lambert Creek 222, 225

East Lambert Creek canyon 225

East Ridge Trail 149

East Staging Area of Carquinez Strait Regional Shoreline 126, 127

EBMUD (East Bay Municipal Utility District) lands 160, 161–64

EBRPD (East Bay Regional Park District) 3

EBSNR Trail (East Bay Skyline National Recreation Trail) 142, 147, 149, 151, 157, 213–14

Eckley Park and Fishing Pier 134

Ecology Trail 269

Ed R. Levin County Park 168, 169–73

Edwards Trail 181, 183

El Corte de Madera Creek Open Space Preserve 232

Elkhorn Peak 102

El Sombroso 194

English Town 209, 210

equestrians. *See also specific areas*
hazards for trail users and 14–15
map legend symbols regarding 13
trail etiquette rules for 14

Erskine, Dorothy 3

Escondido Trail 158

F

facilities. *See specific areas*

Fence Line Trail 229, 230

feral pigs hazard 15

Fifield Ridge Trail 241

Fisher-Hanlon House (Benicia) 116

Fishway Interpretive Site 154

Five Canyons 165–67

Five Corners (Marin Headlands) 28, 29, 30

"The Five Sisters" 48

footwear 16

Fort Funston 249–50, 252–53, 256, 257, 258

Fort Point 273

Fort Winfield Scott Parade Ground 272

Franklin Canyon Road 130

French Trail 152

G

Gary Giacomini Open Space Preserve 50

Golden Gate Bridge
from Presidio Arguello Gate to toll plaza of 267–75
to Tennessee Valley from 25–30
trail over 21–24

Golden Gate National Recreation Area (GGNRA)
from Bolinas-Fairfax Road to State Park Entrance 43–48
description of 7
Fort Funston to Stern Grove 256, 257–60
Mussel Rock to Fort Funston 248–53

open space promoted by 5
from Pantoll Ranger Station to Bolinas-
    Fairfax Road 39–42
Presidio 261–75
from Rancho Sausalito to 29
Sweeney Ridge to Milagra Ridge
    242–47
Golden Spike Trail 153
Gold Rush redwood logging 47, 229, 233
Goodspeed Trail 89
Graham Trail 153
Grass Valley Creek 154
Grass Valley Ranch 157
Greater Vallejo Recreation District 109
Greenbelt Alliance 3, 5
Green Valley Road 102
Green Valley Trailhead 101, 102
Grizzly Peak Boulevard 141, 145
Guadalupe Creek 194
Guadalupe Reservoir 194
Gunshot Fire Road 54

H
Hacienda Trail 210
"Halfway to Hell Club" 122
Hall's Valley 183
Hamm's Gulch Trail 229
hang glider viewing deck 257
Harkins Ridge Trail 237
Harvey Bear Trail 187
Hayfields Trail 76
Hayward Fault 147
hazards information 14–15, 158
Hendrickson Historic Site 85
Herbert Law's quarry 229
Heron Trail 183
Hetch Hetchy Reservoir 246
Hickory Oaks Trail 220, 221
Hicks Road 207, 210
Hiddenbrooke Trail 105, 106–107, 110
Hidden Springs Trail 302
Hidden Valley Trail 170
Highway 121 (Silverado Trail) 91, 93, 94
hikers
    accommodations available along trails
        for 16–17, 233
    clothing recommendations for 15–16
    etiquette for sharing the trails 14

general hazards to watch for 14–15
Mission Peak side trip for 172
historic facts/tours. *See also* Native
        Americans
California and Hawaiian Sugar
        Refinery Company 134
California and Nevada Railroad 142,
        144
County Historic Zoning District (New
        Almaden) 209
early Skyline setters (late 1800s) 213
English Town 209, 210
Fort Funston 249–50, 252–53, 256,
        257, 258
Fort Point 273
Gold Rush redwood logging 47, 229,
        233
Hendrickson Historic Site 85
historic Martinez 125
House of Happy Walls museum (Jack
        London State Historic Park) 77
Inspiration Point 269
Jack London State Historic Park 73–77
John Muir National Historic Site 124,
        127–31
McNear Building 70
Mare Island Naval Shipyard 117
Mission San José de Guadalupe 171
New Almaden Quicksilver Mining
        Company 209
Point Bonita Lighthouse 273
Presidio 261–75
quicksilver (cinnabar) mining 209
redwood forests 47, 146, 150–54, 229,
        233
San Francisco National Military
        Cemetery 270, 274
San Miguel Rancho (now Sunset
        District) 263
Sea Captain's House 97
The Sleeping Lady legend 37
"Summer Capital" 225
touring historic Benicia 113, 114,
        115–16
Hood Mountain 81–82, 83, 87
Hood Mountain Regional Park 83–85
Hornbeck Trail 124
horseback riders. *See* equestrians

Horseshoe Lake
  to Rapley Ranch Road from 223–26
  from Saratoga Gap to 219–22
hostels 16–17
House of Happy Walls museum (Jack
  London State Historic Park) 77
Howarth Park 78, 79
Huckleberry Botanic Regional Preserve
  149
Huckleberry Preserve Nature Trail 149
Huddart County Park 231–34
Hulet Hornbeck Trail 128–29
Hunt Camp Road 50

I

Independent School
  EBMUD lands to 160, 161–64
  to Five Canyons from 165–67
Indian Rock 214
Indian Tree Fire Road 60
Indian Tree Open Space Preserve
  to O'Hair Park from 59–62
  overview of trails in 58
  Inkwells Bridge 50
  Inspiration Point
  history of 269
  from Kennedy Grove to 139–44
  to Skyline Gate from 145–49
  view of 266
I Street (Benicia) 116

J

Jack London State Historic Park 73–77
Jarvis Landing 172
Jewell Trail 43, 48
John F. Kennedy Park 93, 94
John F. Kennedy University 144
John Muir National Historic Site
  Carquinez Strait Regional Shoreline to
    127–29
  history and visitor center of 128
  Mount Wanda Trail in 130–31
  overview of 124
Jones Gulch 228
Jones Point 115
Joseph D. Grant County Park 180,
  181–84

K

K Street (Benicia) 115
Kenilworth Park 71
Kennedy Grove Regional Recreation
  Area 136, 139, 140, 141
Kennedy Trail 194
Kestrel Loop Trail 133–34
Kestrel Trail 105

L

La Casa Grande 209
Lagunitas Creek 50
Lake Chabot 157
Lake Chabot Bicycle Loop 157
Lake Herman Road 110
Lake Merced 258–59
Lake Trail 73, 75
Landfill Remediation Project 273
LaTourrette, Sue 14
Lawndale Trail 82
Lick Observatory (Mt. Hamilton) 183,
  204
Limekiln Trail 194
Lincoln, Robert Todd 270
Little Mountain Open Space Preserve 62
Little Mountain Trail 62
Logger's Loop 158
Loma Alta Open Space Preserve
  to Lucas Valley Open Space Preserve
    from 53–55
  from Samuel P. Taylor State Park to
    49–51
Lomas Cantadas Road 145, 147
London, Charmian 76, 77
London, Jack 76
Long Ridge Open Space Preserve 220,
  221
Loop Trail 190
Los Alamitos/Calero Creek Trail 201–
  206
Los Alamitos Creek 205, 206
Lost Trail 227–28, 229
Loughry Woods 214
Loughry Woods Trail 213–14
Lower Bald Mountain Trail 86
Lower Golden Spike Trail 153

Lower Johnson Road Trail 83
Lower Red Mountain 82
Lucas Valley Open Space Preserve
  from Loma Alta Open Space Preserve
    to 53–55
  trails within 56–57
Lucas Valley Road 53–55
Lupine Trail 147
lyme disease 15
Lynch Canyon Open Space 103–105

M
McCurdy Trail 47
MacDonald Gate Staging Area 153
MacDonald Trail 154
McIntyre Ranch 110
McNear Building 70
McNear, George P. 72
McNear Park 68, 69, 70, 72
McRorie, Toni 82
Meadow Trail 191
Manzanita Trail 137, 138
  maps
    legend used for 13
    provided for each trail 12, 14
Marciel Gate 154
Mare Island Naval Shipyard 117
Marie Dhority Bridge 50
Marina Vista Street 125–26
Marin Headlands
  from Golden Gate Bridge to Tennessee
    Valley 25–30
  from Tennessee Valley to Shoreline
    Highway 31–33
Maritime Academy 122
Marsh Trail 80, 82
Martinez
  to Carquinez Strait Regional Shoreline
    from 123–26
  historic 125
  to summit of Mount Wanda from 130
Martinez Museum 125
Matt Davis Trail 37
Matthew Turner Shipyards Park 115
Meadows Canyon Trail 147
Merganser Pond 84
Merry-Go-Round Trail 189, 190
Metcalf Park

  to Burnett Ranger Station from 199–200
  from Stonegate Park to 195–98
Middle Burdell Fire Road 65–66, 67
Middle Graham Creek 76
Middle Valley Trail 105
Midpeninsula Regional Open Space
  District 193, 194, 237
Milagra Ridge Gate 243–44, 247
Milagra Ridge Preserve 247
Miller Creek 56
Mindego Hill 225
Mindego Ridge Trail 226
Mine Hill Trail 210
Mine Trail 203
Mirador Trail 158
Mission Peak 172
Mission Peak Regional Preserve 168,
  169–73
Mission San José de Guadalupe 171
Miwok Trail 33, 36
Mockingbird Trail 206–209
Monte Bello Open Space Preserve 220
Monte Bello Ridge 222
Monument Peak 173
Moon Gate (Skyline Boulevard) 152
Moraga Fault 147
Mori Ridge Trail 246
Morningside Trail 137
Morocco Road 123, 124, 125
Mott, William Penn, Jr. 7
mountain lions 15
Mount Madonna County Park 188–91
Mount Tamalpais State Park 35–42
Mount Wanda 124, 137
Mount Wanda Trail 130–31
Mt. Diablo, views of 143, 154, 172
Mt. Hamilton 179, 183, 204
Mt. Helen 130–31
Mt. Tamalpais 37, 133, 137, 143, 179
Mt. Umunhum 204, 207
Muir, John 2, 225
Mussel Rock 248, 249, 250–52
Mystic Ridge Trail 102

N
Napa River Ecological Reserve 90, 91
Napa Solano Ridge Trail Loop 3

Napa-Sonoma Marshes Wildlife Area 106

Napa State Hospital 94, 95

National Military Cemetery 270, 274

Native Americans. *See also* historic facts/tours
  Bitakomtara tribe 81
  Ohlone people 153, 197
  Olompali Miwok Indians 66
  Oroysom village of 171
  Pomo Indians 82, 85
  San Pablo Creek valley settlements by 143
  "2 Bits" (military scout) 270
  Wappos tribe 88
  Wintun people 105

New Almaden (County Historic Zoning District) 209

New Almaden Quicksilver Mining Company 209

Nilsson, Karen 11

Nimitz Way 142, 143, 147

No Name Gulch 237

North Bay
  Annadel State Park 78–82
  Golden Gate Bridge 21–24
  Golden Gate National Recreation Area 43–48
  Helen Putnam Regional Park 68–72
  Hiddenbrooke Trail 105, 106–107, 110
  Hood Mountain Regional Park and Open Space Preserve 83–85
  Indian Tree Open Space Preserve 58–62
  Jack London State Historic Park 73–77
  Loma Alta Open Space Preserve 49–55
  Lucas Valley Open Space Preserve 53–57
  Lynch Canyon Open Space 103–105
  McNear Park 68, 70–72
  Marin Headlands 25–33
  Mount Burdell Open Space Preserve 63–67
  Mount Tamalpais State Park 34–42
  overview of 18
  Petaluma Adobe State Historic Park 68, 70–72
  River-to-Ridge Trail 93–94

Rockville Hills Regional Park 98–102

Samuel P. Taylor State Park 43–51

Skyline Wilderness Park 93, 94, 95–97

Sugarloaf Ridge State Park 86–89

Vallejo-Benicia Buffer 108–12

Vallejo-Benicia Waterfront 113–17

Yountville Cross Road 90–92

North Bay Trails (Weintraub) 14

North Ridge Trail 103–4

North Rim Trail 178, 180

North Trailhead (Tennessee Valley) 27

Nunes Ranch (Scow Canyon) 142

O

Oaks Picnic Area 141

O'Hair Park
  to Olompali State Historic Park from 63–67
  from Vineyard Road to 59–62

Ohlone College 169–70, 171

Ohlone people 153, 197

Ohlone Trail 170

Ohlone Wilderness Trail 172

Oil Creek canyon 220

Old Church picnic area 153

Old Mine Trail 190

Old Page Mill Road 225

Old Quarry Trail 67

Old San Pablo Dam Road 141–42, 143

Olompali Miwok Indians 66

O'Neill, Brian 7

Open Space Foundation 100, 101

Open Space Preserve 83–85

open spaces
  Bay Area Ridge Trail development as 7–10
  development of parks and 3–5
  land conservation ethic basis of 2–3
  nonprofit groups role in preserving 5

Orchard Meadow Trail 85

Orchard picnic area 153

Orchard Trail 153

P

Palomares Creek Canyon 167

Panhandle's Fell Street path 265

Pantoll Ranger Station
  to Bolinas-Fairfax Road from 39–42

from Shoreline Highway to 35–37
park entrance fees 11
Peak Trail 170
Peninsula
  Golden Gate National Recreation Area
    243–53
  Huddart County Park 231–34
  overview of the 216
  Purisima Creek Redwoods Open Space
    Preserve 235–38
  Russian Ridge Open Space Preserve
    223–26
  San Francisco Watershed Trail 239–42
  Saratoga Gap Open Space Preserve
    211, 212, 218, 219–22
  Skyline Ridge Open Space Preserve
    218, 219–26
  Teague Hill Open Space Preserve 232,
    234
  Windy Hill Open Space Preserve
    227–30
  Wunderlich County Park 231–34
Peninsula Trails (Rusmore, Crowder,
  Spangle, and LaTourrette) 14
Penitencia Creek 178, 180
People's Water Company of Oakland
  157
Pescadero Creek 221
Petaluma River 68, 70, 71
Petaluma River Trail 71
Peters Creek 221
Phleger Estate 232, 236
Pinole Valley Park 135–37
Platform Bridge Road 43, 46
Point Bonita Lighthouse 273
poison oak 14, 158
Pomo Indians 82, 85
Pond Trail 83, 84–85
Portolá, Don Gaspar de 244–45
Portola Gate 243–47
Portola Redwoods State Park 221
POS (People for Open Space) 7
POST (Peninsula Open Space Trust) 5
Prairie Ridge Trail 105
Presidio
  Arguello Gate of 266

to Golden Gate from Arguello Gate of
    267–75
  Main Post Parade Ground 274, 275
  military museum on 275
  from Stern Grove to 261–66
Priest Rock Trail 193, 194
Proctor Staging Area 159
Pueblo Group Picnic Area 203
Pueblo Trail 203
Pulgas Redwoods forest 233
Purisima Creek 237
Purisima Creek Redwoods Open Space
  Preserve 235–38
Purisima Creek Trail 235, 236, 237

Q
Quarry Road 239
quicksilver (cinnabar) mining 206
Quimby Road 183

R
Ramage Peak Trail 162
Rancho El Corte de Madera 229
Rancho El Sobrante 141
Rancho Los Guilicos 80
Rancho Sausalito 29
Rancho Soscol 111
Randall Trail 47
Rapley Ranch Road 223–26
rattlesnakes 14–15
Razorback Ridge Trail 227
Red Mountain 87, 89
Redtail Trail 157
Redwood Bowl 153
Redwood Canyon 153, 154
Redwood Creek 153, 154
Redwood Creek Trail 35, 36
redwood forests
  Bolinas Ridge logging of 47
  Pulgas Redwoods 233
  Rancho El Corte de Madera site of
    primeval 229
Redwood Regional Park historic site of
  152
Redwood Regional Park 146, 150,
  151–54
Redwood Road 161

Ridge Trail. *See* Bay Area Ridge Trail
Rifle Range Road 162
rift zone lakes 246
Rincon Creek 194
River-to-Ridge Trail 93–94
Robert Sibley Volcanic Regional Preserve
    147, 148–49
Rob Hill Group Camp 271–72
Rockaway Quarry 247
Rockville Hills Regional Park 98–102
Rockville Hills Trail 100–101
Rockville (historic settlement) 100
Rockville Public Cemetery 100
Rodeo Valley Trail 28
Rollye Wiskerson Trail 112
Rolph, James "Sunny Jim" 225
Rose Drive 108, 109, 112
Round Top Loop Trail 149
Rush Ranch 100
Rusmore, Jean 14
Russian Ridge Open Space Preserve
    223–26

S
Saddle Loop Trail 105
St. Brendan's Church 263
St. Ignatius Church 265
St. Johns Mine Hill 107
St. John's Presbyterian Church 266
Solano, Chief 105
Salmo iridia (rainbow trout) 154
Samuel P. Taylor State Park
    from Bolinas-Fairfax Road to 43–48
    to Loma Alta Open Space Preserve
        from 49–51
San Andreas Fault 46–47, 48
San Andreas Fire Road 62, 63, 65
San Andreas Lake 246
Sanborn County Park 211–14
Sanborn Trail 213
San Cristobal Mine 209
Sandy Wool Lake 169, 173
San Felipe Trail 184
San Francisco
    Fort Funston to Stern Grove 256,
        257–60
    overview of 254
    Presidio 267–75

Stern Grove to the Presidio 261–66
Sunset District of 263
San Francisco 254, 256–75
San Francisco Bay Area. *See also* Bay
    Area Ridge Trail
development of parks and open
    spaces in 3–5
East Bay 118, 120–73
heritage of outdoor enjoyment in 1–2
land conservation ethic of 2–3
nonprofit groups preserving open space
    in 5
North Bay 18, 21–117
park entrance fees 11
Peninsula 216, 218–53
San Francisco 254, 256–75
South Bay 174, 176–215
San Francisco National Military
    Cemetery 270, 274
San Francisco Watershed Trail 239–42
San Francisco Zoo 259
San Gregorio Creek 225–26
San Leandro Creek 159
San Leandro Creek Canyon 149
San Lorenzo Creek 166
San Miguel Rancho 263
San Pablo Creek 141
San Pablo Dam 141, 143
San Pablo Reservoir 143
San Pablo Ridge 141, 142, 143
Santa Clara County Open Space
    Authority 177, 179
Santa Clara Valley 213
Santa Clara Valley Parks 204
Santa Teresa County Park 196, 201–206
Santa Teresa Creek 203, 204
Saratoga Gap Open Space Preserve 211,
    212, 218, 219–22
SCA Trail 27, 28
Scow Canyon 143
Scow Dairy 143
Sea Captain's House 97
Sea View Trail 147
The Sea Wolf (London) 76
Sempervirens Fund 5
Senador Mine 209
Sequoia Grove 143

SFWD (San Francisco Water
Department) 4–5
Shady Oaks Park 196
Shafter Trail 47, 48, 50
sheep "fire-prevention team" 138
Ship's Mast Trail 60
Shoreline Highway 35–37
Sibley Preserve (Robert Sibley Volcanic
Regional Preserve) 147, 148–49
Sierra Azul Open Space Preserve 192,
193–94
Sierra Club 2–3
Silverado Trail (Highway 121) 91, 93, 94
Sir Francis Drake Boulevard
to Lucas Valley Road from 53–55
parking close to 43, 46
from Samuel P. Taylor State Park to
Brown Bridge on 49–51
Shafter Trail along 48
Skeggs Point 233
Skyline College Ridge Trail Connection
247
Skyline Community College 246–47
Skyline Gate
to Bort Meadow from 151–54
from Inspiration Point to 145–49
Skyline Ridge Open Space Preserve 218,
219–26
Skyline Trail (or EBSNR Trail) 142, 147,
148, 151, 157, 213–14
Skyline Trail (Skyline Wilderness Park)
95–97
Skyline Wilderness Park 93, 94, 95–97
The Sleeping Lady legend 37
Smith Ridge Fire Road 54
snakes 14–15
Sneath Lane Trail 239, 241, 243
Sobrante Ridge Regional Preserve
135–38
Sobrante Ridge Trail 137, 138
Soda Gulch Creek 237
Soda Gulch Trail 237
Solano County Farmlands 100, 101
Sonoma Developmental Center 75
Sonoma Mountain Trail 73–77
Sonoma Volcanics (rock formation) 101
Southampton Bay 112

South Bay
Almaden Quicksilver County Park
193, 204, 206–10
Alum Rock Park and Boccardo Trail
Corridor 176, 177–80
Castle Rock State Park 211, 213–15
Coyote Creek Parkway North 195–98
Coyote Creek Parkway South 199–200
Coyote Lake-Harvey Bear Ranch Trail
185–87
Joseph D. Grant County Park 181–84
Los Alamitos/Calero Creek Trail 201–6
Mount Madonna County Park 188–91
overview of 174
Sanborn County Park 211–14
Santa Teresa County Park 196, 201–6
Sierra Azul Open Space Preserve 192,
193–94
South Bay Trails (Rusmore, Crowder,
Spangle, and LaTourrette) 14
South Park Drive 141, 145
South Trailhead 25
South Valley Trail 105
Spangle, Frances 11, 14
Sprig Recreation Area 191
Sprig Trail 191
Spring Lake Regional Park 78, 79
Spring Ridge 227–30
Stafford Lake 62
Stafford Lake Trail 61
Stafford Lake Watershed 60, 61–62
Stage Meadow (Stern Grove) 260
Steamer Landing Park 71
Steam Trains (Tilden Park) 148, 149
Stern Grove
from Fort Funston to 256, 257–60
to Presidio from 261–66
Stevens Creek canyon 222
Stile Ranch Trail 203, 206
Stonegate Park 195–96
Stream Trail 152
Sugarloaf Mountain 97
Sugarloaf Ridge State Park 86–89
Sulphur Springs Mountain chain 110
"Summer Capital" 225
Summit Rock 214
Summit Rock Loop Trail 213

Sunnyvale Mountain Picnic Area 211, 212, 213–14
Sunset Boulevard 259
Sunset District (San Francisco) 263
Sunset Trail 258
supply recommendations 15–16
Sutro Tower 263
Sweeney Ridge Trail 244, 245, 246
Sycamore Rest Area 200

T
Tanoak Trail 191
Teague Hill Open Space Preserve 232, 234
Temple Emanu-El 266
Tennessee Valley
Marin Headlands from Golden Gate Bridge to 25–30
Marin Headlands to Shoreline Highway from 31–33
ticks 15
Tie-Camp Trail 190
Tilden Regional Park
from Kennedy Grove to 139–44
to Redwood Regional Park from 145–49
Todd Creek Canyon 213
Todd Quick Loop Trail 178, 180
Todd Redwood Grove 214
Trail Center 203
trails. *See also specific Bay Area trails*
accommodations available along 16–17
clothing and supplies recommended 15–16
etiquette for sharing the 14
general hazards to watch for 14–15, 158
directions to 12
summary information 11–12
on the trail section 12–17
Tres Sendas Trail 152
Trocadero Inn 257, 260
Trout Unlimited 50
Tuteur Family Trust 96, 97
Twin Peaks Boulevard 264–65
Twin Peaks Summit 264
Twin Peaks Tunnel 263
Twin Sisters 102, 105, 106
Two Rocks Trail 158

U
Up and Down California (Brewer) 1
Upper Fallen Bridge Trail 75
Upper Johnson Ridge Trail 85
Upper Lake's dam 101
Upper Razorback Ridge 227–30
Upper Stevens Creek County Park 220
Upper Terrance 265

V
Vallejo-Benicia Buffer 108–12
Vallejo-Benicia Waterfront 113–17
Vallejo, General Mariano 105, 109, 111
Valley of Heart's Delight 203
Valley View Trail 83–84
Verissimo Hills Open Space Reserve 62
Virl O. Norton Trail 193, 209–10
Vollmer Peak 143, 147
Vollmer Peak Trail 147–48

W
Walnut Rest Area 200
Wappos tribe 88
Weather Loop 180
Weintraub, David 14
West Meadow (Stern Grove) 260
West Ridge Trail 152, 153
wheelchair access
Golden Gate Bridge 21
historic Benicia and Benicia Marina 115, 117
Horseshoe Lake 222, 223
Los Alamitos/Calero Creek Trail 205
Purisima Creek Redwoods Open Space Preserve 235
Sunset Trail to Fort Funston 258
on trail around Alpine Pond 223
White Hill 51
White Hill Underpass Trail 49
Whitney, Josiah D. 1
Whittemore Gulch 237
Wildcat Canyon Regional Park 142–43
Wildcat Canyon Road 141, 144, 145
Wildcat Peak 142
Willow Brook Farm 228
Willow Park Golf Course 159, 161
Willow Springs Trail 187
Willow View Trail 159

Wilson, John 80
Windy Hill Open Space Preserve 227–30
Winnett, Thomas 11
Wintun tribe 105
Wolf House ruins 77
Woodchopper Trail 142
Woodcutters Meadow 75
Woods Trail 193

Wood Trail 209
Woodville (Dogtown) 47
Wunderlich County Park 231–34

Y
Yountville Cross Road 90–92
Yountville Park 90

About the Author

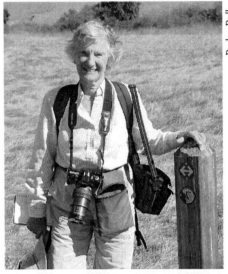

Roslyn Bullas

JEAN RUSMORE grew up in what was once the small town of Anaheim in the county that boasted orange and lemon groves as its namesake. At age 16 she took her first backpacking trip with a cousin up the slopes of Mt. Wilson in the San Gabriel Mountains with some food and a jacket rolled up in a blanket. Her outdoor experience was enlarged through her husband, Ted, whom she met at the University of California, Berkeley. They skied and backpacked with their six children, and all looked forward to their annual Sierra backpacking trip.

When the Midpeninsula Regional Open Space District was established, she and her friend Frances Spangle decided to write a book about the new foothill preserves, *Peninsula Trails*, followed by *South Bay Trails*, both of which are still published by Wilderness Press. When the first segments of the Ridge Trail opened, they wrote pamphlets about each leg. These were later combined and published as the first edition of this book. Since Frances's retirement, Jean has continued to hike and write about new segments of the Ridge Trail.